THE GIFT OF DEATH

. . . and bless'd are those
whose blood and judgment are so well co-mingled
That they are not a pipe for fortune's finger
To sound what stop she pleases.

Shakespeare
Hamlet, Act III ii 72

THE GIFT OF DEATH

CONFRONTING CANADA'S
TAINTED-BLOOD TRAGEDY

ANDRÉ PICARD

A Phyllis Bruce Book
HarperCollins*PublishersLtd*

This book is dedicated to the AIDS care-givers — the parents, children, spouses, lovers, siblings and nurses — who do not allow a disease that robs so many of life to steal away their dignity in dying.

First Edition

Canadian Cataloguing in Publication Data

Picard, André, 1960–
The gift of death

"A Phyllis Bruce book".
Includes index.
ISBN 0-00-255415-1

1. Blood banks — Risk management — Canada.
2. Blood banks — Canada — Quality control.
3. HIV infections — Canada.
I. Title.

RM172.P53 1995   362.1'784'0971   C95-931370-2

95 96 97 98 99 ❖ HC 10 9 8 7 6 5 4 3 2 1

Printed and bound in the United States

CONTENTS

ACKNOWLEDGMENTS

It would not have been possible for me to write this book if I were not a reporter for *The Globe and Mail*. My reporting and that of my colleague Rod Mickleburgh, which all started with an order to the two of us to "put these tainted-blood stories into perspective", provided the core of this account.

My bosses at *The Globe* granted me not only the time necessary to work on the book, but much personal encouragement. One of the strengths of Canada's national newspaper over the years has been the fact that, in addition to looking at issues from a national rather than just a local perspective, it allows its reporters to develop their expertise. I believe our ability to step back and look at the social and political ramifications of tainted blood from a truly national perspective is one of the reasons the story is still in the news.

Much of the credit for the story's longevity must go to my direct boss at *The Globe and Mail*, national editor Sylvia Stead. Her patience, her guidance and, above all, her trusting reporters to "run with the story" ensured that the news was pursued to its natural end. The recognition granted to the newspaper's coverage of the tainted-blood disaster — two nominations for the Michener Award for meritorious public service journalism and a National Newspaper Award nomination for enterprise reporting — is a testament to her daily commitment to news that matters to Canadians.

The numerous references in the Sources section do not begin to give credit to the contribution of Rod Mickleburgh, who is now the *Globe and Mail* correspondent in China. We collaborated on most of the tainted-blood stories that are the basis of this book, and pushed each other to dig deeper. Only the distance that separates us prevented there being two authors. Thanks to e-mail, Rod provided me with regular encouragement during the writing stage, for which I am also thankful.

A book cataloguing a tragedy that unfolded over more than a decade involves, necessarily, a lot of documentary and paper work, and I have collected thousands of pages of material. That would not have been possible without the

countless secretaries, librarians, archivists, access-to-information clerks and fellow pack rats whose thorough record-keeping let me piece the story together
with the kind of detail that memory alone would not have allowed. I am particularly grateful to the librarians at *The Globe and Mail*, and McGill University
medical library for their extra effort.

The Commission of Inquiry on the Blood System in Canada, headed by Mr.
Justice Horace Krever, provided a gold-mine of information, and I was privi-
leged to have Gregory Hamara, the commission's director of communications,
as my courteous and ever-affable guide through the mountains of evidence. I
spent many days at the hearings and many more reading through transcripts,
minutes of meetings and correspondence, and with each passing day my respect
and admiration for the commission staff grew. Their task — to discover the
root causes of Canada's tainted-blood tragedy — was a formidable one, and
they have, in my view, exceeded any reasonable expectation.

Often forgotten in the dynamic of the inquiry process are the lawyers for the
various interested parties. I am particularly grateful to Douglas Elliott of the
Canadian AIDS Society for drawing my attention to the underlying social
causes of this tragedy, and for his guidance as I stumbled through numerous
ethical minefields, and to Dawna Ring of the group Canadians Infected with
HIV-AIDS (Spouses and Children) for her keen eye for detail and for never letting me lose sight of the fact that the scope of the tragedy is too often mini-
mized, that every hemophiliac and transfusion patient has a family and a community that was touched by tainted blood.

I can honestly say that every major institution involved in the blood system
— the Canadian Red Cross Society, the Canadian Blood Agency, Health
Canada and the Canadian Hemophilia Society (CHS) — all of which had as
much to lose as to gain by co-operating with me and granting me access to
their records and people — was accessible and helpful, despite not always being
enthused by the newspaper articles I produced.

Angela Prokopiak, technical information officer at the Red Cross, answered
a countless number of my questions over the years, and was always the model
of professionalism — even when the agency was under a heavy media barrage,
and even when I phoned with queries late on Friday afternoon. At Health
Canada, spokesperson JoAnne Ford was equally professional and courteous,
while Access to Information co-ordinator Yvette Parent speedily and cheerily
shepherded my mountain of requests through the bureaucratic maze. The
members of the Canadian Hemophilia Society who have assisted me in telling
this story over the years are too numerous to mention, though David Page of
Quebec City must be singled out as a constant and invaluable helper, a font of

information and a level-headed analyst. Not only have David Page and other CHS members like Durhane Wong-Rieger, Lindee David and Santo Caira served as the institutional voice for many victims of tainted blood, but their actions as consumer activists have helped ensure that hospital patients who require blood and blood products are safer today than they ever have been.

Any journalist who writes about the healthcare system in general, and about the AIDS epidemic in particular, owes a debt of gratitude to the late Randy Shilts. I first met the San Francisco *Chronicle* reporter at the 1989 International AIDS Conference in Montreal, where, as usual, he blazed a trail the rest of us followed. The author of *And the Band Played On: Politics, People and the AIDS Epidemic* set a standard of quality and dedication that is a model for all journalists writing about AIDS.

From the outset, Phyllis Bruce, my editor at HarperCollins, was convinced that the only way to prevent another tainted-blood tragedy was to understand how and why things went so terribly wrong when AIDS first entered the blood supply in the early 1980s. Phyllis used her extraordinary editing talents not only to focus my energies but, with the help of copy editor Gena Gorrell, to transform a complex and sprawling thesis into a cohesive book.

Writing a book is impossible without the support of your loved ones, and I have been blessed in that regard. My mom and dad forgave me the ultimate in bad-son behaviour — skipping the Christmas visit home. My spouse, Michelle Lalonde, a superb reporter in her own right, not only lent her talents as a researcher and editor but endured, with saintly good humour, my talking about tainted blood almost constantly for months on end. A special thanks also to my dear friend Angus Smith, who served as my one-man focus group, reading early drafts of chapters and offering constructive criticism. Angus is probably the only person who has read the manuscript as many times and in as many forms as I have, and I can only hope that the exercise was not too much for an inveterate book lover to bear.

Above all, my heartfelt thanks must go to the victims of tainted blood and their families, of whom I have met hundreds over the years. I have been deeply moved by the fact that so many people betrayed by deeply cherished elements of Canadian society — the Red Cross, hospitals, doctors and the medicare system — have dared to trust again. I can only hope that I have done their stories justice.

A.P.
Montreal, June 1995

PREFACE

IN APRIL 1994 I WAS INVITED to address a conference of the Canadian Association of Journalists on the topic "Could the media have done a better job covering the tainted-blood tragedy?"

I began my speech with this very harsh assessment: "We journalists are guilty of the same 'crime' as the main players in the blood system — the Red Cross, Health Canada, the Canadian Blood Committee, the provinces, the politicians, medical officers of health, doctors — a failure to inform the public. Like them, we have excuses . . . but, collectively, our mistakes have cost hundreds of people their lives. There can be no excuse for that. We cannot be forgiven. But we can make amends by learning from our failures, by never again repeating them."

More than 1.5 million Canadians who received blood transfusions between 1980 and 1985 were unwitting participants in a lottery of death, and the odds grew worse with each passing month of inaction. The country's 2,300 hemophiliacs, whose blood products are manufactured with the plasma of thousands of donors, were even more at risk: 43 per cent of them contracted the AIDS* virus from the products that were supposed to keep them healthy. Even after public health authorities finally reacted to AIDS, another menace, hepatitis C, continued to infect thousands of transfusion patients and hemophiliacs until testing was introduced in 1990.

Despite the enormity of the tragedy, tainted blood did not become front-page news in Canada until late 1992. In an age when the media examine, in minute detail, everything from murder cases to the deliberately vague pronouncements of politicians, it is unbelievable that the infection of more than 1,200 Canadians with a deadly virus went virtually unnoticed for almost a decade after the first victims started dying.

---

* For the sake of simplicity, the terms "HIV" and "AIDS virus" have been used synonymously throughout the text, although some scientists still question whether HIV is the cause of AIDS. Similarly, the term HIV has sometimes been used to describe the virus in the time period before scientists agreed on the designation, again, to avoid an excess of technical terminology.

Yet there were real barriers to getting to the bottom of the story, among them lack of accurate information. As journalists and members of the public, we are too trusting of the so-called experts; we all too often accept their views, however speculative or self-interested, as the unvarnished truth. When, at the outset of the AIDS epidemic, Red Cross officials said the risks of contracting AIDS from blood were one in a million — coded language for "don't worry" — we took them at their word. The media, in covering health-related issues, remain far too much in awe of institutions and people with fancy titles, and not nearly respectful enough of the needs of patients and their families.

Adding to the problem, perhaps central to it, is the structure of Canada's blood system. It is daunting and impenetrable in its bureaucracy, administered by a combination of the Red Cross and thirteen federal and provincial governments. This overblown and inefficient administration allowed virtually endless buck-passing while a fatal virus spread unchecked. Though countless people, from hemophiliacs through to epidemiologists, expressed concern about the transmission of AIDS via blood, their worries were summarily dismissed because they were mere individuals. Users of blood products, when they raised red flags, were considered hysterical. Transfusion recipients and hemophiliacs were lied to repeatedly by "experts", and the checks and balances that should have been there to protect them failed.

Above all, the full extent of the disaster went unexplored for a decade because of the stigma of AIDS. Ignored as a disease of minorities on the margins of society — homosexuals, drug addicts, prostitutes, Haitians, hemophiliacs — the epidemic wasn't taken seriously by the mainstream media. Many journalists, like the public health officials and politicians, didn't allow themselves to see beyond their prejudices, notably homophobia. In turn, many of the victims were ashamed to speak out, because we treated their disease as shameful.

With scorn as a backdrop, it has not been easy for people with AIDS to step forward. The gay community, where the disease hit first and hardest, responded to the epidemic by building support networks. Their activism changed the health system for the better, though not nearly enough. But the victims of tainted blood didn't have self-help groups, and they were further isolated by the lack of information in the media. Those who did come forward to explain the ravages of blood-borne AIDS were particularly brave.

* * *

It's a very special person who, in the midst of his or her own suffering, can reach out to help others. Yet during the four years I've been working on the tainted-blood story, I have met many, many such generous souls. For most of them it was too late but, rather than die silently, they spoke out in the hope that they would help others. Marc Dagenais was typical of these altruists. In March 1993, just days before the federal compensation plan for victims of tainted blood expired, he welcomed me into his Montreal home to make a case for an extension of government assistance. He was suffering from a case of oral thrush so severe that he could barely speak; I could tell that each word cut his throat like a razor blade. But the pain didn't matter to him. "Right now, I'm living on borrowed time," Marc said, as he showed off pictures of his daughters, Carolyne, ten, Tammy, eleven, and Tina, twelve. "The girls probably won't have a dad in a year. All they'll have left is a wonderful mom and the money the province gives them. Right now, that looks like nothing. And it doesn't seem fair." Marc Dagenais died a couple of months later, at age thirty-six. His girls won't benefit from the provincial compensation plan, but hundreds of others will, in part because of his refusal to be silenced.

In recent years, the news stories about the tainted blood tragedy have had a tremendous impact. The steady stream of revelations about the failings of healthcare officials, and their utter contempt for hundreds of people infected with AIDS, forced the provincial ministers of health to cobble together a $151-million assistance package, and the lingering questions about misdeeds prompted the federal government to order a judicial inquiry into the decisions, and non-decisions, of the administrators of the blood system. The Commission of Inquiry on the Blood System in Canada, headed by Mr. Justice Horace Krever, has provided an important forum for the victims of tainted blood to air their grievances, and an unprecedented opportunity to get to the bottom of this complex story. The commission will also make recommendations on the changes required to ensure that a similar tragedy never happens.

*   *   *

I wish I could have told the story of each of the 1,200-plus victims individually. The hardest part of the editing process has been choosing whose horror story to leave untold. I have tried to present a cross-section: children, women and men from every region of Canada and every walk of life. No community from Newfoundland to British Columbia, and no age group from newborn to senior citizen, has been untouched by the epidemic. Yet too many of us remain smug, convinced that the disease only affects others.

Many victims have asked for anonymity because the stigma of AIDS is still so pervasive. They fear being pointed out in the supermarket, seated apart in restaurants, patronized by physicians and pitied by journalists. In all my professional dealings with people with AIDS, I have attempted to treat them not as lepers, but as people with a story to tell, and I have been rewarded with candour and intimacy. I am convinced that we must make a greater effort to ensure that people with HIV-AIDS be permitted to be full members of society. There can't be diseases of "good" people, like cancer, and diseases of "bad" people, like AIDS. It is abhorrent, for example, that provincial healthcare plans provide free drug therapy to people with cancer but not to those with AIDS. Regardless of the origin of their illness, all Canadians afflicted by fatal disease should be treated with the utmost care and compassion.

It has been difficult to see these new friends die, knowing that many more will die in the months and years to come. But many have said they have two wishes before death: to know why this tragedy really happened, and to have someone apologize for the wrongdoing.

Writing is an often solitary pursuit, and the complexity of the tainted-blood story made my task all the more difficult. When I was struggling, I always tried to remind myself that behind the statistics, the science and the institutions, there were people like Billie Jo Decarie, a little girl who turned six in June — Canada's youngest victim of tainted blood.

For inspiration I turned not only to my memories of Billie Jo swallowing her AZT pills as she coloured, but to a binder I labelled "Krever's List", in which I kept a summary of the testimony of every witness who appeared at the commission of inquiry. (Excerpts from the testimony at the Krever Commission can be found, in italics, at the beginning of each chapter.) The words of Ronald Mitchell, a plain-talking man of few words from Hagersville, Ontario, often popped out at me, because I had heard the feelings expressed so many times, though rarely so poignantly: "I feared death at one time, but I don't fear that no more. But I would really like to see a few answers before I do pass away."

I hope this book helps answer the "why?" for Ronald Mitchell and for thousands of Canadians who have been touched, directly or indirectly, by the tainted-blood tragedy. If my work can bring even a modicum of dignity to those who are dying of AIDS, then it will have been worth the effort.

Yet, as I said in concluding my speech to the Canadian Association of Journalists, we cannot content ourselves with burying the dead. What the media are doing today, rehashing the past failings of the blood system and reporting bland assurances that things are different now, is no better than the days when, blind to crisis, we routinely reported the blood shortages at the Red Cross every Christmas and summer. Nor can we continue to give fawning coverage to every small breakthrough in the molecular biology of AIDS while giving short shrift to the broader legal, ethical, political and social issues at the heart of the epidemic. With the next blood-borne catastrophe possibly just around the corner, we need to add foresight and leadership to our public health arsenal. We cannot content ourselves with writing the obituary for Canada's failed blood system; we must help draft the blueprints for a new, more responsive, more democratic system.

*   *   *

In the final chapter, I make a series of recommendations for change — proposals that are radical and hard-hitting, designed not only to be thought-provoking but to reflect the fact that the response to an unparalleled tragedy cannot be half-hearted.

In offering these conclusions, I don't mean to compete with the findings of the Krever Commission. On the contrary, I hope that my account of the enormity of the tragedy will help convince Canada's health ministers that change can no longer wait, and inspire them to act swiftly and decisively on Judge Krever's recommendations. Letting his report gather dust on a shelf would be the ultimate insult to the victims of tainted blood.

At the same time, we must not allow ourselves to be so disillusioned by the tragedy that we forget all the benefits of blood and blood products, life-savers for more than 300,000 Canadians each year. Nor should we ignore the more than 1.1 million Canadians who give blood each year. "Giving a pint" is one of the purest acts of charity; it is truly giving of oneself to a stranger. Donors like Jean-Guy Duclos, a retired firefighter from L'Assomption, Quebec, who has donated blood and plasma almost five hundred times since he started in 1961, are truly heroes.

I have learned from people like Jean-Guy Duclos that giving blood may hurt a little, but it helps a lot; and I have learned from tainted-blood victims like Marc Dagenais that speaking up for change may hurt a lot, but it too is necessary. More than anything else, it is the undying spirit of caring, the unselfish desire to help fellow citizens in need, exhibited by people like Marc and Jean-Guy, that has inspired me to write this book.

I hope no matter how the blood system changes, how ugly the turf battles get, and how outraged Canadians may be by the news out of the inquiry, that no one will stop giving blood. The soundest part of the structure of our muddled, bureaucratic blood system, the one element that must be retained, is its foundation, the selfless generosity of those who give the Gift of Life.

<u>1</u>

GIFT OF LIFE:KISS OF DEATH
MR. L. AND MR. P.

When desperate ills demand a speedy cure,
Distrust is cowardice, and prudence folly.
Samuel Johnson
Irene

Rose Marie Gillis, New Waterford, Nova Scotia

A coal miner's wife with three young boys, Rose Marie was devastated when her eldest, Everett, was diagnosed with leukemia in 1982, at age five. On Christmas Eve 1985, the family doctor phoned to say Everett was in remission, but a week later called back to say the boy had likely contracted AIDS from tainted blood. As part of his leukemia treatment, Everett had been injected with about two tablespoons of platelets. The boy died in 1988, just days after his eleventh birthday. Before going to the hospital for the last time, Everett insisted on a party and invited singing star Rita MacNeil, whom he had befriended when he was a cancer patient.

"*Everett was very, very sick. He was sicker with AIDS than he was when he had cancer. . . . He wanted a birthday party, but I was kind of hesitant. I was saying, I should wait until he comes home again. It's a good job I didn't because he didn't come home.*

I had a party for him, and [MacNeil] came. She bought him a stereo, and she just made his day. She was fantastic to Everett, and I often thanked her for that because she's a busy lady and she took the time out of her busy schedule to spend a little time with Everett, and that made him very happy. . . .

Her Christmas album says: 'This album is dedicated to the memory of Everett Gillis who at the young age of 11 taught me the meaning of the words strength and courage.'"

(*August 2, 1994*)

THE BOYS ON THE CHRYSLER ASSEMBLY LINE were in a good mood; not only were they cutting out of work early, with the boss's permission, but they were off to do a good deed. As the thirteen of them scrambled aboard the minibus, they joked that the blood would flow not only that afternoon at the clinic in Ajax but at the hockey game in Oshawa later in the evening. When they bounded up the steps to the second floor of the Royal Canadian Legion Hall on November 13, 1984, Mr. L.* and his co-workers were welcomed by a smiling Red Cross volunteer still sporting a Remembrance Day poppy. With the greeting came an offer of juice and a pamphlet entitled "An Important Message to Blood Donors", the first step of the bureaucratic shuffle that is blood donation. First-time donors were shown to the registration table, asked a few stock questions and given donor cards. At the next table, technician Dolores Beaven pricked Mr. L.'s finger to type his blood and test his hemoglobin level. She also handed him a questionnaire and asked some follow-up medical questions, including whether he had read the pamphlet. Mr. L. nodded, even though he could barely read. The veterans, those who had already earned their stripes as donors, were by now lying back on the "bleeding beds" with needles in their arms, flirting with the nurses. Mr. L., a strapping 32-year-old who had recently emigrated from Montreal, joined them. After giving 450 millilitres of blood, he moved to a recovery bed and, after a few minutes, into the refreshment area for Peek Freans and orange juice. The blood donor clinic operated according to a finely honed system: the donors moved in clockwise fashion, with military precision.

By evening, when Mr. L. and his buddies had knocked back a few beers — one of the unspoken benefits of giving blood, the assembly-line workers knew, was that it was a lot easier to get drunk after giving a pint — and laced up their skates for the weekly hockey game, their blood was safely on ice in the freezer

---

* Mr. L. cannot be identified due to an injunction issued by Madam Justice Susan Lang on March 23, 1993.

at the Toronto headquarters of the Canadian Red Cross Society, ready to save lives during the busy holiday season.

Voluntary blood donation is as archetypically Canadian as the pick-up hockey game, and the red cross has been as enduring a symbol as the maple leaf since Canadians were first asked to "make a date with a wounded soldier" during the Second World War. The annual drive by Chrysler workers was just one of hundreds of corporate blood challenges held every month across Canada — feel-good competitions in which everyone from students to factory workers to company presidents willingly rolled up their sleeves and gave a pint to save a stranger.

Kenneth Pittman, a 53-year-old manager at The Bay and self-described "best hardware man in Canada", would have loved to share a few beers with the Chrysler workers that cold November day, but his health didn't allow it. Since his triple bypass in October 1982 he had curtailed his smoking and drinking, but his heart problems had persisted. In September of 1984 he had gone under the knife for another bypass, but months of illness had followed, so the doctors decided to open him up again in December 1984. The surgery was a disaster; Mr. Pittman suffered a heart attack on the operating table, and bleeding that threatened his life. The next morning he was infused with cryoprecipitate,* a fluffy white protein mass that is extracted from blood and helps clotting.

One week after the cryo injection, Kenneth Pittman sat up in his hospital bed and looked at the clock grumpily. Rochelle, his wife, couldn't help but laugh. After all he had been through, Ken was scolding her and the children for being a few minutes late for Christmas dinner. It was strange to be having dinner in the intensive care unit of the Toronto General Hospital instead of at home, but the family was ecstatic to see Ken Pittman looking and sounding so good. They knew he was feeling better because he had mentioned, more than once, how a stiff drink and a smoke would round off the meal nicely. But he would have to settle for singing Christmas carols and telling stories about the holiday fun he had had as a boy in Nova Scotia.

For decades, blood transfusions have been instrumental in bringing people back from the edge of death. That's why they're called the Gift of Life. That Ken Pittman's life-saving operation took place just days before Christmas made it all the more special.

Unfortunately for Mr. Pittman, Mr. L.'s blood was infected with the AIDS virus. This gift of life was a kiss of death.

*   *   *

---

* A cryoprecipitate is any precipitate produced by cooling; in this book, however, it always refers to the clotting factor.

The single unit of blood Mr. L. donated at the Legion Hall was broken down into three parts. Mr. Pittman received component number A96490, the cryoprecipitate. Two other surgery patients also received parts of Mr. L.'s blood during the busy holiday season, the red cells and the platelets. By the time the Chrysler crew boarded the minibus to attend the same Ajax blood clinic in November 1985, two recipients of Mr. L.'s first donation had already died. Mr. Pittman's fate was to suffer a slower death.

Once again the illiterate auto worker breezed through the screening procedure, despite a new pamphlet and questioning about specific symptoms. Luckily for others awaiting surgery, universal testing of blood for the AIDS virus had finally begun two weeks earlier — after lengthy delays — on November 1, 1985. Mr. L. would be one of the first blood donors who tested positive for HIV.

Mr. L. seemed physically quite healthy, just as he had a year earlier. Right before his first donation, in November 1984, he had been discharged from hospital after a hernia operation with a clean bill of health. He had also received high marks on the company physical. His emotional health, however, was wanting. Far away from his hometown of Montreal and his girlfriend, he was lonely and often drowned his sorrows in alcohol and anonymous sex, with prostitutes or women — and men — he met in local strip clubs. Like most Canadians, Mr. L. was unaware that the AIDS era had begun. The Red Cross had done little to warn him; its medical experts insisted that the odds of blood being infected with the AIDS virus were about one in a million, about the same as getting cancer after smoking a single cigarette.

Kenneth Pittman wasn't a gambling man, but his odds were nowhere near as good as the Red Cross scientists predicted. Of the one million blood donations the Red Cross had in 1984, Mr. L.'s was far from the only one infected with the AIDS virus. During a lawsuit many years later, it would be advanced by one of the world's foremost experts on infectious disease that Mr. Pittman's odds of being transfused with AIDS-tainted blood when he lay down on the operating table that day might have been as high as one in four[1] — worse than a game of Russian roulette.

Ironically, on the first roll of the dice during surgery, Kenneth Pittman beat the odds. But the next day, when an intern prescribed the cryoprecipitate to help stem the bleeding in his battered heart, a nurse injected unit A96490.

About two months after Mr. L.'s second blood donation, he received a letter from the Red Cross urging him to see his doctor. He and his common-law wife were tested for the human immunodeficiency virus on January 12, 1986. Mr. L. tested positive; his partner was negative.

Mr. and Mrs. Pittman were not so lucky. It took the Red Cross another eighteen months to contact Toronto General Hospital — now called the Toronto Hospital — to tell them that Mr. L.'s blood had been infected. The hospital, in turn, took from June 12, 1987, until February 24, 1989, to link Mr. Pittman's name to the cryoprecipitate unit number A96490. Mr. L. had actually made the donation forty months earlier.

Sometime in April 1989, Dr. William Francombe, the hematologist in charge of the blood transfusion laboratory at Toronto General, phoned Dr. Stanley Bain to inform him that his patient Kenneth Pittman had received a transfusion that was likely contaminated with AIDS. The North York family physician took note of the information on a Post-it note that he placed on the inside cover of Mr. Pittman's voluminous medical file, and awaited a letter of confirmation. None ever came, nor did he receive any information on how important it was to have his patient tested. Meanwhile, Dr. Francombe wrote to the Red Cross, telling them that the recipient's physician had been contacted. The agency that had collected the tainted blood took no more follow-up action than the hospital that had transfused it.

Dr. Bain had been treating Kenneth Pittman for more than twenty-five years. He had seen him transformed from a healthy bon vivant to someone incapacitated by chronic heart disease and depressed about his fate. The doctor decided his patient was too emotionally fragile to be told of his transfusion of bad blood, so he simply kept him in the dark. Dr. Bain says he examined Mr. Pittman during a routine physical and saw no obvious signs of infection — just as Mr. L. had had no signs of infection when he had donated the poisoned blood. Given that the incubation period of the AIDS virus was known at the time to be as long as a decade, dismissing the possibility because of a lack of symptoms was a dangerously erroneous assumption for a physician to make. General practitioners can't be expected to be up to date on every disease — even one of epidemic proportions — but failure to consult specialists is, at best, sheer arrogance. Dr. Bain not only violated basic ethics by withholding the news from Mr. Pittman, he was also in clear violation of his professional code of conduct. A second violation was failing to report the patient's possible infection to the Medical Officer of Health.

There is no doubt that Mr. Pittman's quality of life would have been improved by a swift diagnosis of AIDS, even though many treatments were still in the experimental stage: he never had the benefit of drugs like zidovudine (AZT); he wasn't given the opportunity to make lifestyle changes that would reduce the chance of contracting an infection; and when he contracted *Pneumocystis carinii* pneumonia (PCP), often a sign that a person with AIDS is on his last legs, he didn't get the chance to say his final goodbyes.

His three weeks in North York Hospital in March 1990 were excruciating. His body, deprived of all immune responses, was racked by infections, including the pneumonia that was ultimately listed as his cause of death. As inexplicable as his own doctor's paternalism was the ignorance of the hospital staff. By then more than four hundred Canadians had contracted AIDS and half of them had died. The symptoms were widely known even to casual readers of newspapers. Months earlier, the federal government had announced a humanitarian assistance package for transfusion patients infected with HIV — hundreds of whom had already been identified and twenty of whom were already known to have died of AIDS. Yet a man with an obvious history of multiple transfusions, who was suffering total collapse of his immune system in a major metropolitan hospital, wasn't diagnosed until his daughter, a nurse, insisted that he be tested for HIV.

Kenneth Pittman was tested for AIDS just days before he died of the disease, although it had taken more than five years to kill him. Rochelle Pittman, his wife and sexual partner of thirty-two years, didn't learn of the diagnosis until three weeks after the funeral.

Her immediate reaction was, "How long do I have to live?"

Dr. Bain responded, "You weren't having sexual relations with him, were you?"

The question, like so many in the tainted-blood saga, came years too late. Dr. Bain had assumed that Mr. Pittman wasn't having sex because he was a cardiac patient (some heart medications dampen sexual drive, but the drug he was taking didn't interfere with erection) married for more than three decades, and depressed. Governments were asking doctors to promote safe sex, but Dr. Bain was too embarrassed even to ask his long-time patient if he was having sex. He just assumed he wasn't.

In fact, the Pittmans had made love just two weeks before Kenneth entered hospital for the last time, in March 1990, by which time he had full-blown AIDS. There is no way of knowing exactly when Mrs. Pittman was infected, but it was almost certainly during this period. Research has shown that HIV carriers are most likely to transmit the disease to their sexual partners when their $CD4^2$ count is low (an indication of high immunodeficiency); this indicator reaches its lowest levels in the first six weeks after infection, and again just before opportunistic infections develop. It was well known at the time that using a condom would dramatically reduce the risk of transmission of the virus, but the family doctor never broached the topic. As a result, Rochelle Pittman, mother of four and grandmother of six, died of AIDS.

For failing to tell Mr. Pittman that he was infected with a deadly disease, and for failing to refer him to a specialist who could have treated and counselled him, conduct judged by the Ontario College of Physicians and Surgeons to be "disgraceful, dishonourable and unprofessional", on March 11, 1993, Dr.

Stanley Bain was handed down a two-month suspension — a meaningless penalty to a man who had already retired — and ordered to complete a course in bioethics. This slap on the wrist is typical of the medical profession's lack of self-criticism concerning tainted blood and AIDS. At the very time he committed the offences against his patient and his profession, Dr. Bain was president of the Ontario College of Physicians and Surgeons. At the height of his profession he was, sadly, leading by example.

Later, in a lawsuit, Dr. Bain would be found negligent for failing to tell Mr. Pittman that he was likely HIV-positive, and assessed 40 per cent liability, while the Toronto Hospital and the Red Cross would share a 60 per cent liability for failing to notify him promptly of the infection. (But the judge found the Red Cross not negligent in its efforts to screen blood and the hospital not negligent in administering it to a patient in need.) The court judged that the lack of diagnosis had cost Mr. Pittman two years of his life.

"No amount of money can ever compensate me and my family for the loss of a husband and father," Rochelle Pittman said the day the landmark judgment was handed down. "Nor will it change the fact that I will likely experience a similar fate."

Mrs. Pittman had sued for $2.085 million — less than the average award in U.S. cases. She was awarded $469,317, while the couple's four adult children shared $45,758. With interest, the total award rose to almost $630,000. The court also ruled that the defendants should pay 60 per cent of Mrs. Pittman's legal costs, about $370,000. Dr. Bain, who was deemed to have been most at fault, didn't have to pay a penny out of his own pocket. His legal costs and the settlement were paid by the Canadian Medical Protective Association, which provides liability insurance to 90 per cent of Canadian physicians.

Madam Justice Susan Lang, of the Ontario Court of Justice General Division, was conscious that, as the first-ever Canadian ruling on a civil suit involving tainted blood, Mrs. Pittman's case was a *cause célèbre*. For that reason, she stressed that the courts were not the appropriate venue for such cases. "It will compound the tragedy of transfusion-associated AIDS if more cases must be decided by the litigation process," Judge Lang wrote in her 312-page judgment. "Litigation is a fault-driven process where each case must be decided on its own merits. It is ill-suited to an expeditious resolution of such tragic situations."

Judge Lang had been under tremendous pressure to write a definitive judgment within a strict deadline, and it was a burden she resented. Guided as much by her social conscience as by legal responsibility — in stark contrast to many of those who dealt with Mr. Pittman's case over the years — she worked day and night to be able to release her ruling on March 14, 1994.

The reason for the haste was that provincial and territorial ministers of health, after years of stonewalling, had offered a compensation package to the victims of tainted blood, but it came with a March 15 deadline. The hundreds of other victims had less than twenty-four hours to digest the Pittman judgment and decide if they would continue fighting or take the settlement.

Throughout the civil suit launched by the Pittman family, Red Cross lawyers repeatedly referred to Mr. L. as an "irresponsible donor" and argued that the organization's efforts to ensure the safety of the blood supply had to be balanced against its duty to ensure an adequate supply, which included not alienating "responsible donors". Mr. L. was precisely the kind of donor they targeted: young, healthy and pushed by workplace peer pressure to give again and again. The agency assumed such people would not carry AIDS. Yet Mr. L. had had sex with at least fifteen different men, and many more prostitutes, making him a high-risk donor. The approach required those at risk not to give blood, but Mr. L., for one, bristled at the thought that someone might consider him homosexual; the failure was that the Red Cross eschewed members of high-risk *groups*, rather than individuals who practised high-risk activities.

Mr. L.'s Gift of Life was no less charitable than that of the other guys on the assembly line, yet he was being vilified, even after his death.[3] The real culprit was a charitable agency that had a virtual monopoly on information about blood-borne infection, but didn't propagate it so that individuals could make informed decisions.

"We have to ensure that something of this magnitude never happens again," Mrs. Pittman told the public hearings of the Commission of Inquiry on the Blood System in Canada. She spoke of the devastation not only of losing a lifelong companion, but of living the horror of a disease that would soon claim her own life. The former People's Jewellers clerk, dressed in a smart suit, stood stoically and told a rapt audience that her husband's death-bed agony was so imprinted in her mind that she couldn't bear to suffer in the same way. She pleaded that the law be changed so people in the advanced stages of AIDS could opt for assisted suicide.

"I'll never forget what his dying was like, the horror of it is etched in my mind. . . When my time comes, when my major organs shut down, I hope someone will help me die with dignity," she said on March 11, 1994. It was four years earlier, almost to the day, that her husband had died — without dignity, and without answers.

Just weeks before her appearance at the public inquiry, Rochelle Pittman had travelled to her hometown, Lunenberg, Nova Scotia, where, thirty-five years earlier, she and her husband had spent their honeymoon. Along the wintry ocean shore, she caught a chill, and developed flu — something HIV sufferers dread. Before long she developed PCP. Unlike her husband, Rochelle was aware of her underlying condition and was treated. Still, the chills that summer reminded her of the way Kenneth shivered during the last year of his life — always cold, always tired, always taking refuge in his blue flannel pyjamas. He had been wearing them at Christmas dinner at the Toronto General, and he was wearing them on that cold March day in 1990 when the family bid him a final farewell. When the doctor disconnected the life support system, a shiver shot up Rochelle's spine. It remained there through her years as an activist, as the public face and voice of HIV-positive women. Rochelle's shivers only dissipated on that warm day in June 1995, when the children gathered around her bed to kiss her goodbye.

2

BLOOD TIES
RED CROSS AND CONNAUGHT

You must begin with an ideal
and end with an ideal.

Sir Frederick Banting

Yves Roy, Ottawa

In 1993, more than a decade after he was transfused with two units of blood to speed up his recovery after elective bladder surgery, the retired civil servant learned that he was infected with AIDS. Sometime during that decade, Yves had also infected his wife Bernadette. Yves says that, like most Canadians, he never bothered to learn anything about AIDS.

"To tell you the truth, I was not interested because AIDS was not the kind of thing that would happen to me—it happens to other people.

Since we discovered we were positive, the quality of our life has been shattered. We had been retired for three years at the time and we were expecting to have a quiet, happy retirement. . . .

Now my health is deteriorating. My immune system is very low so I have to be extra careful. I have absolutely no energy."

(February 22, 1994)

Bernadette Roy, Ottawa

After decades of raising a family and work, Bernadette says the couple was looking forward to taking advantage of the fact that they were spry and healthy, but the AIDS diagnosis destroyed their plans, and robbed her and Yves of happiness.

"I am furious as I sit and watch my husband die, and I know I'm going to follow him, soon after. He doesn't talk. He sleeps all the time. I'm here to look after him, but who's going to look after me? Canada should, because Canada did this to me.

After a lifetime of hard work, we just retired. But our last days on Earth are ruined. He's going to die, and for nothing. He was murdered, and so was I. I want to know why. Why?"

(February 22, 1994) *

TWO OF CANADA'S MOST REVERED INSTITUTIONS in the healthcare field are the Red Cross, the symbol of humanitarianism, and Connaught Laboratories, which became world-famous for the discovery of insulin and many life-saving vaccines. The ties between the two institutions run deep, stretching back decades through Canadian medical history and, in a strange twist of fate, culminating in the tainted-blood tragedy. Their "blood ties" were forged prior to the Second World War, when Dr. Charles Best, who as a medical student was a co-discoverer of insulin, became intrigued by reports that blood transfusion was being used to treat seriously wounded soldiers in the Spanish Civil War (1936–39). There was little doubt that the world was marching inexorably towards war, and medical researchers like those at Connaught were looking for ways to manage the carnage of battle and disease that was an inevitable consequence of armed confrontation.

In the First World War, thousands upon thousands had died of treatable injuries for lack of blood. Eighty per cent of wounds to the leg and the abdomen were fatal; burn victims were consumed by infection; thoracic surgery, to save soldiers who had been gassed, couldn't be performed; all because healthy troops couldn't give enough of the precious liquid to keep their fellow fighters alive. The only alternative available then was a mixture of saline and gum arabic, which helped boost the volume of circulation to treat shock, but did nothing to help wounds clot. Even outside war zones, the lack of organized collection meant that blood was not always available when needed, such as after the Halifax explosion.[1] It was a constant source of frustration for surgeons, and the generals

---

* Yves Roy died of AIDS in May 1995.

leading the troops, that fighters were dying, not for lack of medical expertise, but because of a basic industrial problem — poor supply.

In 1923, whole blood was first fractionated, or separated by centrifuge, into red cells, a red liquid, and plasma, a heavier yellow liquid that was found to be more effective to stem bleeding than whole blood. Dr. Norman Bethune, another Canadian medical hero, pioneered battlefield transfusions fifteen years later, during the Spanish Civil War, but his work was seriously hampered by storage and supply problems. Without refrigeration, red cells and plasma had a shelf life of about ten days, and the fierce fighting made it impossible to recruit the large numbers of donors required.

Back in Canada, Dr. Best, now head of the Department of Physiological Hygiene at the University of Toronto, felt the solution was to come up with a blood derivative that had the same properties, but not the same drawbacks, as plasma. He regularly took blood from his colleagues and students so he could study its characteristics, and by the time the Second World War broke out he had come up with the idea of reducing plasma to a concentrated form. His small-scale experiments, consisting of reducing plasma to serum and treating laboratory animals for shock and hemorrhage, were encouraging, but Dr. Best soon ran out of blood donors. He approached the local Red Cross, an organization well known for its volunteer work, and asked if they could supply a hundred healthy men a week. After consulting with the director of medical services of the Department of National Defence, the director of the Toronto branch of the Red Cross, H.G. Stanton, agreed to co-operate.

The Red Cross, after all, had its origins in providing assistance to wounded soldiers. It traced its beginnings to a battle between Austro-Hungarian and French forces at Solferino, Italy, on June 24, 1859. The fighting was fierce and after only a few hours, with four thousand dead and wounded on the battlefield, the armies' overwhelmed medical corps simply gave up. Henri Dunant, a wealthy Swiss businessman who happened to be visiting the village as a "simple tourist", was appalled by the suffering he witnessed and set out to help the wounded, regardless of their nationality. Villagers, inspired by his humanitarian deeds, joined him, comforting their compatriots and enemies alike. Dunant later wrote a book about the tragedy of war, entitled *A Memory of Solferino*, which was acclaimed among philanthropists and humanists. Gustave Moynier, a lawyer and president of the Geneva Public Welfare Society, was moved by the work and, along with Dunant, created the International Committee for the Relief to the Wounded. At its founding conference in October 1863, the group adopted a distinctive logo, a red cross on a white background — the Swiss flag in reverse. Its first achievement was political: the negotiation in 1864 of the Geneva Convention, a treaty that established basic rules for the treatment of prisoners and wounded soldiers. The group was later renamed the International Committee of the Red Cross (ICRC), and its flag soon came to be synonymous with neutrality, finding its place outside field hospitals where the wounded were treated.

Yet in the beginning not everyone accepted the Red Cross. Army surgeons weren't happy with civilian volunteers, no matter how well intentioned, blundering around battlefields. Florence Nightingale, the legendary nurse who managed almost single-handedly to reduce the death rate in field hospitals to 2 per cent from 42 per cent during the Crimean War, was one of the staunchest opponents of the Red Cross. Nightingale argued that having a volunteer society provide medical supplies and treatment would allow armies to neglect their responsibilities, and she dismissed the Geneva Convention as a ridiculous notion. In the agency's early days there was also widespread mistrust; the Red Cross armband was seen as an easy cover for spies, and the flag of neutrality a means of protecting ammunition stocks. These early growing pains were overcome in a curious way: the Red Cross leadership made every effort to integrate itself into military medical corps, to the point where, when the pacifist movement burgeoned at the end of the nineteenth century, the Red Cross wanted nothing to do with it. Dunant, the pacifist who had founded the humanitarian group, eventually exhausted himself physically and financially, and became disillusioned with the group's direction. When the Red Cross was awarded its first Nobel Peace Prize in 1901 the founder was located in a Swiss almshouse, but faded into obscurity again after attending the ceremony. He died penniless and forgotten in 1910.

The Canadian branch of the ICRC had its unofficial beginning during the North-West Rebellion of 1885. The army's medical officer, Dr. George Sterling Ryerson, hoisted a makeshift Red Cross flag to protect his horse-drawn ambulance. The flag was also flown at the Battle of Batoche, May 9–12, 1885, in what is now Saskatchewan, where comfort was offered to the wounded on both sides.[2] It was not until more than a decade later, however, that Dr. Ryerson, who had risen to the rank of surgeon-general, held the founding meeting of the Canadian branch of the National Society for Aid to the Sick and Wounded, on October 16, 1896. Born, as it was, between the North-West Rebellion and the Boer War, the Red Cross was initially inactive because the society's board of directors felt peacetime work should be left to the St. John Ambulance Association.[3] The first public meeting of the Red Cross wasn't held until over a year and a half later, on May 5, 1898, at Massey Hall in Toronto, as part of a fund-raising campaign for the Spanish-American War. The American army, suspicious of the Canadian group, refused to accept medical supplies, while the Spanish accepted a modest amount. At a time when patriotic fervour was common, the public was a bit unclear on the concept of neutrality and medical aid in time of war. At the outset of the fighting in South Africa, a Red Cross fund-raising drive collected more than $50,000 in cash and copious quantities of clothes and liquor, because people thought of the agency as a medium for delivering parcels to the fighting men.

For many years the group's expenses were paid by its well-heeled volunteer directors. It was not until 1909, when the federal government passed the Canadian Red Cross Society Act, that the agency was incorporated as a charitable organization (its charter made no reference to the collection and distribution of blood, and still does not). The Red Cross remained largely quiescent from 1902 until the declaration of war by Great Britain in August 1914.

Colonel Albert E. Gooderham, national commissioner of the Red Cross, had asked the Department of Physiological Hygiene of the University of Toronto to produce sera, antitoxins and vaccines for Canadian soldiers, and he personally provided scientists with the means to do so. An extremely wealthy man, Colonel Gooderham, who already sponsored many Red Cross activities himself, bought a 58-acre farm outside Toronto, where scientists created one of the finest research laboratories in the world. He named it Connaught Anti-Toxins Laboratory, in honour of his friend the Duke of Connaught, the Governor-General of Canada, whose wife was president of the Red Cross. The two institutions would be intertwined for many years to come.

Connaught Laboratories made its mark by providing the vaccines for Canada's first immunization campaign, against smallpox, tetanus and typhoid; soldiers heading overseas were treated first, then civilians. The Red Cross not only offered medical help to wounded soldiers and civilians during the First World War, but visited prisoners of war, mostly in Germany, ensuring that they were kept in humane conditions and providing them with blankets and other comforts, as well as supplying five hospitals in England and one in France. Due to the close links it had forged with the military and those in positions of power, however, the Red Cross became a vehicle for patriotism, not internationalism. Nowhere was this more evident than in the United States. When the U.S. entered the war in 1917, the American Red Cross distributed a poster of the Stars and Stripes alongside the Red Cross flag with the slogan "Loyalty to one means loyalty to both."[4] A similar attitude existed in Canada, where the Red Cross raised a staggering $35 million during the First World War.

In peacetime, the Red Cross and Connaught continued to play significant roles. The Red Cross helped with the reunification of families and the rehabilitation of wounded soldiers. Its well-organized network of volunteers also became involved in emergency medical and social services for civilians. Red Cross volunteers would invariably be on hand, for example, at any major fire or flood. Similarly, the wartime efforts of Connaught came to have a dramatic influence on public policy. Dr. John FitzGerald, the first director of Connaught, would profoundly change the way Canadians viewed health services. Dr. FitzGerald felt his wartime experience in preventing and controlling contagious diseases should be applied to the civilian population. He convinced the Ontario government not only to conduct wide-scale immunization, but to distribute, free of charge, treatment for diphtheria — a disease that ravaged poor families. In pre-medicare days, poorer Canadians had little access to medical care, including immunizations.

Dr. FitzGerald's views were underlined by an epidemic of influenza that hit Toronto in October 1918, killing thousands of people.* The Red Cross and Connaught were again on the front lines, one coming to the aid of the sick and dying, the other producing a vaccine to stem the deadly outbreak. Dr. FitzGerald used the tragedy and the disillusionment of returning veterans to lobby for greater government involvement in public health, and in the spring of 1919 the federal government created a Department of Health. "At this time when we are suffering from the losses due to the war, and when the value of human life has become of greatest moment, it is fitting that the House and the country should turn attention to considering better measures for conserving the health of our people," Newton Rowell, the country's first health minister, said in the House of Commons. While he welcomed federal involvement, Dr. FitzGerald also recognized that the overlapping public health responsibilities of Ottawa and the provinces were a potential problem. In 1920 he was instrumental in founding the Dominion Council of Health, a group of senior bureaucrats and medical officers of health who tried to co-ordinate public health campaigns nation-wide.

The discovery of insulin in April 1922 trained the eyes of the world on Connaught Laboratories. That same year, the Red Cross decided to expand its functions to include peacetime work. Its first priority was to create an international public health organization whose goal was "the promotion of health, the prevention of disease and the mitigation of suffering throughout the world". The impact in Canada was immediate. The Red Cross sponsored the education of hundreds of young women so they could get Public Health Nursing degrees at universities, and the agency financed, between 1920 and 1938, outpost hospitals and nursing stations all across rural Canada, providing healthcare for almost half a

---

* World-wide, an estimated 25 million people died in the influenza epidemic. Virtually the entire world's population was infected with the disease.

million of the country's poorest citizens. A Red Cross nurse from Bonfield, Ontario, was on hand for the delivery of the Dionne quintuplets in 1934; she cared for the five girls before the doctor arrived, and kept them alive during the early weeks by collecting breast milk from other women in her nursing territory.

Given its key role in the nascent public health system and its close ties to the military, it was natural for the Red Cross to become involved in the supplying of blood. The British Red Cross Society established the first voluntary blood donor service, the Greater London Blood Transfusion Service, in 1921. After the Munich crisis, in the fall of 1938, the British army established its own Blood Transfusion Service. With the help of the Red Cross it also laid the foundations for a volunteer donor network, and, within forty-eight hours of the declaration of war, volunteer blood was being provided to British soldiers. On October 6, 1939, the first airdrop, forty pints of blood, was made at Dieppe, the site of a large military hospital. In Canada, the first volunteer blood donor clinic sponsored by the Red Cross was held at Toronto's Grace Hospital on January 29, 1940; the birth of the Blood Transfusion Service (BTS) went virtually unnoticed.

Dr. Charles Best was determined to solve the problem of providing blood to wounded soldiers. With a $5,000 grant from the Department of National Defence in early 1940, he purchased a drying apparatus that allowed him to reduce plasma serum to powder. It may have been the best investment of defence money in Canadian military history. The bulk of the credit, however, must go to the University of Toronto, which built a one-storey structure as a laboratory and provided the huge quantities of steam heat required for the drying process. Within months, the life-saving powder was shipped off to field hospitals. The first transfusion of volunteer Canadian plasma went to an anonymous British soldier on June 4, 1940, at Dunkirk. "Doctors were so agreeably surprised with its power," the Red Cross said in its annual report, "that it was not long before it was listed as a vital medical treatment. Thus was commenced a new Red Cross service that was later destined to save thousands of lives in the battlefields of Europe."

The dried plasma developed by Dr. Best was a godsend. British researchers had only been able to come up with a filtered blood serum, but it needed to be shipped in special insulated boxes to keep it cool. The powder from Connaught Laboratories was far more portable, didn't require any special storage and had a virtually unlimited shelf life. It was shipped with bottles of distilled water and administration kits (needles, tubing, etc.), making it all the more convenient. Convinced that Dr. Best had developed a miracle product, the military asked the Red Cross if it could collect a mind-boggling 2,000 donations a week, or 100,000 donations a year, to supply Canadian and British troops. There was no tradition of blood-giving, and there was widespread fear that the procedure was painful, so the goal was far too ambitious.

That first year, the Red Cross managed to collect 5,325 blood donations, a substantial increase from the 1,200 units Dr. Best had come up with at his makeshift clinics in 1939. Soon there were regular appeals, such as this one in *The Globe and Mail*: "A hundred men between the ages of 21 and 50 are needed to donate a cupful of blood each, the Red Cross announced yesterday"; the article stressed that the procedure was painless and would take only fifteen minutes. The blood program got off to a slow start given the need for plasma. Nevertheless, Fred Routley, national commissioner of the Red Cross, recognized its importance: "Another wonderful piece of work launched in 1940, though only just now getting under way, is the securing and sending of blood serum, or blood plasma, as it is generally called," he wrote in his annual report. "This method of blood transfusion is now recognized by the medical profession as one of the greatest steps forward in medical science, and the Canadian Red Cross Society is proud to have a part in furthering this remarkable work. . . . It is felt this will constitute one of the most remarkable activities that our society has ever undertaken." That same year, the Red Cross established the Canadian Red Cross Military Hospital in Taplow, England, a "gift of the Canadian people to their fighting forces". The 600-bed hospital, which cost $700,000, was among the first to receive regular stocks of dried plasma.

In October 1940, the Red Cross opened a permanent blood donor clinic at 410 Sherbourne Street in Toronto. It was there that volunteers began the tradition of serving coffee and home-made biscuits, as part of the process of making blood donations pleasant. (At first donors were asked not to eat before donating, but soon juice and soup became the drinks of choice; doctors realized that coffee, because caffeine is a powerful diuretic, caused many donors to faint so it was served only after donations.) Another practice at the time was using local anesthetic on the donor's arm before inserting the needle, which was much larger than those used today. As with many domestic wartime endeavours, the first clinics were operated almost entirely by women, with the exception of a male doctor who did a cursory medical examination and the actual needle insertion. All the material was reused, so needles had to be sharpened, bottles washed and sterilized, and the freshly donated blood treated to keep it from clotting. Those tasks were performed by women volunteers, who were organized into military-style units and fitted with the military-style uniforms of the Blood Corps. Still, women were seen as too fragile to be donors themselves. The no-women policy, however, was forgotten at the Ottawa clinic, Canada's second blood-collection facility, which opened its doors in the winter of 1940. Dignitaries like Princess Juliana, later the Queen of The Netherlands, and Princess Alice, wife of the Governor-General, the Earl of Athlone, were among the first donors, but they remained exceptions to the rule.[5]

Before people could donate blood, their hemoglobin, or iron level, was tested (later in the war, when nutrition standards slipped, donors routinely received iron pills). There was also rudimentary screening of donors and testing of blood to minimize infections from bacteria and viruses. Those with jaundice (later recognized as being, in many cases, a symptom of hepatitis) or a history of malaria were turned away, as were those suffering from the sexually transmitted disease syphilis. While indelicate questions about venereal diseases could be asked openly by army physicians, Red Cross doctors opted to test the blood of civilians and discard the donations infected with syphilis. Statistics on the infection rate weren't kept at the time, but deductions can be made. In 1941, for example, there were almost 36,000 Red Cross donors, but only 33,981 units of blood were used to produce dried plasma, meaning that about five per cent of blood donations were rejected. Still, bouts of jaundice were not uncommon after transfusions. Syphilis became much less of a problem with the commercial production of penicillin at Connaught Laboratories late in 1940, and its widespread availability for civilians in the post-war years.

A greater problem was the lack of sterile conditions at the clinics and in the laboratory. To get the blood flowing from a patient, the nurse would sometimes suck air up the tube. Similarly, blood was often exposed to contaminants during the processing phase. After typing and testing, the blood was placed in a refrigerator overnight and allowed to clot. The next day, the plasma was separated out by centrifuge and many donations mixed together before being filtered. The serum was then frozen solid at -50° Celsius in a mixture of dry ice and alcohol, and transferred to a vacuum cabinet where the serum "boiled" at -10° Celsius, removing all the moisture. Each bottle was then capped and sealed in a tin for transport. The entire process took about five weeks. Dr. Best and his team were constantly on the lookout for bacteria and viruses that could infect the plasma, even equipping the lab with ultraviolet lights, thus exposing themselves to radiation for hours at a time. The biggest culprit by far was airborne coliform, but there were also cases of bacterial meningitis and other illnesses reported after transfusions. All told, the infection rate was about five per cent, with the bulk of cases being jaundice, but the actual consequences of blood-borne disease, the death and illness it caused, are not known.

Since its founding, the Red Cross had depended on corporate and individual donations to fund its many activities. By far the largest single cash sponsor of the blood program was the Toronto Skating Club, which contributed $25,000 in 1941. Walpole Pharmaceutical Company of Perth, Ontario, purchased, in honour of a staff member's son who was missing in action, a house that became home to the Ottawa clinic. By the second year of BTS operations, clinics were open in six provinces, but the logistics of getting blood to Toronto hampered the Blood for the Wounded campaign. Despite demand for dried plasma, particularly in the Royal Navy — burns, common in torpedo attacks, required huge quantities of plasma — Connaught Laboratories was operating at only 50 per cent of capacity. To reach its goal of 2,000 donors a week, the Red Cross knew that it had to set up clinics across Canada — a daunting task, particularly in wartime. About 10 per cent of all wounded required transfusions, and they received four pints each on average. As the number of casualties increased, so did the urgency of the task at hand. An estimated 100,000 donors were required for every 17,000 casualties because substantial yield was lost in the drying process. In 1941, the Red Cross set aside $150,000 to set up clinics in every province, almost three times what the blood program had cost in its first full year of operation.

In 1942, the war hit home in Canada with the bloody, futile raid on Dieppe, which left 1,496 dead and wounded and 1,944 prisoners of war. The massive need for blood that resulted was matched by an unprecedented level of interest in the population at large. Three initiatives introduced into the blood program that year remain key to the service's success to this day: the Red Cross officially accepted women donors, it set up clinics in industrial plants and it established mobile clinics that travelled to towns and villages from coast to coast. The number of donations jumped to 181,091 from 36,000 in a single year. But that was only the beginning. By 1943 Canadians donated a total of 536,311 units of blood to the Red Cross. But the price was high, in both cost and safety. The budget for the blood program jumped tenfold in a single year, to almost $700,000, and the Red Cross experienced its first tainted-blood problem. Thousands of bottles of dried plasma were discarded after soldiers contracted a bacterial infection, but the details were never revealed publicly. The Red Cross annual report of 1943 referred cryptically to "the problem" and indicated that an infectious disease specialist had been hired to resolve it.

But the problem, most likely fecal coliform bacteria, did not disappear. In April 1944 the National Research Council in Ottawa was given ten thousand litres of blood serum that the Red Cross knew was contaminated. The serum went to the E.B. Lilly Company in the U.S., which used it to manufacture albumin, a blood derivative used to treat burn victims (the process of making albumin, which included heat treatment, killed bacteria and viruses). Disposing of the contaminated lot, the equivalent of almost fifty thousand blood donations, did not cause serious hardship because in 1944, for the first time, the number of blood donations topped one million. Despite working around the clock, Connaught Laboratories couldn't keep pace, so a second drying plant was opened at the University of Montreal.

Canadians had every reason to be proud of their efforts. During the final twelve months of the war in Europe, from May 1944 to April 1945, there were an amazing 890,000 blood donations, more than one-third of the 2.5 million donations made during the war. Throughout the war years, Connaught Laboratories produced a total of 436,000 bottles of dried plasma, at a total cost of just under $2 per bottle. Canada provided not only enough for its own soldiers, but plasma for the treatment of 60 per cent of the entire British force as well.

*　　*　　*

Even before it closed down wartime clinics on August 15, 1945 — VJ Day — the Red Cross was considering a move to blood collection for civilians. A survey of Canadian hospitals found that blood collection and transfusion facilities were seriously wanting. In virtually every province, a single burn victim could exhaust the entire blood supply, and entire regions didn't offer transfusion. Further, transfusion was well beyond the means of most patients. In pre-medicare days, patients would pay handsomely for blood — up to $25 a pint, plus administration fees of $5 to $10. Dried plasma like that provided to Allied soldiers cost $40 per bottle. Because whole blood was inefficient compared to today's specialized blood components, surgery would often require twenty to thirty pints of blood. In other words, just the blood required for surgery could easily cost $1,000 — in excess of a year's salary for the average worker. To make matters worse, no government or private insurance plan covered the cost of transfusion, although the benefits were widely known. While it kept the operation quiet, the Red Cross had diverted about 2 per cent of its wartime blood collections to needy civilians, mostly obstetrics cases and women suffering anemia. During the war years, the infant mortality rate fell significantly.

Dr. Stuart Stanbury, director of the Red Cross Blood Transfusion Service during the war years, had grand plans for the BTS and no doubt that his vision of care could set a precedent for free and universal medical treatment. When the plan to make Canada the "first nation in the world to have a complete blood transfusion service organized and administered by a national voluntary organization" was presented to the Red Cross board of directors in October 1945, it was enthusiastically endorsed and granted a $1-million budget for start-up costs. "This great undertaking, if successful, may well pave the way for other major projects vitally affecting the health and welfare of the people of this

Dominion," Dr. Stanbury said. "Blood is a peculiar commodity in that it can only be obtained from human sources. It cannot be manufactured in the test tube, nor is there any adequate substitute. It cannot, and should not, be bought or sold as a commercial commodity for it represents the free gift of one man to another in order that a human life may be saved."

While the director of the Blood Transfusion Service enthused about how free blood would help with the development of new medical procedures such as brain surgery, skin grafts and immunization for children, he also warned that the agency had to take a leadership role to ensure that the blood was disease-free, and that making transfusions safe would be costly. "The Society will assume complete responsibility from the time that the blood leaves the veins of the donor until it enters those of the patient. It follows, therefore, that the safeguarding of human life will necessitate the employment of full-time, highly trained medical and technical personnel," he said.

In 1946, Dr. Stanbury personally negotiated contracts with provincial ministers of health. The agreements called for the Red Cross to provide blood, plasma and transfusion equipment to all hospitals on the understanding that they would not charge patients for the service. Each province agreed to provide a building for the Blood Transfusion Service, including services and maintenance, while the Red Cross assumed all the costs of personnel, transportation and processing blood into plasma. The Department of National Health was asked to underwrite the cost of processing at Connaught, but refused, saying the Red Cross, the country's biggest charity, was "too affluent". Dr. Stanbury also travelled to England, where he hired nine young doctors who would serve as Red Cross medical directors for the next four decades.

On February 3, 1947, the first peacetime blood donor clinic was held, at Vancouver's Shaughnessy Hospital. Dr. Patrick Moore was a young doctor when he stepped on board the *Empress of Britain*, but he was soon medical director of the provincial Red Cross BTS in Vancouver. "We knew nothing of blood transfusion, but we learned on the job," he recalls. The new service soon proved its worth; during the Fraser Valley floods, when a big area of British Columbia was cut off, the Royal Canadian Air Force dropped bottles of blood collected in Vancouver by parachute, saving dozens of lives.

It was an exhilarating time, but the blood program was politicized from the beginning. The medical directors were ordered to stage clinics everywhere, regardless of cost; the idea was to keep the Red Cross branches, which had in excess of one million full-time volunteers by the end of the war, active. It didn't matter that there was more blood collected than there was demand; after ten

days outdated blood was shipped by train to Connaught Laboratories, where it
was processed into dried plasma.

Later in 1947, blood transfusion centres opened in Edmonton and Calgary,
and the next year there was one in Charlottetown. The choices were strange
ones, motivated again by politics, not by demand for blood. The giant Toronto
BTS opened officially on Valentine's Day, 1949, followed by those in Montreal
and Hamilton. That same year, an amendment to the Red Cross charter
allowed it to carry on peacetime charitable activities officially. In 1950,
Winnipeg and Saint John started collecting volunteer blood; in 1952, so did
Regina and Saskatoon.

The expansion was rapid and ambitious, but soon costs were spiralling out of
control. By 1952 a "radical retrenchment within the Society became necessary"
according to the annual report because the blood program was eating up virtually all the money donated to the Red Cross. In fact, only the advent of the
Korean War allowed the blood program to stave off financial collapse. The
Department of National Defence awarded the Red Cross a grant of $230,185
to produce ten thousand bottles of dried plasma for its field hospitals. The
beauty of the contract was that almost all the plasma was already in stock at
Connaught and, because all soldiers were ordered to give blood, Red Cross
reserves were replenished quickly. The contract renewed the close ties between
the Red Cross, Connaught Laboratories and the armed forces. The blood
products provided to soldiers in Korea had another distinguishing feature: they
were irradiated to kill bacteria and the hepatitis virus.

In 1954 Connaught Laboratories built Canada's first blood fractionation
plant, funded entirely by federal and provincial grants — a plant designed to
produce the blood derivative gamma globulin for the prevention of paralytic
polio, which had hit 8,000 Canadians in a 1953 epidemic. The Red Cross was
on the front lines of the endeavour, collecting an extra 200,000 blood donations. In the end, Connaught produced 90,586 vials of gamma globulin, but
the product was rendered obsolete by the development of the Salk vaccine in
the United States. Connaught began producing the Salk vaccine but the fractionation plant didn't go to waste; the Red Cross continued to collect blood
from all army recruits, and it was used to produce vaccines like human anti-
tetanus serum, and vaccinia immune globulin (VIG) for smallpox.

While the good deeds continued, so did the financial woes. In October
1956, George Aitken, chairman of the national executive committee of the Red
Cross, wrote the prime minister, premiers and federal and provincial health
ministers stating that the "Society is no longer in a position to continue to
finance the Canadian Red Cross Blood Transfusion Service from charitable

funds alone and, unless the federal and provincial governments assist in financing the service on a regular basis, the Society must regretfully withdraw from
this programme." That year the BTS budget was almost $2.5 million — more
than the blood program had cost during the entire Second World War. Only
three provinces — Alberta, New Brunswick and Ontario — responded to the
plea, with grants totalling $177,873 in 1957.

In April 1958 the Red Cross submitted a brief to the Council of Health
Ministers — the representatives of federal and provincial health ministers —
requesting support from the new hospital insurance plans, the beginnings of
national medicare. After much negotiation, the health ministers agreed to pay
30 per cent of the technical and professional costs of providing whole blood,
while the Red Cross would cover donor procurement costs. The Red Cross also
began charging hospitals for fractionating blood and manufacturing specialized
blood products; the hospitals paid cost plus 10 per cent, which the Red Cross
received to cover financing and handling charges. With the 30 per cent formula, however, revenue from government was still far less than the cost of
procuring donors, so the Red Cross reallocated many of its collection costs to
the professional and technical part of the budget. As a result, government
grants skyrocketed from just over $175,000 in 1957 to almost $700,000 the
next year, and to almost $900,000 in 1960. For six years the Red Cross hadn't
opened a single new BTS centre, and it had dramatically cut back on mobile
clinics, but now the government funding allowed the expansion of the blood
service. New centres were built in St. John's, Ottawa and London, with government grants covering only 22 per cent of the costs of the network.

May 22, 1961, was one of the most important days in the history of the Red
Cross Blood Transfusion Service. On that Friday, Dr. Stanbury made an urgent
plea to the Royal Commission on Health Services — established by the
Diefenbaker government to evaluate the healthcare system — warning that,
without adequate government financing, the Red Cross would be forced to
withdraw from the blood program. His arguments ran the gamut from the
purely emotional to the coldly financial.

"Without question this gigantic national humanitarian effort was responsible
for saving many lives on the battlefields as well as in the bombed cities of
Europe," Dr. Stanbury began. Yet 46 cents of every charitable dollar collected by
the Red Cross was going to the blood program, he said, and it had a shortfall of
almost $700,000 a year. The bulk of Dr. Stanbury's presentation focused on the
money the Red Cross had saved patients and provincial governments over the
years. During the period from 1947 to 1960, he argued, a total of 1,810,288
patients had been transfused with 3,029,524 bottles of blood, all of it free of

charge. The Red Cross had spent just over $28 million on blood services in its first thirteen years of operation. At prevailing rates in Canadian hospitals, those transfusions would have ordinarily cost patients $75,738,100 and an additional $6,920,765 in service charges, Dr. Stanbury continued. He also argued that Canadians had an emotional attachment to the Red Cross because 35 bottles of volunteer blood were collected per thousand population, compared to 13.6 per thousand in the mixed profit- and non-profit system in the United States and 22 per thousand in the United Kingdom, where the government paid 100 per cent of the blood program. Dr. Stanbury also noted that, with the planned opening of the Quebec City BTS centre in 1961, the Red Cross would be providing blood to all but four of the hospitals across Canada, and that new medical break-throughs like heart surgery and the "artificial kidney" (dialysis machine) would mean a big increase in demand for blood. Further, the blood program had become quite efficient in recent years, with the net cost of a bottle of blood falling to $2.83 in 1960 from $5.29 just three years earlier.

"We believe it has been satisfactorily established that the voluntary system of blood donations operated by a private charitable agency, such as the Canadian Red Cross Society, is admirably suited to meet the blood transfusion requirements of Canadian hospitals," Dr. Stanbury told the public hearings. "It is their sincere hope that this Royal Commission will recognize the serious financial dilemma facing the Canadian Red Cross Society and recommend to the federal and provincial governments the provision of necessary financial assistance which would enable the Society to continue this vital humanitarian service."

The plea bore fruit. The royal commission, headed by Mr. Justice Emmett Hall — who, coincidentally, was president of the Saskatchewan branch of the Red Cross at the time — sang the praises of the blood program. The federal and provincial governments agreed to a new funding formula: they would cover 45 per cent of technical costs of the Blood Transfusion Service, or $1.3 million. The next year government support jumped again, to 60 per cent of technical costs. Sadly, 1962 also marked the year that Dr. Stuart Stanbury died. During more than two decades at the helm, during war and peace, he had been the heart and soul of the blood program, a scientist whose social conscience was a driving force in the push for universal healthcare. In his final annual report Dr. Stanbury had urged the charitable agency to ease itself out of the blood program and take up new challenges. But, as the Red Cross came to be identified increasingly with blood, the agency became less open to change, and more reluctant to surrender control of its cash cow.

* * *

In the early days of the blood program, safety was not a major concern. After the war, most hospitals returned to using whole blood, or liquid plasma. Hemolytic reactions, the body's rejection of the blood, occurred in 5 to 10 per cent of cases but were rarely fatal, so they were seen as an acceptable risk, as they are today. Infectious diseases were not viewed as a serious problem either, though a fair number of transfusion recipients contracted hepatitis. Even though cases were rare, the Red Cross continued to test blood for syphilis, and in 1958 it began rejecting donors who had ever had jaundice, after the federal Food and Drug Act was amended requiring them to do so. (Previous to that, only donors who had had jaundice or malaria in the previous year were excluded.) Until the late 1950s, the major safety risk remained airborne bacteria. Although blood from a hundred donations was pooled into gallon jars in a sterile room for shipment, there was still the risk of contamination because the system was "open", the bottles and tubing were not only exposed to air, but reused. In 1959 the Red Cross began using disposable bottles and tubing, but with the advent of new products that necessitated the pooling of multiple units of blood, the risks of infection continued. In 1962, for example, hepatitis reached such epidemic proportions that some blood donor clinics were shut down.

The next year, the Red Cross experienced its second major contamination of blood products. For years its outdated plasma had been sent to Connaught for fractionation and, under an agreement with the Department of National Defence, an extensive inventory of the blood product albumin (used to treat burns) had been stockpiled, in case it was required for treating victims of a nuclear attack. In 1963 the Red Cross was given permission to distribute some of the albumin, which had been stored for between three and five years, to hospitals. There were hundreds of reactions to the product, so it was withdrawn, but not before 5,375 vials were injected into patients. In his annual report, the scientific advisor to the blood program, Dr. John Phair, expressed relief that no one had died.

In 1964, when a bottle of Red Cross blood or blood products was being transfused every minute of every day in Canada, Red Cross scientists took a step that would markedly improve the safety of blood and blood products: the introduction of plastic bags to replace glass bottles. The move would cut down substantially on the rate of contamination — which, they revealed for the first time, was actually about 25 per cent. The problem with plastic bags was that, while they revolutionized the medical and safety aspects of blood collection and distribution, they cost substantially more than bottles, and money was tight. Despite the fact that as many as one in four bottles of blood was contaminated with some bacteria or virus, it would take two years for governments to come up with money for the move, and four full years before the new product was fully phased in. That kind of foot-dragging allowed a large number of transfusion recipients to be infected by hepatitis. Meanwhile, government funding of the Red Cross climbed steadily higher, with Ottawa and the provinces picking up 67.5 per cent of the blood bill in 1965 and 75 per cent the next year.

The plastic bag brought not only greater safety, but far more flexibility. The new bag allowed the Red Cross to easily derive specialized blood products from donations of whole blood, such as platelets for leukemia patients and cryoprecipitate for hemophiliacs. The plastic bag also allowed blood collection centres to perform plasmapheresis, a technique in which whole blood is collected from a donor and fractionated on the spot; the blood plasma is collected in the plastic bag, while the red cells are immediately reinjected into the donor. While it is a more time-consuming process, plasmapheresis is far less draining on the body, and donors can return weekly. It is also more efficient, because more plasma is required than whole blood. In addition, it allows scientists to derive plasma from people with special antibodies and create vaccines.[6]

The Red Cross plan was to carry out plasmapheresis in Canadian prisons, in conjunction with Connaught Laboratories, to produce thousands of litres of plasma for the manufacture of vaccine sera, albumin and concentrate for hemophiliacs. With $75,000 in grants from Health and Welfare Canada and Corrections Canada, the Red Cross purchased state-of-the-art plasmapheresis machines, and trained staff. But the program never got off the ground because government scientists were troubled by the high rate of hepatitis infection in prisons. The Red Cross then approached the Metropolitan Toronto Police and Canadian Forces Base Borden for plasmapheresis donors, but they were refused because the procedure was too time-consuming, so the key element in making Canada self-sufficient in plasma, foundered. Meanwhile, the private blood collection business flourished. Canadian Bio Plasma, a division of Ortho Pharmaceuticals Company, bought plasma from Toronto University students for $15 a pint. Another company, Plasmapheresis Laboratory Limited, bought plasma from patients at Toronto East General Hospital and sold it to Ortho Pharmaceuticals, which in turn sold it to Connaught Laboratories. The laboratory was owned by Dr. George Miller, head of the Red Cross Blood Transfusion Service, which publicly opposed all commercialization of blood; when Dr. Miller retired in 1973, he became a paid consultant to Connaught, the company his successor said threatened the very survival of the Canadian blood program. When Dr. Roger Perrault took over as head of BTS, he candidly said Canada's blood system was 15–20 years out of date, and he vowed to modernize.

Having purer blood and more plasma was important because of various medical advances like blood concentrate, open heart surgery and organ transplants. The immune suppression that is induced to avoid rejection of organs, for example, made transfusion patients susceptible to the slightest impurities, and the risks were enormous because, at the time, surgeons used an average of twenty-four units of blood for heart surgery. Similarly, the pooling of plasma for the manufacture of blood concentrate increased the rate of contamination exponentially; one tainted donation would be mixed in with many pure ones. The biggest problem faced by the Red Cross during Canada's Centennial year, however, was the prospect that the demand for blood would not wane in the foreseeable future.

Demand was growing because blood was being over-prescribed. A full 95 per cent of transfusion patients were receiving whole blood, though hematologists suggested that only 40 per cent should be getting red cells, and the balance should get various specialized blood components derived from plasma. With one of the best volunteer blood collection systems in the world (43.8 units donated per 1,000 population, a rate double that in the U.S.), Canada was using more blood per hospital bed than any other country in the world, largely because it was free and accessible.

The agency's response to the ever-growing demand was to launch recruitment drives in high schools. The push to enlist teenage boys as young as sixteen to the cause — girls under eighteen were considered unfit as donors — demonstrated how the Red Cross remained rooted in its military tradition. "By indoctrinating the youth at an impressionable age, the adult of the future was guaranteed as a voluntary blood donor," the blood recruitment service explained in its 1967 annual report.

Despite the cavalier use of blood and increasingly expensive moves to expand collection, government support for the blood program increased to 82.5 per cent in 1967, then up to 90 per cent in 1968. By then, government grants were $5.7 million — as much as the entire blood program had cost only two years earlier.

In 1969, the Red Cross was broadsided by something totally unexpected and unprecedented: public criticism. At the time, Nigeria was waging a genocidal war against secessionists in Biafra, and the Red Cross decision to provide medical help to both sides provoked protests at blood donor clinics around the world, including in Canada. While the protests cost, at the most, a few hundred donations out of nearly a million, the Red Cross decided to step up its public relations campaign.

The following year, there were three important developments at the Red Cross. For the first time in the history of the blood program, donations actually dropped.

As well, the Red Cross made its first attempt at computerization, to facilitate the filing, recording and recalling of donors. "As mistakes in the computer field can be costly, the whole programme is proceeding with caution," Carel Endert, chairman of the donor recruitment committee, noted in his report. But the most notable event of 1970 was that the Red Cross began testing blood for hepatitis B, a project that was not fully implemented until January 1972. The delay again had to do with money; at $1 per unit, the new safety measure cost $1 million a year.

The Red Cross ended the practice of collecting blood in penitentiaries in 1972; it was the first time in its history that it had excluded a particular social group (aside from women) from donation. The move came after it was revealed that the hepatitis infection rate was ten times higher among prisoners than among the general population. Still, the agency was apologetic in its annual report. "This should not be interpreted as a social judgment against any group of donors as there is no difference in the quality of the blood between racial and ethnic groups. It is simply a fact of life that some life styles are more prone to produce hepatitis carriers than others." The high-risk activities for hepatitis included drug use and anal sex, but the Red Cross was a little too genteel to make those connections publicly, just as it would be when AIDS came along years later.

In its twenty-fifth anniversary year, the cost of Canada's blood program topped $10 million, with $8 million coming from public coffers. In a quarter-century the program had grown from a small charitable venture into a multi-million-dollar business. It was firmly entrenched not only as a key component of the healthcare system but as the heart of the Red Cross in Canada, and the charitable agency had no intention of letting go.

While the Red Cross continued to expand, its old partner, Connaught Laboratories, had fallen on hard times. In 1972 the University of Toronto sold the money-losing laboratory to CDC Life Sciences Inc., a subsidiary of the Canada Development Corporation. John Evans, president of the university at the time, said the sale was acceptable because the Crown corporation would be more than a commercial enterprise, and more sensitive to the public interest. Relations between the Red Cross and Connaught had, in fact, been strained for some time, because the fractionation plant was producing substandard blood products.

The executive of the Canadian Hematology Society appointed a committee to investigate Canada's blood program that year. The blood specialists were concerned about the growing number of Canadian hospitals and individuals who were buying blood products on the open market. The committee concluded that while the Red Cross Blood Transfusion Service was a "sound structure and a valuable national resource", it wasn't doing the job as well as it could. "The major objective of the Transfusion Service should be to supply the total need for blood and blood products (therapeutic and diagnostic) in Canada. This does not necessarily imply that the Red Cross should produce all such products."

The response of federal and provincial health ministers to that report, the first independent look at the blood program, was to establish the Federal-Provincial program and Budget Review Committee in 1974. The committee's first act was to increase financial support to the Red Cross, to cover 100 per cent of technical costs and 40 per cent of donor recruitment costs. Aside from a small contribution of funds to recruitment, the blood program was no longer a charitable activity; the Red Cross was essentially working on contract to the country's health ministries.

The next year, 1975, the gross inadequacies of Connaught's fractionation facilities began coming to light after an inspection by the Bureau of Biologics (the first since 1969, it was prompted by a series of articles in *The Globe and Mail*). Stuart McInnes, vice-president of Connaught, said in an internal memorandum that the fractionation facilities "would be closed if it were subjected to an inspection" and estimated that more than $300,000 in renovations were needed "to reduce severe and costly contamination problems." At the time, about 50 per cent of the plasma Connaught received from the Red Cross was lost because of contamination problems within the laboratories. Still, after a quick paint job, federal health inspectors gave Connaught a passing grade and it continued to receive volunteer plasma, though the Red Cross remained irked by the wastage.

The Red Cross and Connaught had another falling-out the following year, after CBC's "the fifth estate" revealed that the newly privatized company had sold more than $500,000 worth of powdered albumin to a Montreal blood broker in 1974, at a time when there were severe shortages in Canada. Since 1963, the year the Red Cross and Connaught had signed a fractionation contract, almost $7 million worth of blood components had been sold into the U.S., with the Red Cross getting a 10 per cent "royalty" on the sales — a commercialization of volunteer blood that violated the most fundamental Red Cross principles but one which earned the agency $689,827. The federal government finally outlawed such exports in 1976, in its first timid regulation of the blood system.

The Red Cross, like Connaught, had the full support of government, which was willing to overlook problems to support Canadian agencies. The Red Cross also had an enviable contract, unwritten and open-ended; the provinces paid the bills, the agency answered to no one. In such an arrangement lay the seeds of the disaster that would strike the Canadian blood supply less than a decade later.

3

BOYS WHO BLEED
HEMOPHILIA AND TRANSFUSION

> . . . the voice of thy brother's blood crieth
> unto me from the ground.
>
> Genesis 4:10

Kama Steliga, Lilooet, British Columbia

Before Kama married her husband, Lyle, they talked about the risk of AIDS. He is a mild hemophiliac who used factor concentrate only because it allowed him to play hockey. Lyle was tested for the AIDS virus in early 1986, and assumed he was fine. The couple married and had two children. In 1991, the results of his positive AIDS test were found in Lyle's medical file; no one had called with the news.

"I'd like to present a picture of how AIDS has affected our children and will affect our children. We have a son who is five and a daughter who is three . . . Regardless of their status as being negative, the effect this disease has had on our lives will be incredible. The loss, the pain will be life-long. They are very young now. When I look in their faces there is a tremendous amount of emotion. . . .

There is pain when our son asks me if Daddy's coming home from the hospital or if he's going to heaven. There is pain when he asked his dad one night: "Where will you be when I wake up in the morning?" He wanted to know if Lyle would be there or if he would be in heaven. They are losing their father in a physical sense but they are losing so much more: bedtime stories, kisses, hugs, being there for them when they need him. . . .

This tragedy in the blood supply was preventable. To think that my children's lives are so affected by these decisions and by this infection. The impact is multi-generational. My mother-in-law is losing a son, I'm losing the man that I love, my children are losing their father and our grandchildren are losing their grandfather. It doesn't stop just with asking Lyle how the disease affected him, or how it is affecting me as his wife.

The larger issue is the fact that it affected the kids and their father. That relationship is a cornerstone and a foundation of a healthy childhood and on into life. They were stripped of it and that makes me hurt for them. It also makes me very, very angry."

(March 31, 1994)

WHEN ED KUBIN TALKS ABOUT the certain death that awaits him, you can sometimes catch a glimpse of the boy lacing up his skates on a cold Prairie day in the winter of 1953. Impending death, like coming of age, brings a certain glint to a man's eyes, the mixture of fear and determination that you find in the look of a soldier as he readies himself for battle. Ed Kubin has those soldier's eyes when he tells of the 11-year-old boy stepping onto the rink in St. Vital, Manitoba. For months the young hemophiliac had prepared for the moment, skating cautiously, grasping his father's waist, with pillows tied to his arms and his backside, conscious that the slightest misstep could prove fatal. Bleeders weren't supposed to skate, let alone play the rough-and-tumble game of hockey; they weren't supposed to go to school either. Their lot in life was supposed to be quiet resignation. Yet, despite the precautions, only one in ten hemophiliacs of Ed Kubin's generation lived past adolescence.

Charles Kubin wasn't there to witness his son's achievement that day, but he would have been proud. If there was one thing he'd learned from the war, it was that you didn't sit back and wait to die. No matter how desperate the situation, you fought, and when there was a break in the fighting you let loose. During the war, Charles Kubin had had his life saved by a blood transfusion after a serious motorcycle accident. Grateful for a second chance at life, he had gone on to marry and to pass on his wild spirit to his two sons. The boys also inherited a genetic disorder from their mother that made them dependent on blood transfusions.

Undaunted, Charles Kubin decided his sons would live their lives to the fullest. Ed and his older brother, Barry, both went to regular school, and they never hesitated to duke it out when other boys taunted them in the schoolyard. Ed even had a paper route. Like so many Prairie boys, he wanted to be the next Gordie Howe. When the moment of truth came — when he took those wobbly first strides onto the rink, he was almost oblivious of the searing pain in his limbs. Momentarily freed of the stigma of his affliction, he soared around the ice as if the blades were winged. For a few fleeting moments he was just like the other boys, chasing the puck and stickhandling clumsily in a bid for glory. Then, without warning, he was broadsided by a check that sent him crashing into the boards. As he dragged himself from the ice, young Ed knew he was headed for hospital — again.

* * *

Hemophilia is a hereditary disorder that affects one in every five thousand males[1]; it is passed on in skip-gap manner, meaning that women are carriers but are very rarely affected directly. (Von Willebrand's disease, which is lumped in with the hemophilia family, is not a genetic disorder but a protein deficiency that can affect men or women.) Hemophiliacs lack a coagulation factor in their blood. There are thirteen clotting factors but, like the majority of hemophiliacs, Ed and Barry had Factor VIII deficiency.[2] Contrary to popular belief, bleeders do not bleed more profusely than others, nor do they have thinner blood; but the absence of the coagulation factor means that their blood doesn't clot properly so their bodies can't repair cuts and bruises, and they can bleed uncontrollably.

Ed Kubin didn't cut himself when he fell to the ice but, even at his young age, he knew the greatest danger was internal bleeding. The slightest bump could cause muscles and joints to swell up tremendously, and they would feel like they were being tightened in a vice; it might even prevent vital organs from functioning properly. Sometimes severe hemophiliacs — those with no clotting factor at all — suffer from spontaneous bleeds; the body's normal functioning can provoke internal hemorrhaging, something that is unbearably painful. As a result, hemophiliacs of Ed's generation were tethered to emergency rooms.

The word "hemophilia" is derived from the Greek *haima* (blood) and *philia* (love). The bleeding disease was first described in written records more than two thousand years ago. By the fifth century it was already recognized as an inherited disease that affected males; rabbis decreed that boys were to be exempted from the rite of circumcision if they had brothers or uncles who had died during the procedure. For centuries, hemophilia was one of those mysterious diseases that haunted humanity. What made it particularly notable was the myths and rituals that revolved around the magical powers of blood.

Long before scientists understood the life-giving properties of blood, pagan farmers sprinkled the red liquid on their fields to ensure a fruitful harvest, and warriors painted themselves in blood to make themselves invincible on the battlefield. The Egyptians believed bathing in blood was therapeutic. The Greeks introduced the practice of blood-letting to rid the body of illness, while the Romans drank blood to cure disease. One of the earliest references to transfusion in literature is in Ovid's *Metamorphoses*, where Jason pleads with Medea to restore the youth of his father, King Aeson, which she does by "cutting the old man's throat, letting all of his old blood out of him", then she "filled his veins with a rich elixir". There are several passages in the Bible referring to blood that to this day form the basis for denial of transfusions on religious grounds. For example, in Acts 15:29 it is written, "That ye abstain from meats offered to idols, and from blood, and from things strangled, and from fornication: from which if ye keep yourselves, ye shall do well."

During the Renaissance, physicians practised astrological blood-letting, convinced that diseases could be cured and powers conferred by bleeding on specific days of the lunar calendar. The operations were often performed hundreds of times on a single patient; one woman in Prague was bled more than seven hundred times, and each procedure was dutifully recorded. In the fifteenth and sixteenth centuries, surgeons were people who did blood-letting. In fact, barber-surgeons travelled from village to village, often advertising their services of bleeding and haircutting by wrapping bloody sheets around a white pole — the origin of the barber pole. (During the First World War, American barbers added blue stripes to their poles as a patriotic gesture.) By the time blood-letting was abandoned as a therapy, the practice had killed more people than all the wars in recorded history combined.

In 1616, there was a major breakthrough in hematology, the science of blood, when William Harvey discovered that blood circulates in the body. So controversial was his finding that it wasn't published until 1628. Even then the Royal College of Physicians in London insisted that blood moved "to and fro", not in a continuous route, until the discovery of capillaries some forty years later provided visual proof that arteries and veins were connected. Blood became a favoured interest of scientists in the years that followed, and many of them experimented with the effects of injecting all kinds of fluids (such as milk, ale and opium) into the bloodstreams of animals. Some scientists argued that a dog transfused with a lamb's blood would grow wool and hoofs and bleat instead of bark, or that a man who received another's blood would lose his soul. Richard Lower, an Oxford physician, performed the first successful blood transfusion between two dogs in 1666. The next year, Jean-Baptiste Denis, physician to

Louis XIV of France, administered the first recorded human blood transfusion, injecting half a pint of lamb's blood into a sick 15-year-old boy who subsequently recovered. Soon after, Dr. Lower transfused blood from a lamb into a man, then from one man to another. The events were recorded in the diary of Samuel Pepys, who suggested it might be a good idea to give the Archbishop of Canterbury — who was too Catholic in his ways for Pepys's taste — a transfusion from a Puritan. Dr. Lower, for his part, suggested that "good blood" should be used to replace "lost or bad blood", but it wasn't used in this logical manner until much later. Dr. Denis continued to experiment until one of his patients received a fatal transfusion of calf's blood in 1668. The Faculty of Medicine of the University of Paris exonerated the physician of murder, but banned blood transfusion in France. England and Rome followed suit. As a result, the practice of transfusion fell into disrepute until the late nineteenth century, when the physiological and chemical effects of injecting blood became better understood.

In 1803, U.S. scientists determined that hemophilia could be transmitted from an unaffected mother to her son, but it would be several more decades before blood transfusion was attempted as a treatment for hemophilia. The presence of hemophilia among Queen Victoria's descendants, who married into virtually all the royal houses of Europe, not only aroused the interest of the medical community but spawned the appellation "royal disease". Along with this term came the notion that hemophilia was the result of inbreeding, and that hemophiliacs were weak and effeminate. The stereotype of weakness was further fuelled by Alexei Romanoff, son of Nicholas II, the last tsar of Russia, and grandson of Queen Victoria. The young hemophiliac heir was carried everywhere by bodyguards, and was seen as too feeble to succeed his ineffectual father. As a result, the court was subjugated by the monk Rasputin, setting off a series of events that led to the Russian Revolution and the overthrow of the tsar. Alexei and his family were shot by the Bolsheviks in 1918.

Blood transfusion as it is practised today had its beginnings in early nineteenth-century England. Dr. James Blundell, an expert in abdominal surgery who recognized the need for transfusions in people suffering severe blood loss, began treating patients with incurable diseases with human-to-human transfusions in 1818. He didn't succeed until 1829, when he treated a woman who had had severe blood loss during childbirth with eight ounces of blood. But the practice was still very risky at the end of the century; many times, patients died not from the underlying injury but from an allergic reaction to the transfusion itself.

The discovery of the existence of blood groups in 1901, by Austrian researcher Dr. Karl Landsteiner, was the key breakthrough that allowed transfusion to be incorporated into medical practice, but there were still reactions that doctors couldn't explain. As well, blood collected from a donor would coagulate unless it was transfused directly, arm to arm, to the recipient. That difficulty was overcome just before the First World War, when sodium citrate was discovered to be an anti-coagulant with no side effects. This allowed Dr. Oswald Robertson, an American army surgeon, to create the first known blood bank, which served for the treatment of casualties of the Battle of Cambrai in November 1917. When the Red Cross established the first volunteer donor program in London, in 1921, donors were listed and called upon when needed, and got to know the recipient when they went to donate. In the Soviet Union doctors took a startlingly different approach, routinely bleeding cadavers and using the blood for surgery. In 1923, a full seventy-five years after hemophiliacs first received transfusions, researchers identified blood plasma as a more efficient form of treatment. Plasma would allow mild hemophiliacs, such as Canada's Governor-General, the Duke of Connaught (and Queen Victoria's son), to lead relatively normal lives.

Hematology had progressed tremendously by 1940, the year that researchers began producing dried plasma at the University of Toronto. Dr. Landsteiner discovered the missing part of the puzzle; in addition to the four basic blood types —A, B, AB and O — there was another element, dubbed the Rhesus (Rh) factor. Matching the donor and the recipient on Rh factor as well as blood type virtually eliminated the danger of hemolytic reaction.

*   *   *

During their childhood, Ed and Barry routinely spent almost three months of every year in the St. Boniface Hospital, most of the time in excruciating pain. In those days it could easily take a gallon of blood to stem a bleed; it was infused into the boys, drop by drop, while they were strapped to a board to keep them still. Painkillers were rarely prescribed because of the fear that bleeders would develop a tolerance, and perhaps an addiction. The boys were allowed an occasional Aspirin; doctors would learn later that this had only worsened their condition by further inhibiting clotting. The approach the medical profession took to hemophilia was crude but reasonably efficient: clinical observation, and intervention only if life was threatened.

Ed Kubin's father had never been a practitioner of the "do nothing" school. A University of Manitoba instrument technician who supplemented his income by working as a watchmaker, he did what the doctors recommended, treating the boys' bleeds with ice, splints and immobilization. But he also devised all manner of elaborate contraptions to ease the suffering of his sons. Their beds, designed to raise and immobilize various body parts, looked like something out of a science fiction movie. When their joints were too dangerously swollen for them to walk, he dragged them around the house on a pillowed cart. Charles Kubin was the working man's version of Alfonso XIII, the King of Spain who ordered all the trees in the royal garden padded with pillows to protect his princely sons, Alfonso and Gonzalo.

In the days before medicare, however, there was no cushioning the costs of hemophilia treatment. As a veteran Charles Kubin was entitled to an acre of land, which he subdivided and sold to pay his sons' exorbitant medical bills. Before the Red Cross blood program came into existence in 1947, blood cost $25 a unit, and that didn't include the cost of hospitalization and medical treatment. Between them, Ed and Barry needed hundreds of transfusions a year — well beyond the means of a man who earned $75 a month. But there was an alternative. Hospitals would provide a free pint of blood to a patient whose family could replace it with two fresh pints. As a result, Charles Kubin became adept at organizing his own blood drives, rounding up neighbours who would give a pint. But money was so tight that the proud father would have to bring in empty milk bottles to get the fare for the trolley ride to the hospital.

The arrival of the Red Cross blood transfusion service in Winnipeg in 1950, with its thousands of volunteer blood donors and its principle of free blood, was a godsend, one to which Ed Kubin owed his life time and time again. The introduction of medicare just a few years later was another answered prayer, though hemophiliacs continued to repay debts to family doctors for twenty years after free universal healthcare coverage was guaranteed by law. By the time they reached high school, Ed and Barry Kubin were being treated with blood plasma, and no longer had to be strapped to wooden boards to have whole units of blood injected into them to treat cuts and bruises.

Barry Isaac was also a war baby. When he was born in Calgary in 1942, he was healthy. Like most baby boys of the era, he was circumcised. The bleeding was so profuse that he almost died; in fact, the doctor transfused his own blood into the boy to save his life. When Barry was ten days old, his parents learned that he was a hemophiliac. The news came as a shock; like 40 per cent of hemophiliacs, he was born into a family with no known history of the disorder. In 1946 Barry's parents took him to the world-famous Mayo Clinic in Rochester, Minnesota, but the only thing the doctors there could suggest was that the removal of his spleen might prove useful — a recommendation typical of the unsophisticated treatment of hemophiliacs at the time. (As the spleen destroys worn-out red cells and platelets, it would become overburdened due to the number of transfusions a hemophiliac receives, and the organ itself would hemorrhage dangerously.) All his parents' friends had their blood typed and cross-matched, in case of an emergency.

In 1954 Barry hurt his neck and, ignoring his mother's warning that he was a severe hemophiliac, doctors performed a tracheotomy. In the following days Barry drained the blood banks in Calgary, Edmonton and Vancouver, using fifty pints daily for nine days. At one point, he had four bottles of blood being pumped into different parts of his body simultaneously. This was a risky exercise; when that much blood is pumped into the body, there is a danger of the lungs filling with fluid and the patient literally drowning while lying in the hospital bed — a fate that had befallen many hemophiliacs over the years. But Barry didn't drown, because the blood was spewing out of him as quickly as it was being infused. One nurse who tried to comfort the boy said the hospital room looked like an abattoir. Finally an experimental product, fresh-frozen plasma, was flown in on ice from Saskatoon, courtesy of the RCAF. At last, the bleeding was stopped. When he left hospital almost a month later, Barry weighed only seventy-five pounds but he had sprouted six inches to five foot ten. Like most hemophiliacs, he spent much of his time in a wheelchair because his joints were very fragile. The only physiotherapy at the time was trying to lift five-pound weights, an exercise that proved a struggle and often provoked new bleeds.

The next year, the seeds would be sown for a system that would avoid such unnecessary suffering for hemophiliacs. Pushed by his dynamic patient Frank Schnabel — founder of the Canadian Hemophilia Society — Dr. Cecil Harris opened the first hemophilia treatment clinic, at St. Mary's Hospital in Montreal. Schnabel envisaged a series of clinics from coast to coast, where people with bleeding disorders could get specialized care and state-of-the-art products. They would no longer have to argue with doctors about the gravity of their condition, and they wouldn't have to wait for hours in emergency rooms for treatment while the bleeding caused serious damage to their muscles, joints and vital organs.

When Connaught Laboratories' gamma globulin was overtaken by the more effective Salk vaccine, Connaught scientists looked for other blood products to manufacture. In 1958 they turned their attention to freeze-dried anti-hemophilic globulin (AHG). At the time, Factor VIII — the clotting factor that most hemophiliacs lack — had yet to be isolated; it was thought that the important element in plasma was fibrinogen, a globulin that also helps blood clot. AHG, a concentrated form of fibrinogen, was manufactured by pharmaceutical companies in the U.S. and Europe. In fact, Swedish doctors began using the new product as a prophylaxis, or preventive treatment, in 1958, and hemophiliacs showed dramatic improvements in health and mobility. But Connaught's efforts were marred by technical setbacks, and the AHG they produced was outlandishly expensive. Thus, in Canada, AHG was reserved primarily for severe hemophiliacs who required surgery.

In April 1960, Toronto teenager William Rudd became the first Canadian hemophiliac to get prophylactic treatment with AHG, and Connaught promised that affordable concentrate would soon be available to everyone. Most hemophiliacs continued to be treated with transfusions of whole blood and plasma, though big-city hospitals made a switch to the more efficient fresh-frozen plasma that had saved Barry Isaac's life. In a single year, the use of fresh-frozen plasma jumped 35 per cent.

The major breakthrough in hemophilia treatment, however, came in 1964, when Dr. Judith Pool, a post-graduate student at Stanford University, discovered a cryoprecipitate by chance. The researcher was thawing frozen plasma when she noticed unusual crystals forming on the top. On a whim, she scraped some off and tested them; the crystals were almost pure fibrinogen (and were, she would learn later, rich in Factor VIII). In tests it soon became obvious that a tiny bit of cryoprecipitate was more effective than dozens of units of blood, and about thirty times more potent than fresh-frozen plasma. The easy process of freezing and thawing plasma meant that the cryoprecipitate would cost a fraction of what concentrate did. It was licensed for sale in Canada in 1965.

The Red Cross, by its own admission, kept the news of the concentrate to itself. "AHG has not been used extensively as anticipated," the agency reported to its members in 1965, "although the Society has not broadcast its availability due largely to the difficulty in obtaining donors for the supply of plasma." The Red Cross told the federal government that it couldn't provide an adequate supply of the new concentrate until its plan to conduct plasmapheresis in federal penitentiaries was approved. In the meantime, the available concentrate went to the newly established pediatric hemophilia clinic at Toronto's Hospital for Sick Children, whose goal was to allow a new generation of hemophiliacs to live normal lives. Most adult hemophiliacs were still being treated with whole blood, plasma and fresh-frozen plasma, and suffered crippling arthritis and multiple health problems.

Luckily for hemophiliacs, Dr. Pool's cryoprecipitate moved from the laboratory to hospitals within months. The Red Cross, which over the years had lost many medical directors because of its autocratic rules, had finally begun to decentralize some laboratory services, and a number of BTS centres had new centrifuge machines, which were needed to separate red cells from plasma, the base ingredient for the production of blood products. The centrifuges, in conjunction with the much-anticipated introduction of the plastic bag for blood collection, meant cryoprecipitate could be easily manufactured almost anywhere in the country, and by early 1965 it was being used to treat hemophiliacs in Toronto, London, St. John's and Calgary. Better still, the treatment was preventive, not just for bleeds.

The next year, when cryoprecipitate was made available in Winnipeg, Ed Kubin's ties to the emergency room were loosened dramatically; he married and got a new job. While he still had to go to the hospital for treatment, it was much quicker and painless. Kubin had even heard of AHG, a product that would allow him to treat himself — something revolutionary for a man who not long ago had had to be strapped to a board to be transfused.

These were heady times for hemophiliacs; with their new-found freedom came cautious whisperings that a cure might some day be discovered. Frank Schnabel, the visionary who had done so much to blaze a trail into mainstream society that many hemophiliacs would follow, speculated in the group's newsletter about the implications of being able to alter the molecules of the DNA gene for sufferers of the hereditary disease. His musings were dismissed as science fiction by the medical community, but the discovery of the genetic causes of hemophilia would, within a generation, bring treatments that even Schnabel could never have imagined.

For most Canadian hemophiliacs, however, reality wasn't as rosy as the promised sci-fi future. Their treatment lagged years behind that in the U.S. and Europe. Frank Schnabel did what had previously been unthinkable: he publicly criticized the Red Cross, suggesting that new scientific developments meant they should lose their monopoly over the blood business. Citing lack of treatment facilities for hemophiliacs, chronic shortage of concentrate for their care, and the risk that the lure of profits would lead to the commercialization of the Red Cross BTS, Schnabel called for "government participation in blood transfusion services in Canada". The system, he said, in his opening address to the Canadian Hemophilia Society annual meeting in 1966, wasn't responsive to the needs of users, and as a result people were dying. "One can accept a death when one appreciates that everything possible has been done to save the life. When we realize, however, that a life has been lost unnecessarily because of an absence of or inadequate supply of concentrate, this we cannot accept."

Barry Isaac's situation typified what was wrong with the system. In 1966 he was still being treated with transfusions of fresh-frozen plasma. Even though concentrate had been licensed, it wasn't made available because of the cost. Medicare had still not come to Alberta, so Isaac was on welfare to ease the burden of medical bills. He had never been allowed to go to school because the authorities had thought it was too risky to have a bleeder around. At age twenty-two he could barely walk a block, and was often confined to a wheelchair. When he moved from High River to Calgary, he started being treated with cryoprecipitate. Within two years he was not only walking easily, but was a student at the University of Alberta. No longer tied to a hospital bed for half the year, he started to lead a normal life. His only hospital stays were voluntary, for surgery to repair ravaged joints and the arthritic knees that virtually all hemophiliacs suffered, as well as regular visits for injection of cryoprecipitate: Monday, Wednesday and Friday, four bags each time.

*   *   *

By the mid-1960s, freeze-dried factor concentrate that pooled the Factor VIII from up to 20,000 blood donations — this was a refinement from AHG, which was made from pooled fibrinogen — was widely marketed by U.S. pharmaceutical companies. Hemophiliacs and doctors loved the new product because it was completely portable. The powder, like that produced for the treatment of soldiers during the Second World War, needed only to be mixed with distilled water and infused. People with the blood disorder would no longer have to go to the hospital to be treated for minor bleeds. Almost immediately, however, researchers found that the new product provoked negative reactions in patients. At first these were dismissed as general reactions to receiving blood — something to which hemophiliacs were fairly accustomed — that were somehow enhanced by the potency of the concentrate. But in 1967 a number of scientists published research revealing that the new concentrates were contaminated with the hepatitis virus. The infection rate was virtually 100 per cent, because a single unit of plasma infected with hepatitis B could contaminate the whole lot of concentrate. Red Cross scientists had known for years, ever since they began lobbying for the plastic bag to replace the blood bottle, that one out of four units of blood was infected with some contaminant.

While hepatitis B infection could lead to devastating liver disease, doctors judged the risk acceptable. At the time, many hemophiliacs suffered from crippling arthritis and many had livers and spleens that had already been damaged by the massive quantities of blood and plasma pumped into their bodies. Besides, their life expectancy was still less than thirty years on average. This willingness of the authorities and hemophiliacs themselves to value blood supply above blood safety would come to shape policy decisions by doctors and the compliance of recipients many years later, long after the problem of bleeding had been resolved.

In 1967 the Canadian Hematology Society published a report that echoed some of Schnabel's concerns from a year earlier. The lack of availability of concentrate was "tragic", the blood specialists said in calling on the federal government to make construction of a fractionation plant a priority. Given their history and reputation, and the fact they were the only company licensed to sell concentrate in Canada, Connaught Laboratories seemed like the natural site for a commercial fractionation plant, one that could manufacture all the blood concentrates needed in Canada. Hemophiliacs were clamouring for the products that would make their lives so much easier; use of cryoprecipitate jumped to 131,651 units in 1969, up from 17,609 units just five years earlier.

At a meeting on May 26, 1969, the BTS committee of the Red Cross discussed the issue of treatment of hemophiliacs. Scientists knew that aggressive prophylactic treatment with either cryoprecipitate or factor concentrate could virtually eliminate the crippling effects of joint bleeds. They also knew that almost 100 per cent of hemophiliacs exposed to concentrate were infected with hepatitis B. Yet they decided that the "present policy of distribution of fractionation products should remain the same." In other words, they would do nothing to encourage the use of cryoprecipitate and nothing to discourage the use of concentrate. Just as important, they would do nothing about contaminated blood and blood products. In place of action, they issued reassuring words. In his annual report, for example, Dr. Ian Johnston, chairman of the BTS committee, stated, "It is our conviction that the hemophiliac in Canada is receiving excellent attention both from the point of view of prevention of episodes and the treatment of actual bleeding crises."

In 1970 — on the initiative of Dr. Patrick Moore, who had been promoted from the Vancouver BTS to head the National Reference Laboratory — the Red Cross began testing blood for contamination with the hepatitis virus. The test, the first new one since the agency had begun testing for syphilis in 1940, was introduced in Vancouver, then in Toronto. In the first year, 281,571 units of blood were tested for the hepatitis-B surface antigen, and 8,949 tested positive — a 3 per cent infection rate. "At this stage, it is not possible to achieve 100 per cent efficacy in detecting hazardous units of blood," Dr. John Partridge, head of the BTS, wrote in a report, "but the service has a moral obligation to eliminate carriers of a virus wherever possible." Still, it wasn't until January 1972, five years after articles about contamination of blood concentrates had first appeared in medical journals, that all of Canada's blood was tested for hepatitis B.

While government funding of the Red Cross had increased steadily over the years, there were still a number of blood products that the agency didn't provide. Instead, hospitals purchased them from U.S. pharmaceutical companies on the open market, an approach that was tacitly accepted by the provinces even though it undermined the whole philosophy underlying a national blood system. The federal Department of Health and Welfare seemed unaware of this arrangement; in a survey conducted by the International Society of Blood Transfusion, federal officials stated categorically that no blood products were imported into

Canada. Dr. Cecil Harris, who still ran the hemophilia clinic at St. Mary's Hospital in Montreal, was startled by that answer. He raised the issue of imported blood products at a meeting of the executive committee of the Canadian Hematology Society, which agreed that there was "evidence of a gap between what the Red Cross Blood Transfusion Service now accomplishes and what it could accomplish." The committee of hematologists found that more than $2.5 million in blood products were being imported into Canada, and felt that, over the long term, this threatened the blood program.

It was this concern, more than any worries about safety, that prompted federal and provincial health ministers to establish a committee overseeing the blood program in 1973. It wasn't until the next year that the ministers asked the Red Cross to set up a quality control program to ensure the safety and equitable distribution of blood products, in particular the ones most used — Factor VIII concentrate and platelets. In 1974, just over 6 per cent of blood donations were deemed unsuitable for transfusion. The Red Cross had always welcomed just about anyone as a donor, but in June 1975 it established the Ad Hoc Committee on Donor Selection to establish guidelines and, for the first time, introduced a donor questionnaire. Ron George, then president of the Canadian Hemophilia Society, made it his priority to push not only for more, but for better-quality concentrate. Most hemophiliacs had been infected with hepatitis B by concentrate, many of them had had violent reactions immediately after infusion. Little did they know that some of the plasma used to manufacture the miracle product was purchased from blood brokers who collected the raw material in so-called "vampire operations" in Haiti, Latin America and Africa (where the desperately poor would get as little as $1 for a pint of blood), bought outdated stocks from U.S. blood banks and even purchased blood drained from corpses in the Soviet Union.

Supply was a priority for hemophiliacs, as much as safety. Despite more than a decade of universal medicare, treatment facilities varied widely from one province to the next. Homecare programs were available in Vancouver, Montreal and Toronto, but in 1976 the majority of Canadian hemophiliacs still had to go to the hospital for injections of cryoprecipitate. In Alberta, factor concentrate was not even covered by the provincial drug plan.

That year, Barry Isaac — the boy too feeble to be a student — was a man heading to England to begin his second year of doctoral studies. While he could keep cryoprecipitate in the refrigerator at home, it wasn't practical to transport and store it in bed-and-breakfast accommodation. Isaac got a prescription for Factor VIII concentrate from his doctor; the one-month supply, which he packed in a single suitcase, cost him $1,200. The trip was a revelation. For the first time in his life, hemophilia was little more than a minor inconvenience. Across Canada, hemophiliacs had similar eye-opening experiences; concentrate revolutionized their lives, and everyone was clamouring for the miracle product.

The Red Cross saw the demand for the concentrate not as a nuisance but as an opportunity. The agency had taken to heart the Canadian Hematology Society's recommendation that it supply all blood and blood products in Canada. In October 1975 the Red Cross commissioned Dr. John Watt, scientific director of protein fractionation for the Scottish National Transfusion Service, to carry out a study of Canada's blood collection needs and fractionation capacity. Not surprisingly, he concluded that Canada could be self-sufficient in production of albumin and most factor concentrates if a fractionation plant was built as an integral part of the Red Cross BTS. The Red Cross proposed to the federal-provincial funding body that it build, within five years, a fractionation plant with a 350,000-litre capacity. A consultant pegged the cost at $20,813,000 and estimated that the state's investment would be repaid in six years.

Connaught Laboratories had, since 1955, routinely fractionated outdated plasma into the blood components albumin and gamma globulin, but it didn't have the facilities for large-scale production of factor concentrate. In fact, in 1973 and 1974 federal inspectors cited Connaught for violating a series of regulations regarding the quality of its factor concentrate. The Canadian Medical Association also warned that the plant was in desperate need of repair. Dr. Andrew Moriarty, vice-president of Connlab Holdings Ltd. (the parent company of Connaught), conceded that expanding the fractionation facilities — the oldest in North America — would be a "waste of time" and that a new plant should be built from scratch. His concerns were dismissed.

In a letter dated September 24, 1976, Marc Lalonde, Minister of Health and Welfare, said the Red Cross proposals conformed to three basic principles that were the pillars of Canada's blood system: 1) protection of the voluntary blood donor system; 2) national self-sufficiency in blood products; and 3) free supply of blood products. Within two months, federal and provincial deputy ministers of health had established the Ad Hoc Committee on Plasma Fractionation. They gave the Red Cross a green light to proceed with a more detailed study of the ambitious plan, and solicited briefs from commercial firms interested in fractionation. Topping the list, of course, was Connaught Laboratories.

The Red Cross and Connaught had been partners in providing quality health-care for Canadians for decades, dating back to the First World War. For the first time, they were competitors. Only one of them would build the plant — unless they could work together, which seemed increasingly unlikely given their differing visions. The newly privatized Connaught saw the plant as a business opportunity, one that could launch it into the same league as its competitors in the international pharmaceutical field. The Red Cross saw it as a way to consolidate its control over the blood system, to administer everything from the collection of blood through to the manufacture and distribution of blood products. As they jockeyed for position, the Red Cross refused to renew a long-standing contract to supply plasma to Connaught; directors of the laboratory lobbied the Ontario government, urging it to exert control over blood donations collected in the province. The donors of blood and recipients of blood products — the people most vitally involved in the blood system — took a back seat to this quest for business success. Blood collection and transfusion was no longer a humanitarian endeavor; it had become a cut-throat business.

4

DEATH TOUCHES DOWN
AIDS IN CANADA

The beginning of health
is to know the disease.

Cervantes
Don Quixote

Lorraine Olson, St. Albert, Alberta

As someone who lost a loved one to AIDS suddenly and unexpectedly, Lorraine, whose husband Tom, a hemophiliac, died in January 1994 at age 35, has a wish list.

"*First, I wish everyone here could have known Tom. He was a wonderful man. I also wish that everyone here knew what it was like every morning waking up and wondering what a new day would bring, whether it would be pneumonia or cancer or meningitis or any of the strange diseases people with AIDS are able to get. To wonder if you have days or weeks or months left together.*

I wish brothers didn't have to watch brothers die and cousins didn't have to watch cousins die. I wish this never happened, and I wish it never happens again. I wish I could have had one more day with Tom, so I could have said goodbye. I'd give up everything if I could just have him back right now."

(*April 22, 1994*)

ACQUIRED IMMUNE DEFICIENCY SYNDROME — or AIDS, as it has come to be known — had made many furtive visits to North America over the years, but it touched down for good on an Air Canada flight from Paris in early 1977. Epidemiologists at the U.S. Centers for Disease Control years later identified "Patient Zero" as Gaétan Dugas, a handsome and sexually adventurous flight attendant with Canada's national airline. He had been at the party to end all parties in New York City on July 4, 1976, when thousands had gathered to celebrate the U.S. Bicentennial and the coming of age of the gay liberation movement. Ironically, that festive event marked the beginning of the AIDS epidemic, and Mr. Dugas became a modern-day Typhoid Mary. The flamboyant flight attendant liked to be the life of the party, whether he was in a Paris discothèque, a San Francisco bathhouse, cruising the beach at the Club Med in Port-au-Prince or on a rare weekend at his home base in Halifax. In June 1980 he visited a Toronto doctor to have an unseemly purple spot looked at, but the unusual skin cancer, Kaposi's sarcoma, wasn't diagnosed until Dugas visited a doctor in New York City's Greenwich Village who was familiar with the symptoms of the emerging "gay cancer".

Officially, the first Canadian diagnosed with the strange new disease was a 43-year-old homosexual man from Windsor who, like Dugas, was a regular customer of the gay bathhouses in New York, San Francisco and Haiti. That was in January 1982, only six months after *Mortality and Morbidity Weekly Report*,[1] a publication of the U.S. Centers for Disease Control, reported on the strange outbreak of two previously rare diseases. The article, "Kaposi's Sarcoma and Pneumocystis Carinii Pneumonia among Homosexual Men — New York City and California", detailed similar symptoms among twenty-six young, otherwise healthy men, including Dugas, who had been diagnosed in the previous thirty months. That all the sufferers were gay men indicated that the immune breakdown that allowed the two diseases to flourish was "not an isolated phenomenon". Physicians with gay patients already knew this; the purplish Kaposi's lesions, usually seen only in elderly Jewish men and cancer patients whose immune systems were suppressed by radiation therapy, had first begun showing up on sexually active gay men in 1979. They would soon become a sure sign of what was termed Gay-Related Immune Deficiency (GRID), just as the suffocating PCP, a disease seen only twice in the U.S. in the dozen years prior to 1979, would soon become a leading killer of gay men.

At first, GRID was believed to be some strange combination of cytomegalovirus, which is a generally benign, and Epstein-Barr virus, which would later be called "yuppie flu". There was a popular theory early on that the new disease was somehow triggered by "poppers", amyl or butyl nitrite inhalers that were popular with gay men because they enhanced orgasm. But a second, distinct wave of the mysterious disease was spreading in the American Haitian community, in heterosexuals as well as bisexuals. Since March 1981, doctors in New York City had also been faced with an outbreak of PCP among intravenous (IV) drug users. What was certain was that the new disease could be sexually transmitted, like hepatitis. That junkies were being hit hard was a good indication that, whatever the infectious agent was, it was also spread by blood.*

*   *   *

The exact origins of AIDS are unknown, but it is not an entirely new disease, as most people believe. The virus is thought to have had its beginnings in equatorial Africa, around Zaïre, where it remained relatively contained until rapid urbanization and an economically driven rise in prostitution in the early 1970s.[2] From there it likely travelled to France and to Haiti, countries where educated, French-speaking blacks were recruited for work by post-colonial African governments. Sex tourists brought AIDS to North America after jaunts to Paris and Port-au-Prince, and then transported the disease back again.

According to Mirko D. Grmek, one of the world's foremost medical historians, retrospective studies trace AIDS back to 1940. At least sixteen cases published in American medical journals (including two in Canada) and fifteen more in leading European scientific journals between 1940 and June 1981 fit the present clinical definition of AIDS. In February 1952, a 28-year-old male identified only as R.G. was admitted to hospital in Memphis, Tennessee, with "viral pneumonia" that degenerated into total immune breakdown. David Carr, a seaman in the Royal Navy, died on August 31, 1959; his body was so riddled with unusual diseases that British doctors retained tissue samples, and they later tested positive for the AIDS virus. Carr, like many of the early cases, travelled repeatedly to Africa from 1955 to 1957 and almost certainly visited the bordellos of port cities. In 1959, blood serum drawn from an anonymous patient in Kinshasa, Zaïre, was preserved because his symptoms were so unusual; it later tested positive for the AIDS virus. That same year, a New York City merchant

---

* Viruses, which often die in contact with air, are not spread by dirty needles *per se*. Rather, junkies tend to withdraw a bit of blood and then reinject it with the drug, because that gives more "kick".

sailor died of the unusual symptoms of immune collapse; epidemiologists observed that the man was of Haitian origin and travelled regularly to Africa. Also in 1959, a 36-year-old carpenter identified only as G.Y. died at Toronto General Hospital of an extremely severe case of PCP. "We have no clue as to where the infection started," a group of University of Toronto pathologists wrote, in analysing the case for the *American Journal of Clinical Pathology*. They noted that the man had been hospitalized five times in the year prior to his death with various aches and pains, as well as sudden weight loss, fever, chills and night sweats. G.Y. is believed to be the first case of AIDS in Canada. The first documented case of a woman with AIDS was in the U.S. in 1964. A Norwegian sailor fell ill and died in 1966 with previously unseen respiratory ailments, and his wife and the youngest of his three daughters suffered the same fate; all their tissue samples were preserved and subsequently tested positive for HIV. Retrospective tests on the blood samples of Robert R., a 15-year-old St. Louis boy, confirmed that he had died of AIDS in 1968; what is unusual about the case is that, while the boy had had a number of homosexual experiences, he had never left the U.S. While outbreaks of disease were not recorded and tracked in Africa the way they were in the Western world, Belgian scientists have traced an AIDS case to the Congo in 1962, and several Zaïrean and Burundian AIDS patients who died prior to 1975.

The beginnings of the pandemic, however, are generally identified with a notable increase in Kaposi's sarcoma in central Africa around 1950. By the 1960s the rare cancer hit not only the odd sailor, but whole groups of African migrant workers in the region. In Kinshasa in 1975, health officials were struck by a marked increase in resistant diarrhea characterized by severe weight loss, which is now recognized as "wasting syndrome". Soon there were strange outbreaks of diseases like meningitis and oral thrush in Zambia, Uganda and Rwanda as well as Zaïre. By the late 1970s, well-to-do Africans and expatriates were travelling to Paris for medical treatment. Relative peace and more affordable travel also meant business was booming in the bordellos, particularly along the highway that links Kinshasa to Kampala, in Uganda — a route now dubbed "the AIDS Highway".

The hedonism that characterized gay life in the late 1970s and early 1980s lent itself to the propagation of sexually transmitted diseases; almost 90 per cent of active homosexuals had been infected by hepatitis B and cytomegalovirus by the time the AIDS virus entered the picture. A person like Gaétan Dugas could easily have dozens of sexual encounters during a weekend layover in Paris. Similarly, a sex tourist could have hundreds of sexual contacts during a two-week vacation in Port-au-Prince. Studies found that about one-third of young Haitian men had engaged in homosexual sex with foreign tourists, out of economic necessity — like the prostitutes of Kinshasa. As a result, AIDS spread quickly to the general population in Haiti.[3] The use of *piqûristes*, untrained practitioners who treated patients by injecting various substances, often with unsterilized syringes, also contributed to Haiti's dubious distinction as an AIDS hot spot.

Not surprisingly, the first known case of transfusion AIDS in the world was recorded in Haiti; Claude Chardon, a 31-year-old French geologist working in the country, received blood after his arm was amputated in a serious traffic accident in September 1978. After Chardon died in October 1982, his tissues were among the first identified as being infected with the AIDS virus. Researchers were able to track down the eight blood donors, and all of them seemed to be in good health — an important early clue that carriers with no symptoms could pass on the disease. There are indications that blood products may have been infected even earlier. An 18-year-old Pittsburgh hemophiliac who received a single treatment with Factor VIII concentrate in early 1978 was later found to be infected, but his case wasn't reported in a medical journal until late 1983. This case is not proof, however, that AIDS had arrived in North America. Into the 1980s, brokers in the unsavoury business of blood-banking — including one in Canada — were known to purchase low-cost blood in unregulated and unsanitary Third World "vampire shops", and sell it at a profit in the U.S. and Europe.

By January 1982, the U.S. Centers for Disease Control (CDC) were already investigating the first reported case of GRID in a heterosexual hemophiliac, a 69-year-old resident of Miami who had died of PCP a few months earlier. The only possible source of his infection, it seemed, was the Factor VIII blood concentrate that he had infused, on average, four times a month for the previous eight years. CDC epidemiologist Dr. Bruce Evatt immediately recognized the implications: if the deadly new illness was blood-borne, every hemophiliac and transfusion recipient was at risk. The CDC began tracking requests for the drug pentamidine, the only known treatment for PCP, and Dr. Evatt followed up on the hemophilia cases. In the July 16, 1982, edition of *Mortality and Morbidity Weekly Report*, the CDC reported three more cases of GRID in hemophiliacs and stated that they "suggest possible transmission of an agent through blood products". Epidemiologists knew this was just the tip of the iceberg.

In Canada, "gay cancer" was viewed as doubly marginal. Not only did the disease appear to strike only gay men, but it was largely confined to the U.S. Yet on March 27, 1982, *Canada Diseases Weekly Report* — Health and Welfare Canada's equivalent of *Mortality and Morbidity* — published its first report of the new disease. The 43-year-old Windsor man had likely been infected in 1979 during his rounds of San Francisco bathhouses, or on his annual visit to the beaches of Haiti. A couple of weeks later, in April 1982, a 20-year-old hemophiliac, Danny Parabicoli, visited his doctor in Toronto because he was experiencing severe breathing problems. He had been inexplicably ill for several years, and for months had been suffering night sweats, swollen lymph glands and dramatic weight loss; now his lungs were infected with histoplasmosis, an infection caused by inhaling the spores of a fungus. He didn't have the tell-tale Kaposi's blotches, but he had all the other signs of GRID. The disease was spreading in Canada, not only among homosexual men but among Haitians, intravenous drug users and hemophiliacs.

Because blood products were filtered to remove bacteria, fungi and proto-zoa, scientists were left with little doubt that the infectious agent was a virus, tiny enough to slip through the filter. In an update about the spread of GRID in hemophiliacs, Dr. John Bennett of the CDC described the new disease as a "sexually transmitted viral infection . . . the causative agent could be either a common virus producing new effects as a result of certain environmental fac-tors, or one of several novel agents, e.g., mutant or recombinant strains of human or animal pathogens." In the spring of 1982, there was no doubt that blood concentrates were infected with the strange new disease. The only ques-tion was whether it would kill hemophiliacs the way it did homosexuals.

On July 27, 1982, the Centers for Disease Control invited blood bankers and hemophiliacs to an emergency meeting in Washington to warn them that the new disease was blood-borne and to urge suppliers and users of blood products to take precautions. Blood bankers balked at the idea of restricting donations, saying the virus theory was unproven, while the scientific advisors to the National Hemophilia Foundation said hemophiliacs would not stop using concentrate, a product that allowed them to lead normal lives, unless there was more concrete proof of the dangers. In fact, the only consensus that emerged from the meeting was that the disease should be renamed Acquired Immune Deficiency Syndrome, in recognition that it wasn't restricted to gay men. That summer, when the epidemic moved into mainstream society, the lay press began to take notice of AIDS. The news articles were a strange mixture of alarm and reassurance: alarm at the fact that a killer disease seemed to have struck humanity, but reassurance that it seemed to be restricted to certain "high-risk" groups. The clinical characteristics of AIDS had been identified, and the warnings began about the dangers of the strange new virus entering the general population. Even though an epidemic was under way, it didn't set off any alarm bells; rather, the general population — and most public health officials — took comfort in the mistaken belief that one needed a sexual, racial or genetic predisposition to contract AIDS.

The Canadian government reacted swiftly to the CDC warning; just days after the Washington meeting, Alex Morrison, deputy minister of Health and Welfare, asked senior scientists to determine the risks to hemophiliacs. On August 6, 1982, Dr. John Furesz, head of the Bureau of Biologics of the Health Protection Branch, prepared a briefing note about AIDS for Health and Welfare minister Monique Bégin. The document, believed to be the first official acknowledgment that blood products could pose a danger to hemophiliacs in Canada, reads, in part: "Recently, three cases of AIDS were reported in hemophilia patients. Patients with hemophilia are under continuous treatment with a blood plasma fraction, called antihemophilic factor (AHF). There is a theoretical risk that an unknown transmissible agent present in AHF products may be responsible for AIDS in these patients. . . . The Bureau of Biologics requested that the CRC [Canadian Red Cross] alert all physicians in BTS centres to increase surveillance of hemophilia patients for AIDS and co-ordinate laboratory studies if cases are reported." At the time there had been more than four hundred AIDS cases in the U.S., including gay men, Haitians, IV drug users and hemophiliacs. In Canada there had been only eight cases — one in Windsor, one in Vancouver and six in Montreal. Five of the men were homosexual, and one a recent Haitian immigrant. Six of the eight were already dead.

Just days after that briefing note, a 56-year-old hemophiliac was admitted to Montreal General Hospital with breathing problems and a number of unrelated problems that pointed to immune deficiency. The ill health, the man told his doctor, had begun almost immediately after the infusion of blood concentrate for a severe elbow bleed in April. First there had been a rash, then a fever, weight loss, chills and night sweats. The flu-like symptoms — which many years later would be identified as seroconversion illness, the first sign of infection — sounded suspiciously like AIDS, but the patient was a heterosexual. The doctor referred the case to Dr. Christos Tsoukas, an intern studying the effects of foreign proteins such as manufactured insulin, on the immune system, specifically, their ability to alter the T4 count. Dr. Tsoukas was intrigued by the idea that concentrate might also alter the T4 count — a key indicator of immunity — and doubly so when he realized this could be a factor in AIDS.

His patient was Frank Schnabel — founder of both the Canadian Hemophilia Society and the World Federation of Hemophilia, and one of the first hemophiliacs in Canada to use factor concentrate. The man who had opened so many doors for those suffering from the disease would be one of the first victims of tainted blood.

The Red Cross responded to the Bureau of Biologics' request for more surveillance and investigation by setting up a committee to examine the issue.
After a number of informal meetings the Ad Hoc Committee on AIDS, a virtual who's who of Canadian AIDS specialists, met at the Toronto headquarters
of the Red Cross on December 2, 1982. According to the minutes of the meeting, they discussed the growing number of infections among hemophiliacs in
the U.S.: "This has raised concern that intravenous blood products may be a
route of transmission of the agent responsible for the development of AIDS. If
this is indeed true, it would have serious and far-reaching implications with
respect to the donation and distribution of blood and blood products." At the
same meeting, the scientists discussed a new study out of the University of
Wisconsin that "suggests that hemophiliacs on Factor VIII concentrate therapy
have reduced cellular immunity whereas this appears not to be the case in
hemophiliacs treated only with cryoprecipitate." That was logical if the new
disease was, as suspected, a blood-borne virus; concentrate was manufactured
by pooling parts of up to 20,000 blood donations, while cryo was derived from
the plasma of between one and ten donors.

Switching patients to the safer product wasn't raised as a possibility; in fact,
prevention wasn't an issue at all. The bulk of the meeting was dedicated to
discussion of how to get funding for a research project that would track AIDS
in homosexual men and hemophiliacs to determine what could be expected in
the heterosexual community. "The epidemic nature of this disease, now
involving groups without a homosexual lifestyle, is of great concern," read the
application for funding prepared later that month. "The possible transmissibility of blood products is even more disturbing and has implications for
the National Transfusion Service and the public at large. In view of our recent
identification of the problem in Toronto and the apparent increase in
frequency of reporting, we think the epidemic wave is beginning here as well."
The request for $100,000 would be turned down because researchers missed
the application deadline by one day.* An epidemic was beginning, but rules
were rules.

Although the researchers discussed the case of the Montreal hemophiliac
suffering from AIDS, no notice was given to the Canadian Hemophilia Society,
many of whose 2,000 members were at risk of contracting the new disease.
The society's representative at the meeting was the chairwoman of the
group's medical and scientific advisory committee, Dr. Roslyn Herst. She was also

---

* The research was eventually funded by the Medical Research Council, a federal government funding agency, which gave Dr. Philip Gold (and his colleague Dr. Christos Tsoukas)
$741,000 over three years.

deputy medical director of the Toronto branch of the Red Cross, and no doubt more aware than others of the implications of AIDS for the blood program.

Days after the meeting, Dr. John Derrick, a senior advisor who was the Red Cross's point man on AIDS, sent an "information letter" to that agency's medical directors that summarized the latest scientific evidence about the disease. In particular, he raised the issue of infection of hemophilia patients in the U.S., noting that those with AIDS symptoms all used large quantities of factor concentrate. Two of the seven hemophiliacs confirmed to have AIDS were children, he added, so "children with hemophilia must now be considered at risk for the disease. In addition, the number of cases continues to increase, and the illness may pose a significant risk for patients with hemophilia." In fact, he revealed that the "death of one hemophilia A patient has been definitely attributed to AIDS". (Today, the official statistics make no mention of a Canadian hemophiliac dying of AIDS in the fall of 1982. But a diagnosis of AIDS, more than any other disease, has political and social baggage attached to it; as a result, the disease is chronically under-reported, and sometimes deliberately not reported to public health officials.)

The same week that Dr. Derrick sent out his information letter, Dr. Alfred Katz, biomedical services director of the American Red Cross, was sending out his own memo to U.S. medical directors. "It is highly likely that AIDS is transmissible via blood and antihemophilic factors," he wrote. "Our situation has all the earmarks of a lose-lose one." Rather than recommend urgent measures to reduce the spread of AIDS via blood and blood products, Dr. Katz called on his colleagues to shoot the messenger. "We must do everything we can to refute the findings" of the CDC and Food and Drug Administration (FDA), the U.S. regulator. Unfortunately for the Red Cross and other blood bankers, the evidence that AIDS was spread by blood and blood products was mounting daily. On November 5, 1982, the Centers for Disease Control urged doctors and hospitals to adopt "universal precautions" in dealing with AIDS patients. In other words, healthcare workers were to assume that the bodily fluids of all patients were potentially infectious, and were to begin wearing latex gloves and carefully avoid needle pricks. Unfortunately, hemophiliacs and transfusion patients would not benefit from similarly enlightened precautions.

In 1982, four U.S. babies between the ages of two months and four years were reported to be suffering from AIDS. Three had been born to AIDS-infected mothers (all of them IV drug users) and the fourth to an asymptomatic Haitian woman. The cases provided further evidence that the disease was transmitted by blood, but researchers could not say with certainty if the infectious agent was passed on during pregnancy, at birth or afterwards, for example during breast-feeding. On

December 10, 1982, *Mortality and Morbidity Weekly Report* published the case of a 20-month-old baby in San Francisco who had developed AIDS after a transfusion. In an editorial note, U.S. government scientists stated, "This report and continuing reports of AIDS among persons with hemophilia raise serious questions about the possible transmission of AIDS through blood and blood products." Those who doubted or didn't want to believe that AIDS was blood-borne had an out: the baby had needed six complete transfusions in the first six days of her life to treat Rh-incompatibility, and that could have seriously compromised her immune system. By the time the case was published, however, the donor of the platelets the baby had received had himself developed AIDS symptoms.

On December 11, 1982, *Canada Diseases Weekly Report* published the first results of a pilot study on AIDS in hemophilia patients — the study funded by the Medical Research Council. Although the AIDS virus had not yet been identified,[4] the testing showed that 70 per cent of Canadian hemophiliacs who had used large amounts of factor concentrate (more than 40,000 units a year) were already showing signs of cellular immune deficiency, compared to only 5 per cent of hemophiliacs who were not using the product. Notably, none of the thirty-two men in the study group had had his treatment changed, nor had they been informed of the abnormal state of their immune symptoms. *The Medical Post*, a weekly paper distributed to Canadian doctors, in its colourful style, warned prophetically that "hemophilia patients may be sitting on a time bomb". The paper quoted Dr. John Shuster, a professor of medicine at McGill University, warning that gay men shouldn't give blood and that hemophiliacs should reduce their use of blood products to the bare minimum.

The tragic tale of tainted blood in Canada is, above all, a story of opportunities missed. Had health officials acted wisely on the information they had in 1982, hundreds of infections would have been avoided. While it's true that AIDS was still not entirely understood, the warning signs were clearly there: the infection of hemophiliacs and of transfused babies. Unfortunately, the officials entrusted with the responsibility for keeping the blood system safe ignored the red flags. Instead of fighting the epidemic, they practised what one observer later described as "malicious inertia".

*   *   *

In the next months there were several key meetings to discuss the threat of blood-borne AIDS. Hemophilia groups in the U.S. and Canada were pushing for a series of AIDS prevention measures; blood bankers were reluctant to take any action that would cost them money, but eventually they bowed to consumer pressure. After the Red Cross announced plans to screen donors in early March 1983, the outcry was such that it quickly backed off.

On March 31, 1983, Artibano Milito, an unmarried 28-year-old mill worker from Prince Rupert, British Columbia, became the first hemophiliac whose AIDS death was widely reported. He died without ever being told the real diagnosis and, when his family learned after the autopsy that he had not died of cancer, they were angry. The source of infection wasn't in doubt. In 1979, 1981 and 1982, Milito had received a single infusion of Factor VIII concentrate, and at those times he had suffered increasingly bad bouts of swollen lymph glands, fever and rashes, all early symptoms of AIDS. Still, the rumour mill had it that the real reason for his death was that Milito was gay. One month before he died, the mild hemophiliac was refused surgery because the Red Cross feared the blood products required carried too great a risk of AIDS transmission. "Surgery on [Milito] would require large doses of Factor VIII, and the Red Cross is not releasing quantities unless it's an emergency because of the dangers of transmitting AIDS," wrote Dr. Michael Noble, a hematologist at Royal Columbian Hospital. Curious as it was, the Red Cross would not release products for surgery that hemophiliacs across the country, unaware of the risks, were injecting into their bodies every day.*

In July 1983, the 73-year-old wife of the Miami hemophiliac who had died some 18 months earlier succumbed to AIDS. Her death was a portent of a whole new area of concern, the risk to spouses and lovers of hemophiliacs and transfusion patients. The lack of concern for the women threatened by the new disease, which had affected men almost exclusively until that time, would lead to dozens of deaths that were easily preventable. The U.S. blood-banking industry had a different worry: the bottom line. Blood donations were falling markedly — due in part to the erroneous belief that donors, not recipients, could contract AIDS — and the blood bankers responded by calling on their friends in Washington. On August 1, Dr. Joseph Bove, chair of the transfusion committee of the U.S. Food and Drug Administration and the American Association of Blood Banks, told congressional hearings that public concern about transfusion AIDS was misplaced and blamed the situation on hysterical media. "Even if — and it is still a big if — a small number of AIDS cases turn out to be transfusion-related, I do not believe this can be interpreted to mean

---

* In June 1983, a study by the U.S. National Institutes of Health estimated that hemophiliacs were ten times more likely to contract AIDS than homosexuals. The odds were as follows: 1 in 1.5 million for the general population; 1 in 10,000 for homosexual men; 1 in 1,500 for Haitians; and 1 in 1,000 for hemophiliacs.

that our blood supply is contaminated," Dr. Bove testified. He said a person was twenty times more likely to die of an appendectomy or hernia than of transfusion AIDS.

The Canadian Red Cross Society, fearful of losing donors, took a similar tack: they calculated that the danger to transfusion patients was one in a million. Publicly, the Red Cross put an even rosier interpretation on the shocking reality of blood-borne AIDS. In August 1983, in a brief to public health authorities, the Red Cross stated that "there is no evidence that blood is any less safe now than prior to the appearance of AIDS."

The best that can be said is that the Red Cross naively believed that the voluntary nature of Canada's blood collection system would shield it from the ravages of diseases like AIDS. While the argument — good people don't get bad diseases — is attractive on the surface, it has no scientific basis. There was no reason to believe that AIDS would spread more slowly in Canada's gay community than in its U.S. counterpart, particularly considering that U.S. epidemiologists had singled out as Patient Zero a man who was sexually active in several Canadian cities. Second, blood for transfusion is collected almost exclusively from volunteer donors in the U.S., as it is in Canada. Finally, at least half the blood products distributed to Canadian hemophiliacs were made from U.S.-source plasma, undermining the Red Cross's safety argument and, if anything, adding to the need to act urgently. As Ed Kubin wrote in a letter to Canadian Hemophilia Society president Ken Poyser on August 18, 1983, "Each time a hemophiliac receives a treatment, he wonders if the infusion will give him AIDS." Kubin said the organization should demand an independent investigation into the safety of factor concentrate, but the CHS didn't want to make waves.

The number of cases of blood-borne AIDS continued to grow, slowly but relentlessly. In August 1983 *The New England Journal of Medicine* published the case of a baby girl in Montreal who had contracted AIDS during a transfusion in October 1982. One of the five units of blood components she had received at birth was traced to a gay man with a history of multiple sex partners who was himself suffering early symptoms of AIDS infection. Dr. Normand Lapointe, an immunologist at Ste. Justine Hospital in Montreal, said the baby's case left "no doubt" that AIDS could be transmitted by blood. That month the federal government took its first tentative step against the epidemic, announcing the creation of the National Advisory Committee on AIDS (NACAIDS) — a group that was to advise the Minister of Health, Monique Bégin, on "appropriate action and initiatives to combat AIDS in Canada". The impetus for the creation of the expert panel was not epidemiological but political: Bégin's riding had the highest concentration of Haitians in the country, and they were angry. At one of its first meetings, on November 9, 1983, NACAIDS members — including Dr. Roger Perrault, head of the Red Cross blood program, and Dr. John Furesz, head of the Bureau of Biologics — were told that one-third of hemophiliacs were showing symptoms of AIDS. But there was little they could do. The AIDS budget for all of Canada was $1.49 million over four years; in its first year, NACAIDS was allocated a paltry $3,800.

In November 1983, researchers at the Mayo Clinic published the details of a case of a 53-year-old man who had been infected with AIDS during a blood transfusion in November 1980. He had been transfused with seventeen units of blood components during open-heart surgery, and had developed AIDS symptoms twenty-nine months later. The case was important because it demonstrated not only that transfusion AIDS had been a threat for many years, but that the long latency period meant there could be many undetected cases. (Later, researchers would learn that an 80-year-old man in Edmonton had been the first patient to contract transfusion AIDS in Canada, during minor surgery in May 1980. He died only months later of the strange combination of cytomegalovirus and PCP, but the connection wasn't made until the blood donor died of AIDS many years after.)

By the time thirty-eight AIDS experts from around the world gathered at the World Health Organization headquarters in Geneva on November 22, 1983, for the first meeting on the international implications of the AIDS epidemic, the disease had been reported in thirty-three nations on five continents. The most serious discussion at the meeting was about Factor VIII concentrate because European delegates were convinced that this was an area where the epidemic could be slowed. Nine European nations had already banned imports from the U.S., but Canada echoed the U.S. line that there was no conclusive proof that AIDS could be transmitted by blood. Dr. Alistair Clayton, head of the Federal Centre for AIDS, told the meeting that Canada had recorded fifty AIDS cases to date. One dead hemophiliac, and a handful of others who were ill, wasn't proof enough.

The next month, Dr. Dale Lawrence at the CDC published an article saying that the mean incubation period of AIDS was 5.5 years, not two years or less, as previously believed.* That meant that someone exposed to the virus could develop symptoms within six months, or — a more frightening possibility — could go eleven years without any signs of the disease. There were already 3,000 Americans known to be infected with AIDS, including thirty-nine confirmed cases of transfusion AIDS.

---

* Articles in scientific journals now place the average incubation period at fourteen years.

In December 1983, a subcommittee of the U.S. House of Representatives released the findings of an investigation into the response to the AIDS crisis. "Tragically, funding levels for AIDS investigations have been dictated by political considerations rather than by professional judgments of scientists and public health officials who are waging the battle against the epidemic," said Ted Weiss, chairman of the Intergovernmental Relations and Human Resources Subcommittee. "The inadequacy of funding, coupled with inexcusable delays in research activity, leads me to question the Federal Government's preparedness for national health emergencies, as well as the Administration's commitment to an urgent resolution of the AIDS crisis."

Canada was one step behind the U.S. in terms of the spread of AIDS, giving it a window of opportunity. But it was two steps behind in terms of a realistic response. There was still no plan except "wait and see". Health and Welfare Canada closed out the year by refusing another request for it to fund research on blood-borne AIDS, this one from scientists at the University of Toronto.

* * *

By the end of 1983, scientists in the U.S. and France had both discovered the virus responsible for AIDS, but it would be April 1984 before an official announcement was made. Despite lack of agreement on the name of the virus there was ample knowledge about the disease and its modes of transmission to take action. As *The New England Journal of Medicine* wrote in a January 1984 editorial, "Doctors can no longer assure their patients that they will not contract AIDS from a transfusion." Yet, in Canada, doctors gave that very assurance every day. The Canadian Medical Association, the Red Cross and public health authorities issued no warnings. In fact, in March 1984 Health and Welfare distributed hundreds of thousands of pamphlets in supermarkets about the dangers of AIDS; the risk of contracting AIDS from a transfusion, the pamphlet said, was two in a million. At the same time, NACAIDS published a four-page supplement that was distributed as an insert to *The Medical Post*, saying there was "no conclusive proof" that AIDS was blood-borne. In both the U.S. and Canada, the gay community undertook education campaigns promoting the use of condoms. But safe sex messages would not appear in media campaigns and school curricula for many more years.

In March 1984, a full sixteen months after the CDC urged the implementation of "universal precautions", the Irwin Memorial Blood Bank in San Francisco became the first to screen blood for AIDS by "surrogate testing" blood donors for signs of exposure to hepatitis B. (Virtually everyone with AIDS symptoms had previously been infected with hepatitis B, so it was a good indicator of risk.) The measure added 10 per cent to the cost of blood products but, as a study by Dr. Thomas Spira of the U.S. Centers for Disease Control would show later, eliminated 88 per cent of HIV-positive blood donations. Four other California blood banks, including the Red Cross in San Jose, followed suit, citing not improved safety but "competitive pressure". In Canada the Red Cross had a monopoly, so competition wasn't a factor; surrogate testing was rejected.

Other innovative measures were proposed to make factor concentrate safer. Some manufacturers had begun to pasteurize blood products to kill the hepatitis virus, and it seemed reasonable that given all the other parallels between hepatitis and AIDS — both were sexually transmitted and blood-borne — that heat treatment would make the products safer. Yet, once again, the new products cost more, so the technology was written off as unproven. One unassailable fact was that very few women were infected with AIDS; William Mindell, a senior official with the City of Toronto Department of Health and a volunteer with the Canadian Hemophilia Society, suggested that factor concentrate be manufactured with plasma collected from female donors only. His proposal was dismissed out of hand; the Red Cross, he was told, did not discriminate.

Dr. Gail Rock, medical director of the Ottawa branch of the Red Cross Blood Transfusion Service, developed a method that could have dramatically increased the volume of Canadian source plasma, widely believed to be safer than U.S. plasma. When plasma is collected, the bag is already primed with a small amount of anticoagulant: Dr. Rock found that dextrose, the customary anticoagulant, reduced the yield of Factor VIII substantially; by replacing the dextrose with heparin she was able to double the yield. Dr. Rock also proposed that plasmapheresis donors be injected with DDAVP (desmopressin), a drug that increases Factor VIII in the blood — a process that would double the yield without harming the donor. By combining her two ideas, Dr. Rock calculated, Canada could be self-sufficient in plasma for the manufacture of concentrate. And to be even safer, all hemophiliacs could be treated with cryoprecipitate; if the plasma for the manufacture of cryo was boosted with DDAVP, each hemophiliac could be treated with the donations of three donors instead of the 20,000 whose plasma went into concentrate. By the beginning of 1984, AIDS was already the leading killer of hemophiliacs in the U.S., but all those innovative proposals were ignored. Canadian authorities opted to do nothing but institute timid screening measures.

On April 23, 1984, Dr. Robert Gallo of the U.S. National Cancer Institute dramatically announced the discovery of human T-cell leukemia virus type III, or HTLV-III, as the cause of AIDS. (The Americans had simply ignored an earlier but lower-key announcement by the Pasteur Institute in France that they had discovered that lymphadenopathy-associated virus, or LAV, was the cause of AIDS.) Health and Human Services (HHS) Secretary Margaret Heckler gave the scientific breakthrough a political spin. "Today's discovery represents the triumph of science over a dreaded disease," she said. "From the first day that AIDS was identified in 1981, HHS scientists and their medical allies have never stopped searching for the answers to the AIDS mystery. Without a day of procrastination, the resources of the Public Health Service have been effectively mobilized." While politicians and their appointees crowed about the swift discovery of the AIDS virus, the fact is that the task was relatively simple. Had the search been a priority at the outbreak of the epidemic, the virus would probably have been discovered in 1982, and many, many deaths avoided.

Even before the discovery of the virus was announced, scientists at the Centers for Disease Control were conducting testing on high-risk groups, using LAV. (In the end it turned out that LAV and HTLV-III were one and the same; the compromise "human immunodeficiency virus", or HIV, would be the name that stuck.) The real achievement of the National Cancer Institute had been in replicating the virus in industrial quantities. The institute's laboratories were churning out hundreds of gallons a month; it would be needed to test blood for AIDS antibodies.[5] The goal was to have a commercial test on the market within six months. In the meantime, researchers began testing members of high-risk groups and trying to determine the extent of the epidemic in the general population.

Soon the American Red Cross reported that 1 in 500 donors nation-wide tested positive for the AIDS virus. At a New York City drug clinic, 87 per cent of intravenous drug users tested positive. Researchers in San Francisco tested the blood of gay men who showed no signs of AIDS or ARC (AIDS-related complex), and found that 55 per cent of them tested positive for AIDS; among New York City gays, the infection rate was 38 per cent. Tests on hemophiliacs who had no symptoms of AIDS revealed that 72 per cent were infected; among those who infused Factor VIII more than once a month, the infection rate was 90 per cent.

These frightening numbers left epidemiologists alarmed and despondent. The term "epidemic" didn't begin to describe the situation among high-risk groups. Plotting the rates of infection on graphs painted a picture of impending devastation. There was no longer a shred of doubt that AIDS was spread by bodily fluids, and that the virus was more certain to infect people if they were exposed to blood than if they were exposed to semen.

Strangely, these dire warnings didn't prompt blood bankers to institute emergency measures. They put their own spin on the statistics: the large number of people infected but without symptoms could only mean that the disease was less lethal than previously believed. So, despite infection rates of 50 to 75 per cent among those exposed to blood-borne AIDS, the wait-and-see approach continued. Never mind that, in the U.S., more than 5,000 people had contracted AIDS and 2,300 of them were dead. Never mind that about 150 Canadians had contracted AIDS, and more than half of them were dead.

After the AIDS virus was discovered in the spring of 1984, the Red Cross published a new pamphlet for blood donors. Though for the first time it mentioned AIDS, no reference was made to the symptoms or the high-risk activities associated with the disease. Donors were not asked about their sexual practices, or their drug-using habits; they were simply asked if they were in good health. Clinging desperately to the notion that voluntary donations precluded contamination of the blood supply, blood donor clinics conducted business as usual.

It was also business as usual for Gaétan Dugas. A senior official at the U.S. Centers for Disease Control phoned Dr. Tim Johnstone, British Columbia's chief epidemiologist, and urged him to act against Dugas, who steadfastly refused to change his sexual habits. Dr. Johnstone felt he was powerless to act, as did medical officers of health in Ontario, Nova Scotia and Quebec, where the flight attendant lived between 1979 and 1984. Public health officials did not confront a man whose sexual adventures endangered others just as they failed to tackle the spread of AIDS through the blood system. If nothing else, Patient Zero should have shattered the illusion that AIDS was an American problem.

Despite his advancing illness, Dugas still cruised Vancouver's gay bars, but he would soon return to his native Quebec City. He died there on March 30, 1984.

5

LETHAL INDIFFERENCE
"HOW MANY DEATHS DO WE NEED?"

> . . . Small official notices had been just put up about the town, though in places where they would not attract much attention. It was hard to find in these notices that the authorities were facing the situation squarely. The measures enjoined were far from Draconian and one had the feeling that many concessions had been made to a desire not to alarm the public.
>
> Albert Camus
> *The Plague*

Pamela Schwarze, Ladner, British Columbia

AIDS is a disease that kills slowly and, in the latter stages, requires around-the-clock care. Pamela's spouse, John Mervyn, was a hemophiliac infected with the AIDS virus, and she says people simply don't realize the ravages of the disease.

"When people hear about AIDS or HIV, they don't always know what it involves and the extent of infection or disease. It makes me need to say what we've gone through, what John has gone through. I will only run a quick list, I won't bore you with all of the details.

John has greatly increased epileptic seizure activity, grand mal seizures because of AIDS. He has continual nausea and vomiting. He had to undergo surgery to remove two large abscesses in his legs. He went through a period of toxic dementia caused by drugs. He has had middle ear infections that required surgery and caused chronic damage. He has CMV retinitis which has destroyed his right eye. The chemotherapy for that caused kidney failure.

He had congestive heart failure and nearly died. He has mycobacterium avium, which is tuberculosis of the bone marrow and he no longer produces red blood cells and white blood cells that help him stave off infection. We have had to inject him for over a year and a half for that, as well as an IV two or three times a day. He has ITP, which is like a cancer in which he has no platelets left. Not only does he have no Factor VIII to stop clotting, he doesn't have platelets.

John had PCP and had to go through two bronchoscopies and an open-lung biopsy for that, which is quite serious for a severe hemophiliac. He has peripheral neuropathy which makes it difficult for him to walk, and even for his feet to be touched. As a hemophiliac, of course, he has hepatitis B and hepatitis C. . . . He has had constant problems with neutropenia, so we have to be afraid of colds because one could kill him.

He can't work, obviously. I had to quit school twice, the last time when I was six weeks away from getting my teacher's certificate. We've had to beg for welfare for what we need and now the government wants my $35,000 worth of student loans back and I wasn't even able to finish because John is infected."

(March 31, 1994)

THE WAY TO BEAT BACK AN EPIDEMIC, Don Francis knew, was to move swiftly and mercilessly to cut off the transmission routes. Working with the World Health Organization a few years earlier, he had done just that in equatorial Africa to stop the spread of Ebola fever, a virus that is one of the deadliest diseases on the planet. By the time the leadership of the U.S. public health agencies sat down in Washington for a tête-à-tête with the main players in the blood-banking industry on January 3, 1983, however, it had been a full year since the first confirmed case of a hemophiliac dying of AIDS, and several long weeks since the publication of evidence that the San Francisco baby had contracted the disease after a transfusion.

Dr. Francis, a 40-year-old epidemiologist with the U.S. Centers for Disease Control and co-ordinator of the CDC's AIDS Laboratory, was restless before the meeting. At the height of the Reagan era, trying to get money to fight a disease that was killing homosexual men and drug addicts was enough of a struggle. Now the CDC was stepping on the toes of major pharmaceutical companies and a beloved charitable organization by asking them to change the way they collected and distributed blood and blood products. The reaction was hostile; the political beasts were far more cunning and savage than those in the jungles of Africa. An hour into the gathering, during which the blood bankers scornfully rejected the notion of blood-borne AIDS and laid out an endless series of excuses for conducting business as usual, Dr. Francis snapped.

Outraged by the repeated insinuations that not enough people had died of blood-borne AIDS to warrant spending money, he pounded his fist on the table and screamed, "How many people have to die? How many deaths do we need? Give me a threshold of death that you need in order to believe that this is happening, and we'll meet at that time and we can start to do something."

The outburst was greeted with stony silence, and at the day's end the meeting adjourned with agreement on nothing — a result Dr. Francis would later describe as tacit endorsement of negligent homicide.

The meeting was not a total waste of time, however. The dire warnings by the epidemiologists that the deaths of a handful of hemophiliacs were only the beginning startled users of factor concentrate, and prompted preventive action by U.S. non-profit blood bankers, the American Association of Blood Banks, the American Red Cross and the Council of Community Blood Centers. While prefacing their warning with the disclaimer that transmission of AIDS by blood transfusion was still unproven, these bodies issued a joint statement on January 13, 1983, which endorsed screening donors for symptoms of AIDS and avoiding recruitment among high-risk groups. (One of the most successful blood drives was at the annual Gay Pride parade in San Francisco.) But at the same time the American Red Cross and other non-profit blood bankers rejected screening out specific groups like homosexual men, citing civil rights concerns, and rejected calls for surrogate testing of blood donations for hepatitis B, arguing that the link between hepatitis and AIDS was unproven. At a meeting just after the statement was issued, Canadian Red Cross medical directors endorsed the approach wholeheartedly.

The next day, *The New England Journal of Medicine* published a strongly worded editorial recommending a "radical change" in the treatment of hemophiliacs because of the dangers of AIDS. Associate editor Dr. Jane Desforges wrote that, despite the inconvenience, hemophiliacs being treated with factor concentrate should be switched to cryoprecipitate. "The fact that hemophiliacs are at risk for AIDS is becoming clear. . . . Physicians involved in the care of hemophiliacs must now be alert to this risk. Preventing the complications of the present treatment may have to take precedence over preventing the complications of hemophilia itself."

The same day *The New England Journal of Medicine* published its views, the U.S. National Hemophilia Foundation issued a series of recommendations for the prevention of AIDS in hemophiliacs. Operating on the assumption of its scientific advisors that a high percentage of concentrate was contaminated, the foundation called on all manufacturers to eliminate the problem at the source. They suggested five complementary tactics for the blood-banking industry: contacting leaders of high-risk groups to urge voluntary deferral of blood donations; questioning donors specifically to determine if they were members of high-risk groups; using questionnaires to identify people with symptoms associated with AIDS; developing an AIDS education program for all physicians; and immediate evaluation of surrogate testing for AIDS using a core antibody test for hepatitis B (anti-HBc). Eliminating the blood of those testing positive for hepatitis B should thus eliminate most AIDS-tainted blood. It was widely known that homosexual men with multiple partners and intravenous drug users who shared needles had almost universally been exposed to hepatitis B, as had most hemophiliacs using factor concentrate. In fact, because of these similarities in modes of transmission, many researchers assumed early on that AIDS was caused by a virus.

As long as the AIDS virus hadn't been discovered, blood bankers had been able to argue that the theories about modes of transmission were unproven, an excuse that was used time and time again to justify inaction. When it was convenient, however, the same arguments that had been rejected as alarmist were used to assuage concern. The hepatitis-AIDS link, for example, caused a false sense of security; many doctors assumed that, as with hepatitis, only a fraction of people exposed to AIDS would die, while many others would develop antibodies that would leave them immune. In Canada, as in the U.S., blood was already being tested for hepatitis-B, since 1972 in fact, but the wrong test was being used. Blood donations were tested for the hepatitis surface antigen, proof of active hepatitis B infection, rather than for the core antibody which indicated previous exposure. The reality was that blood bankers were reluctant to institute the core antibody test not because the link was unproven but because it would cost them money. Not only would an additional test cost a couple of dollars per unit, but it would result in the loss of tens of thousands of donations; fewer than three in a thousand donors tested positive for the surface antigen, but an estimated 6 per cent had hepatitis-B antibodies.

While they rejected the surrogate test, by early 1983 the U.S. blood banks were already instituting screening procedures, largely due to competitive pressures. Among the measures proposed, the easiest and cheapest was to reduce donations from high-risk groups, the so-called 4-H club (homosexuals, heroin addicts, Haitians and hemophiliacs; soon there would be a fifth H, hookers). What all the members of the club had in common, aside from their higher-than-average risk, was that they were in some way uninfluential or marginal members of society. This was no coincidence; the pharmaceutical companies whose blood and blood products were beginning to infect people with AIDS needed scapegoats. "To reassure the public, 'innocent' groups were omitted from the club of the damned," says medical historian Dr. Mirko Grmek. Scientists had already catalogued others at high risk: the children and heterosexual partners of these "high-risk" people, and recipients of blood transfusions. The unspoken and homophobic notion that there were innocent and guilty carriers of AIDS — that AIDS was as much a sociological phenomenon as a medical one — would contribute to much inaction over the coming decade.

*   *   *

In Canada the similarly unjustifiable notion that, because "good" people gave blood voluntarily and "bad" people did not, the blood system would be shielded from AIDS was a key factor in the tragedy. For example, Dr. John Derrick, the Red Cross official responsible for dealing with AIDS, attended the meeting of the U.S. National Hemophilia Foundation in January 1983 but reported back that the group's recommendations did not apply to Canada because the Red Cross here didn't pay for blood donations. Yet Dr. Derrick, who had worked previously at the New York Blood Center and had regular contact with U.S. blood bankers, knew that more than half the blood donations in the U.S. were also from unpaid volunteers, and that more than half the blood products used in Canada — which were manufactured using paid plasma — were purchased in the U.S.

The scientific advisors to the Canadian Hemophilia Society, who did not agree with Dr. Derrick, waded into the debate a few weeks after their U.S. counterparts. On February 7, members of the CHS's Medical and Scientific Advisory Committee (MSAC) drafted a series of recommendations to reduce the risk of AIDS in the blood supply. Among their suggestions were the following to the Red Cross Blood Transfusion Service:

a) serious efforts should be made to exclude blood donors who might transmit AIDS, including:

1. an education campaign to promote self-exclusion by donors belonging to high-risk groups, such as male homosexuals and Haitian immigrants, with the co-operation of the leadership of these groups;

2. specific questions on the blood donor questionnaire to detect symptoms associated with AIDS, such as swollen lymph glands, night sweats or unexplained fever or weight loss;

3. evaluation and implementation of laboratory tests that would identify individuals at high risk of AIDS transmission.

While the Red Cross was skeptical about the dangers of blood-borne AIDS, it immediately began investigating the MSAC recommendation to screen out high-risk donors. The Canadian system, with its monopoly control and centralized decision-making, lent itself perfectly to screening. A couple of weeks earlier, at a meeting of the Ad Hoc AIDS Group, Dr. Roger Dodd, a senior advisor to the American Red Cross, had expressed his envy at how easy the Canadian Red Cross had things; it could afford to turn away donors without losing market share to competitors, and with virtually no impact on the bottom line; further, new tests and measures to make up for shortages would be paid for by sponsoring governments. On the other hand, the Canadian system was very susceptible to the vagaries of public opinion. The Red Cross was obsessed with never offending a donor, and reluctant to acknowledge any association between AIDS and blood, lest donors imagine that AIDS could be contracted from making a blood donation.

Just three weeks after the MSAC memorandum, the Centers for Disease Control issued a list of recommendations "whose clear intent is to eliminate plasma and blood potentially containing the putative AIDS agent from the supply", including screening out high-risk donors, limiting transfusions to a bare minimum and developing safer blood products. In a long preamble to the recommendations, the U.S. scientists not only implied that AIDS was caused by a viral agent but said it was virtually certain that it was blood-borne. They noted that AIDS infections paralleled hepatitis B infection patterns and warned that the "pool of persons potentially capable of transmitting an AIDS agent may be considerably larger than the presently known number of AIDS cases."

Within days, on March 10, 1983, the Red Cross took its first formal action against AIDS, issuing a press release asking homosexual and bisexual men with multiple partners to abstain from giving blood, along with newly arrived Haitian immigrants and intravenous drug users. The request was eminently reasonable. At the time, 61 per cent of identified AIDS cases were among homosexual men, and 37 per cent among recently immigrated Haitians. But a key component of the MSAC recommendation — that leaders of high-risk groups be contacted to support the initiative — was largely ignored.[1] Dr. Derrick had spoken only to *The Body Politic*, a gay newspaper, and editor Edward Jackson was skeptical: "We're concerned that this might stigmatize the gay community," he said in response to the announcement. When the U.S. non-profit blood bankers drafted their position they invited the National Gay Task Force and the National Hemophilia Foundation to the meeting, and obtained their immediate endorsement. But when the news of the Canadian Red Cross position came out the next day — and it was widely reported, without the qualifications of "multiple partners" and "newly arrived immigrants", that gay men and Haitians were carriers of the new disease — it was the first the leadership of these groups had heard of it, and they were outraged.

Dr. Antony Alcidor, a pathologist and president of the Haitian Physicians' Association, said the singling out of one nationality "hit like a bomb" and was "socially devastating". The association met the next morning and fired off a telex to Monique Bégin, saying that AIDS statistics were skewed and that the Red Cross hadn't considered the consequences of its action. The Haitian community was particularly miffed because it had been given no prior notice of the "high-risk" designation. In any case, Dr. Alcidor had organized a blood donor clinic specifically for Haitians some months earlier and had attracted only one person. There was no tradition of blood donation in the community, there were no Canadian statistics on the extent of AIDS infection among people of Haitian origin, yet the whole community was being vilified for having "bad blood". Leaders of gay groups were equally infuriated. *Rencontres Gaies*, a Montreal-based magazine, likened the Red Cross to "Nazis who would have us wear a pink triangle". The reaction to screening was excessive, but there was a real fear that exclusion from blood donation was the thin edge of the wedge. There was already talk in British Columbia's Social Credit government of shipping people with AIDS and sexually active gay men to Bentinck Island, and across the country in Nova Scotia, there was a persistent rumour that a similar quarantine station was planned for McNab Island. Both islands had previously been used as leper colonies.

For the first time in its existence, the revered Red Cross felt the sting of sustained and pointed public criticism. Complaints of discrimination were filed with human rights commissions, and boycotts of clinics were launched by gay and Haitian organizations. Civil rights, rather than safety of the blood supply, became the issue.

In the same press release, the Red Cross had announced plans to question donors, not about their sexual preferences or national origin, but about symptoms associated with the new disease, and to launch a public information campaign about AIDS. At the time there were eight diseases mentioned by name in the pamphlets handed out to potential donors, but AIDS was not among them. But because of the outcry, plans for symptom-specific questions and an education campaign were dropped — the most blatant example till then of political concerns overriding sensible medical policy decisions.

On March 24 and 25 the medical directors of the Red Cross blood transfusion centres met in Toronto to discuss the brouhaha. Dr. Derrick opened the meeting with a brief summary of the AIDS situation, blaming the disease on the "extremely permissive social behaviour evident in some areas of the United States"; he was still convinced that the epidemic was an American problem. The medical directors were looking for guidance on donor deferral; many said some of their regular donors were known to be at high risk for AIDS, while some claimed a noticeable increase in high-risk donors. Dr. Roger Perrault responded by saying that blood collected from high-risk donors was not to be singled out, and that the only diagnostic question permitted was "Are you well?" Then the directors formed a new committee, the AIDS Working Group. The majority of members weren't medical people. What was needed, they decided, was not swift action but reassuring words. It was to become a familiar response.

At the March 29 meeting of the AIDS Working Group, the thorny issue of discrimination complaints to the human rights commission was raised. Red Cross lawyer Michael Worsoff was asked, "What would be the legal aspects if an issue is made of the right of donors to give blood?" His answer, according to the minutes of the meeting, was the following: "It is not a matter of the donor having a right to donate blood. Rather, it is a case of the Red Cross having both a moral and legal obligation to assure the safety of the blood it accepts for processing and distribution. The evidence of possible unacceptability of the blood does not have to be conclusive, the decision can be made on a basis of 'reasonable doubt' as to its suitability. With reference to the AIDS problem in particular, the premise is not that the CRC has to justify beyond any scientific doubt that there is a link between designated 'high risk groups' and the development of AIDS since, if there is even a possibility of transmission via blood, the CRC has the moral and legal obligation to protect the recipient above all." Yet, immediately after Worsoff's legal opinion, the AIDS Working Group decided that the existing questionnaire — which made no mention of AIDS, its symptoms, high-risk groups or high-risk activities — was adequate. Acting on reasonable doubt would result in lost blood donations, so the problem was better not discussed; wishful thinking would substitute for screening, and official silence for information.

In July the Red Cross held a press conference, in conjunction with the AIDS Committee of Toronto, to reiterate its stand on voluntary deferral. The person doing the talking was Dr. Roslyn Herst, deputy medical director of the Toronto BTS, and her speech was low-key, designed to "counter the fear of AIDS based on rumours and distorted reporting". The goal was threefold: not to offend gays, not to inflame homophobes and, above all, not to alarm donors. Dr. Herst let slip that "unofficial" Red Cross policy was to urge all gay men to refrain from donating blood, a position that was "clarified" in a press release the next day. What Dr. Herst didn't say was that she had quietly ordered that blood collections in predominantly gay areas be stopped, as well as gay-sponsored donor clinics. The move was made without fanfare because gay men were big blood donors, accounting for an estimated 15 per cent of donations. The Judy Garland Memorial Bowling League, a group of rather flamboyant gay men, for example, had given blood on a number of occasions. While the vast majority were more discreet, the voluntary donation was, for some, a way of feeling like full members of society, of countering the public image of promiscuity and "dirty deeds". Gay men tend to live in urban areas, where blood collection is centred. They had been actively courted as blood donors in the mid-1970s, when researchers were developing a vaccine for hepatitis B. (Vaccines are usually extracted from blood that contains antibodies to a disease, and many gay men had hepatitis B antibodies because of their exposure.)

Hepatitis had left a certain legacy of distrust in the gay community. The hepatitis B vaccine that was developed would save tens of thousands of lives in the Third World, but the community would get little or no credit. In Canada the vaccine was made available to healthcare workers, police officers and firefighters who were at risk of contamination on the job, but it was refused to gay men who wanted to avoid transmission by sexual contact. So the same men who voluntarily gave blood for the development of the vaccine found themselves, years later, forced to pay to purchase it.

* * *

Like Dr. Herst, medical directors across the country implemented screening measures on the sly, in direct defiance of the do-nothing policy at head office. One medical director added a question at the bottom of the donor questionnaire — "Have you had any unexplained night sweats, swollen glands, etc." In Manitoba, Dr. Marlis Schroeder attended an AIDS forum held at Club Happenings in August 1983 and said bluntly that sexually active gay men shouldn't donate blood. She was not jeered but praised. In fact, a group of Winnipeg gay activists, using their own money, assembled and distributed pamphlets and posters that provided safe-sex tips and told gay men that it was "not acceptable" to donate blood.[2] It is not a coincidence that Manitoba, despite a proportionally large gay community, has the lowest rate of transfusion AIDS in the country.

The Vancouver gay community also distinguished itself by its activism to counter transfusion AIDS. Vancouver doctor Brian Willoughby was among the first to warn that the new disease was blood-borne, telling *The Body Politic* in November 1982 that gay men shouldn't give blood. Over the years he was instrumental in convincing high-risk patients not to donate, urging them to get the word out and "find a lesbian to take your place". Despite the fact that the Social Credit government refused a request for $200 from AIDS Vancouver to print the education pamphlets — the word "condom" was considered too vulgar — pamphlets and posters reading "Don't give blood" were distributed to bathhouses and gay bars. As in Manitoba, the simple initiative had an obvious impact: while British Columbia has the highest per-capita AIDS rate in Canada, the infected donor rate — two in a thousand after testing was instituted — was less than half the national average. This was a remarkable achievement considering that the community was fighting an epidemic with volunteers, many of whom were suffering from AIDS themselves. It is also a sad reminder of how tainted blood could have been kept out of the system, had the Red Cross and public health officials dedicated just a fraction of their considerable resources to prevention.

In St. John's, Red Cross medical director Dr. Richard Huntsman approached a staff member at the hospital who was openly gay and was put in touch with the Gay Association of Newfoundland and Labrador. Within days he met the group's executive. "We struck a bargain; they would not donate if we did not discriminate," he recalls. The medical director was later invited to join the board of the Newfoundland and Labrador AIDS Committee. While he came from the military background that the Red Cross favoured, Dr. Huntsman's disobedience of orders was a model of professionalism and common sense, and one that saved lives.

In Saskatchewan, Dr. Brian McSheffrey simply looked up "gay" in the phone book and arranged a meeting with community leaders to discuss the problem. Once they understood the risks of blood-borne AIDS, they readily agreed to voluntary deferral of donations. But what was to be done about the many blood clinics in office settings, where closeted gay men would give blood rather than divulge their secret? The blood transfusion service developed euphemisms for donors to indicate that they would like their blood destroyed. Nurses could be asked that the donation be used "for research purposes only", or if the nurses themselves had a hunch someone was a high-risk donor they would "put the unit into quality control". This was a crude version of a system developed in New York City called "confidential unit exclusion (CUE)", where all donors were given the option of designating their blood for "research purposes" rather than for transfusion. The infection rate among CUE units was many times higher than in the general supply, but in Canada the Red Cross worried that well-meaning people who were not at high risk would also choose to support fictitious research efforts, and waste good blood. In Saskatchewan, where Premier Grant Devine was on record as saying that homosexuals were no more deserving of human rights protection than bank robbers, official efforts to work with the community were non-existent.

In Edmonton, local physician Dr. Barbara Romanowski set up an STD clinic right in the Pisces bathhouse, where, among other things, gay men were urged not to give blood, but the service was discontinued after police raided the bathhouse. There would be no contact between the Red Cross and the gay community until the introduction of testing for the AIDS virus years later. The Edmonton BTS — which also oversees the collection and distribution of blood in remote Arctic communities, where blood is collected from "walk-in" donors and transfused directly into patients without testing — had a simple approach: "When in doubt, defer." But in the big city, where state-of-the-art facilities existed for the questioning of donors, and the supply of donors was less limited, that sensible policy wasn't instituted, even at the height of the AIDS epidemic.

In Halifax, the home of Patient Zero, Gaétan Dugas, from 1979 to 1983, and in Quebec City, his birthplace, Red Cross medical directors didn't deign to cross the threshold of local gay groups to discuss voluntary deferral. Dr. Côme Rousseau, the medical director in Quebec City, wrote to his staff that all persons who appeared to be in good health must be accepted as blood donors. "The policy is succinct, clear and explicit. It must be obeyed to the letter, without prejudice," he wrote. In Montreal, which had by far the highest rate of infected donors, the local medical director also followed orders from head office and took no initiative to screen donors. Dr. Raymond Guévin had no contact with gay groups, despite the fact that they were easy to find. Controversial raids on local gay bars like Truxx had sparked an outcry, and community leaders considered the high-risk designation another attack on their civil rights. Complicating matters was the language issue; just as the Red Cross insisted that AIDS was an American problem, French-speaking gays insisted the AIDS was limited to anglophones.

As the crowning touch, the Red Cross not only had its permanent blood transfusion centre on the periphery of the Gay Village, but conducted regular blood donor clinics at Berri de Montigny Métro station (now Berri-UQAM) from 1978 onwards. The clinic was in the heart of the Gay Village, and in the red-light district as well; it was just beside the Université du Québec à Montréal, home of a substantial Haitian student body; and located in close proximity to the largest community of heroin addicts in the country. It was the veritable headquarters of the "4-H Club" — but because the Red Cross BTS didn't discuss matters of safety with its own blood donor recruitment personnel, let alone with the affected communities, the clinic operated for years.

Some medical people, aware that voluntary deferral wasn't working, found ways of instituting informal, unscientific screening as a concession to safety. In Montreal, Dr. Guévin encouraged nurses to use their "flair for intuition" to reject a blood donation they thought might be from a member of a high-risk group. In Vancouver they tagged the donations of "suspect" donors with green tags, not a long way from pink triangles. Nurses in the Toronto area, which has the biggest gay community in the country, were given similar instructions, though they didn't seem particularly adept at spotting sexually active homosexuals by their appearance. Robert M.*, an employee of a popular gay bar, was ideally situated to be aware of news circulating in the community but knew nothing of the voluntary deferral policy. There were no ads in the gay press, and no pamphlets and posters in Toronto's numerous bars and bathhouses. In the five years prior to the summer of 1983, Robert M. had sex with more than a thousand men, but said he never encountered any information that might call into question the acceptability of his blood. "I was healthy, so I figured I'm not going to cause anyone any harm. I was doing this out of the goodness of my heart," he said before his death. Robert M. donated blood thirty-two times before the Red Cross began testing blood for the AIDS virus. He was never asked anything more than "Are you in good health?" He thought he was.

Years later, Douglas Elliott, a lawyer for the Canadian AIDS Society, asked one of the Red Cross medical directors at a public inquiry, "How do you guess whether people are gay? Do you ask them about their record collections or where they go to drink?" The pseudo-scientific approach of trying to identify homosexual men based on a stereotype of what "they" looked like, rather than through a forthright questionnaire, underlines the hypocrisy of the Red Cross. It was somehow considered ethical to allow someone to donate blood in good faith and then covertly discard it — but it wasn't considered appropriate to conduct screening out in the open, or even to conduct an education campaign to warn the general public that AIDS is transmitted by blood.

Dr. John MacKay, the Red Cross medical director in Saint John, was also a company man. He didn't even bother to look up "gay" in the phone book because he considered it wrong to stray from orders. As he put it, "The Red Cross was founded on the battlefield. It has always existed in a sort of paramilitary structure, and I very profoundly believe it should continue to function by a single common standard. In discussions with various authorities at National, I had been reminded of that very forcefully. It is not the role of the individual medical director to attempt to establish standards higher than those imposed by

* A court order prevents identifying him by name.

National." Dr. MacKay's view, held by a number of medical directors, points to another attitude that was prevalent in the Red Cross at the time — that standards were somehow a maximum level of action, rather than a minimum. Uniformity was interpreted as meaning "take no initiative". James Noble, the chair of AIDS Saint John, was a blood donor at the time, and because he has a rare blood type he was called regularly by the Red Cross. One day he approached the clinic nurse and said he was a member of a high-risk group and would rather not give blood. "I was told to donate anyway, because it was important that they get A-negative blood," Noble says.

New Brunswick provides another example of the role homophobia played in the tainted-blood tragedy. Richard Hatfield, premier of the province from 1970 to 1987, was a homosexual. As a frequent visitor to New York, he was well aware of the AIDS epidemic in the gay community. Hatfield gave generously to AIDS New Brunswick as a private citizen, but the politician, outspoken and progressive on so many issues, remained strangely silent about AIDS for fear of drawing attention to his private life.

A similar situation existed at the head office of the Red Cross, where two of the four senior administrators of the blood transfusion service — Dr. John Derrick and Dr. Derek Naylor — were gay men. Like Hatfield, Derrick made regular trips to New York to visit gay bars but remained closeted at home. At the same time he was writing memos saying he didn't know how to contact gay community leaders, and refusing to meet members of "interest groups"; later, he tried to have members of gay groups removed from an AIDS advisory committee because of their "disruptive behaviour". The open secret of Derrick's sexuality strained relations with gay activists at a time when their co-operation could have made a big difference. Gay leaders were able to work with heterosexuals like Dr. Schroeder and Dr. Huntsman, but distrusted initiatives by closeted homosexuals like Dr. Derrick.

Randy Shilts, author of *And the Band Played On*, eloquently summarized the problem in explaining why a senior director of the U.S. National Institutes of Health, a closeted gay man, systematically refused to join the fight against AIDS:

> It was a truism to people active in the gay movement that the greatest impediments to homosexuals' progress often were not heterosexual bigots but closeted homosexuals. Among the nation's decision makers, the homophobes largely had been silenced by the prevailing morality that viewed expressions of overt hostility towards gays as unfashionable. In fact, when not burdened by private sexual insecurities, many heterosexuals could be enlisted to support gays on the basis of personal integrity. By definition, the

homosexual in the closet had surrendered his integrity. This makes closeted homosexual people very useful to the establishment: Once empowered, such people are guaranteed to support the most subtle nuances of anti-gay prejudice. A closeted homosexual has the keenest understanding of these nuances, having chosen to live under the complete subjugation of prejudice. The closeted homosexual is far less likely to demand fair or just treatment of his kind, because to do so would call attention to himself.[3]

Dr. Derrick's hidden homosexuality had a negative impact on his work. He was the consummate Red Cross employee, having started as a member of the Canadian army medical corps during the Second World War and having created the blood products division in 1975. But his profound denial of his own sexuality was translated into a profound denial of the breadth of the AIDS epidemic. Dr. Derrick insisted that the risk of transfusion AIDS was one in a million; he stubbornly stuck to a wait-and-see approach, and demanded ever more scientific proof before instituting new screening measures. And his inaction on AIDS was exploited by others for their own ends.

Sadly, the Canadian Hemophilia Society didn't build any more bridges with the gay community than did the Red Cross. With some notable exceptions, hemophiliacs suffered from "homophobia-phobia"[4]; they were obsessed with not having a link made between homosexuality and hemophilia. This fear was deeply rooted. In the days before blood concentrate, most hemophiliac children weren't allowed to participate in sports, and their disease left them fragile and "effeminate"; few had escaped the painful schoolyard taunts of "hemo-homo". In the U.S., relations between hemophiliac groups and gay groups were strained as they fought publicly about the screening issue; in Canada, the two groups hardest hit by AIDS simply didn't communicate at the outset of the epidemic.

Aside from the screening of individual donors to determine if they were members of high-risk groups — or engaging in high-risk activities, which is what screening measures focus on today — other measures could have made a real difference in Canada. U.S. commercial plasma fractionators not only screened donors, but stopped collecting altogether in major urban areas like New York, Miami and Los Angeles. The Red Cross, in the U.S. as in Canada, balked at the notion of slowing collections in urban centres. In fact, in the years before the introduction of concentrate there had been a marked shift towards collections in cities, to cut costs. Worse yet, because the donor recruitment and blood transfusion divisions of the Red Cross operated virtually independently of one another, some of the busiest clinics in the country continued to operate in the gay neighborhoods of Toronto, Montreal and Vancouver, at a time when medical directors were urging gays to refrain from giving blood.

It took until April 1984 for the Red Cross to update the pamphlet it handed out to blood donors — a full year after Toronto's Hassle Free Clinic published a no-nonsense AIDS pamphlet — and then the changes were so subtle as to be absurd. By then, French and American researchers had discovered the AIDS virus and the incubation period and progression of the disease had been well documented, but the Red Cross was still pussyfooting around the issue, insisting that donors be asked general health questions. Finally, a year later, the questionnaire was changed to include symptom-specific questions; but by that time surgery patients were already dying of transfusion-AIDS.

In the summer of 1985, prompted by fears the federal government would make testing of blood donations for HIV mandatory, the Red Cross changed its approach and made a determined effort to meet gay community leaders and AIDS organizations. Dr. Derrick admitted grudgingly that without the co-operation of the gay community mandatory testing would have a hard time getting off the ground, and he desperately wanted to avoid the negative publicity that had followed the call for voluntary deferral a couple of years earlier.

There could no longer be any denial about AIDS. On October 2, 1985, the actor Rock Hudson died, and the reality of the AIDS epidemic became palpable in mainstream society. The AIDS statistics tacked onto the end of news stories suddenly took on a human dimension. In the U.S. more than 12,000 people had already died of AIDS. In Canada, 435 cases of AIDS had been diagnosed — including 329 homosexual men and 14 recipients of blood and blood products — and half of those had already died. Many more thousands would die because public health authorities had opted to hide behind statistics that would soon collapse like a house of cards, refusing to take the steps necessary to slow the epidemic. As long as there was no public outcry, their political masters were content to substitute bland reassurance for leadership. It took a closeted gay actor — one who, ironically, had been a famous "heart-throb" — to shake them out of their lethal indifference.

6

BLOOD MONEY
THE FRACTIONATION DÉBÂCLE

Surely every medicine is an innovation;
and he that will not apply new remedies,
must expect new evils.

Francis Bacon
Essays: On Innovation

Jeff Lee, Estevan, Saskatchewan

A drywaller and father of four children, Jeff learned he was infected in 1986, but kept his diagnosis secret for many years. A hemophiliac who was ostracized as a child, he decided to go public after a discussion with his kids about discrimination against people with HIV-AIDS.

"My eldest daughter talked to me about the stigma attached to HIV and AIDS. She asked why it was there and why people were scared, and stuff like that.

I said: 'Well, because it's such a scary disease. People don't know exactly what's going on, and they all relate HIV and AIDS to gay men.'

She said: 'How are things ever going to change?'

So, I said: 'Well, obviously, people are going to have to go out and start talking about it.'"

(May 24, 1994)

SERGE AND STÉPHANE LANDRY were born on July 16, 1976, less than two weeks after the U.S. Bicentennial celebrations. It was eleven months before doctors realized that the twins were hemophiliacs. By the boys' first birthday AIDS had taken root in North America, but the "gay plague" was probably the farthest thing from their parents' minds. You didn't worry about such things in Moncton, New Brunswick. What Normand Landry remembers most about that first visit to the hematologist is two of the other patients in the waiting room: one a boy of fifteen, unable to straighten his legs because of the damage bleeds had caused to his knees; the other a man of thirty, though he looked much older, hunched over and confined to a wheelchair by crippling arthritis.

What the father had seen, Dr. Sheldon Rubin explained, was not the future that awaited Serge and Stéphane, but the painful fate they had narrowly avoided. In this day and age, Normand Landry learned, the hereditary disease was no longer debilitating; it was little more than an inconvenience. For the first three years of their lives Serge and Stéphane, who were moderate hemophiliacs, had to be taken on occasional visits to the local hospital for injections of cryoprecipitate to treat the bumps and bruises of childhood. While concentrate that could be administered at home had been on the market for several years, it was not among the products provided free of charge by the Red Cross. On request, the agency would purchase the products and bill hospitals for them, tacking on a 10 per cent handling fee, but most hospitals that wanted factor concentrate purchased it directly from pharmaceutical companies along with other prescription drugs. It was this practice that had alarmed the Canadian Hematology Society way back in 1972, when it recommended that the Blood Transfusion Service supply the "total need for blood and blood products in Canada".

The blood fractionation plant that the Red Cross proposed building would have a capacity of 350,000 litres, and would require a $21 million investment and $5 million more to operate each year. Although it was expected to make Canada self-sufficient in blood products within two years, there was a problem: the Red Cross still didn't have a plasmapheresis program that could provide enough raw material to achieve that goal. The prison-collection idea had been rejected, and there was no alternative on the table that would provide anywhere near 350,000 litres of plasma annually. Connaught Laboratories, which was still hoping to be involved in the plant despite its feud with the Red Cross, was proposing that the supply of raw material be increased through payments for plasma donations, as in the U.S.

Pressure to resolve the fractionation void was mounting. Governments saw opportunities for high-technology jobs, while doctors and patients were clamouring for the easy-to-use concentrate that was already widely available in the U.S. and Europe. In 1976 the Red Cross purchased 2.7 million units of Factor IX, and demand for the product doubled within a year. Most hemophiliacs were deficient in Factor VIII and were using cryoprecipitate, while those outside urban centres were still transfused with plasma — a treatment that was horribly out of date and inefficient.

Leaders of the Canadian Hemophilia Society wanted the new generation, boys like the Landry twins, to benefit from concentrate, so they pleaded with governments to resolve the bickering between the Red Cross and Connaught and get the new products into their homes. Still, their pleas were tempered with concern. Blood-borne diseases spread rapidly as plasma was pooled for processing into concentrate, which was why almost all early users of blood concentrate were infected with hepatitis. Though the Red Cross had begun testing blood for hepatitis B in 1970, that did little to stop the infections; the concentrate was, in large part, imported from the U.S. and made with commercial plasma, or a mix of U.S. and Canadian plasma. A single unit that slipped through screening could infect the entire lot. Besides, hepatitis B wasn't the only problem; non-A-non-B hepatitis (now called hepatitis C) was also blood-borne, and there was no test available to detect it. The concern, expressed in a CHS newsletter at the time, was that "we are trading a devil we know — uncontrolled bleeding — for one we don't know — transfusion-transmitted diseases."

Between the two extremes, disease-free but inefficient plasma and effective but infected concentrate, lay a practical alternative, cryoprecipitate. Made by pooling only a handful of donations, it was rarely contaminated and was thirty times more effective than plasma for treating bleeds. The problem with cryoprecipitate was not therapeutic but bureaucratic; most hospitals insisted that the product be infused on site. So a ridiculous routine was repeated daily in hospitals across the country: a hemophiliac requiring treatment for a bleed would make his way to the hospital, be admitted through emergency, go to the fridge and take out as many packs of cryo as he figured he would need,* and then sit there in pain, watching his limbs swell, until an intern found time to do

---

* Cryo was generally prepared in plastic packs of eighty international units, and a hemophiliac could use anywhere from one to a hundred or more packs, depending on the severity of the bleed.

the infusion. In the summer of 1977 the CHS did its first registration of hemo-philiacs; 1,639 hemophiliacs were interviewed and the major complaint was that emergency room waits were interminable. For people with blood disorders, poor care was the norm.

The beauty of concentrate was that it was issued with syringes that allowed self-infusion at home or at the office. The risk of hepatitis, when users were even aware that it existed, was seen as a trade-off for freedom.

*   *   *

In October 1977 the Red Cross signed its first contract to have Canadian plasma manufactured into Factor VIII and Factor IX; plasma from volunteer donors would be frozen, shipped by refrigerated truck to a plant in North Carolina and transformed into a white powder, and the vials would be shipped back for use by Canadian hemophiliacs. The deal, with the Hyland Division of Travenol Laboratories, was a modest one, providing fewer than 300,000 units of Factor VIII — the vast majority of concentrate purchased by the Red Cross was made from commercial U.S. plasma — but it infuriated Connaught, which could see a big money-maker slipping away.

So, after nineteen years of promises, Connaught Laboratories announced that it would conduct trials with its Factor VIII concentrate. Because it no longer had a contract with the Red Cross, however, Connaught began paying plasma donors. This violation of a fundamental principle of the nation's blood system outraged both the Red Cross and the Canadian Hemophilia Society, who felt it could prompt the collapse of the volunteer system, but it was tolerated by governments. (In fact, pharmaceutical companies have long paid and continue to pay donors who have specific antibodies in their blood, for plasma used to create vaccines.) This made the Red Cross even more determined to build its own non-profit plant, using volunteer-only plasma.

In 1978 the Red Cross made it a priority to produce fresh-frozen plasma, the blood component required to manufacture concentrate. Still, it managed to provide enough raw material for only half of Canada's concentrate needs. In a single year Factor VIII use jumped ninefold, to over twenty million units. The Red Cross goal was to achieve 100 per cent Canadian production of concentrate by 1983. Its arguments for self-sufficiency were given credence in 1978 when a giant plasma collection plant in Nicaragua was destroyed by rebels prompting U.S. shortages.

In 1979, Serge and Stéphane Landry were, like most other hemophiliacs, placed in a homecare program. They were part of a new generation of hemo-philiacs who would keep vials of powdered blood concentrate in the refrigerator, to mix with distilled water and infuse whenever it was needed — either in response to a bleed, or as a prophylaxis, for example when they were heading out to play soccer with the other kids after school. Many doctors were leery of the miracle product, but they had seen patients suffer so much over the years that they didn't want to deny them the benefits concentrate offered.

While the users of blood products were finally free of the shackles of their disorder, the Red Cross found itself unusually constrained by its political masters. The provinces had, only a couple of years before, set up a funding review mechanism for the blood program. In 1979, they set up the Ad Hoc Committee on Blood and Blood Products, headed by Gary Chatfield, Alberta's deputy minister of health, to examine the security of supply of raw materials and manufactured blood products. In September of that year the committee made a number of recommendations to the federal-provincial conference of the ministers of health. The bulk of the report was "motherhood" — a reaffirmation of the voluntary blood collection system and the principle of free blood, as well as yet another reminder of the need to be self-sufficient in blood and blood products. The Chatfield Committee said that only non-profit operations should be permitted to process Canadian blood but called for a small contract to be awarded to Connaught so that its abilities could be better evaluated. The report justified the contradiction by adding, "In order not to exclude Connaught Laboratories, the Committee recommends that the Federal government review and consider changing Connaught's corporate status and its present profit-motivated objectives." Still, the bottom line for Chatfield and his colleagues was that Canada should aim for self-sufficiency in production only if the cost of domestic production was comparable to that of foreign fractionation of Canadian plasma. The lingering problem, noted federal health minister John Crombie, was that the ageing Connaught Laboratories was badly in need of repair. He didn't bother mentioning what his officials had told him — that the Red Cross and Connaught, the supplier and the manufacturer, had developed a "continuing unstable and antagonistic relationship".

On April 5, 1979, Connaught was awarded a licence by the federal Bureau of Biologics to produce Factor VIII concentrate. To mark the occasion, there was a ceremony where Dr. Roger Perrault, head of the Red Cross Blood Transfusion Service, presented a vial of the new product to Major Jack Barr, president of the Canadian Hemophilia Society. There were smiles all around, at the event that symbolized the emancipation of Canada's hemophiliacs.

The smiles masked the end of an era of innocence. Blood had become big business.

*   *   *

The Red Cross was no longer just a charitable organization that collected and distributed blood; it had become a manufacturer of blood products. Its longtime ally, the privatized Connaught, was now a competitor and a hindrance. Provincial governments, which had long left the Red Cross to go about its business, also took a sudden interest in the blood system, seeing the large-scale production of concentrate as a job-creation tool. Ontario was the most aggressive, convinced that fractionation could save the legendary Connaught. The solidarity of the war years, the gathering together for a common cause, was a thing of the past. Health and Welfare Canada was the only major player in the blood system that didn't realize things had changed drastically; despite the dramatic scientific advances and the new threats of diseases like hepatitis, it continued to treat the Red Cross and Connaught with a reverence unworthy of a regulator. As a result, there was no one to establish the rules.

In June 1980 the Red Cross signed a thirty-two-month, $9.1-million contract with Cutter Biological (a division of the U.S. pharmaceutical giant Miles Inc.) to produce factor concentrate. Connaught had bid $14 million for the same work even though it didn't have adequate production facilities. Yet three months later, Ontario health minister Dennis Timbrell* demanded that the Red Cross cancel its contract with Cutter and award it to Connaught, because of the need for self-sufficiency. He insisted that Connaught had the technology in place to produce commercial quantities of factor concentrate, a position that was, at best, wishful thinking. What really angered Timbrell, however, was that the Cutter contract was seen as a gambit to drive Connaught out of the blood business so the Red Cross could build its own plant. On September 29 the provincial ministers of health, at the urging of Ontario, formally rejected the proposal the Red Cross had made four years earlier to build its own fractionation plant. "There will be no further consideration given to a plant to be built and operated by the Red Cross," Timbrell said. "It simply isn't needed. We have the facilities and the potential to process blood plasma in Canada already." The ministers ordered another study to determine who would get the lucrative fractionation contract, but in the meantime ordered that business be split between Cutter and Connaught. The Ad Hoc Committee on Plasma Fractionation, headed by Dr. Chapin Key, British Columbia's deputy minister of health, once again called for a non-profit policy but recommended that "at least two separate fractionation plants should be developed in Canada, even though there would probably be an associated financial

---

* His deputy minister, Allan Dyer, was a former employee of Connaught.

penalty." The committee concluded that self-sufficiency would take at least three years to achieve because of the need to renovate and upgrade Connaught's facilities, and conceded that foreign imports would probably have to continue for practical reasons.

Dr. Key was the first government official to zero in on the fact that the Canadian Red Cross simply didn't collect enough plasma to provide the raw material for domestic production. Connaught had quietly begun to pay for blood, buying from Dominion Biologicals, a plasmapheresis centre near Dalhousie University in Halifax. Other entrepreneurs got in on the act: the Canadian Plasmapheresis Centre in Ottawa paid donors $8 per unit and a $6 bonus after eight bleeds; Canadian Bioplasma, which advertised in the University of Toronto student newspaper *The Varsity*, paid $15 per donation. The new business was totally unregulated, and the Red Cross, which for years had been pushing for the provinces to invest in plasmapheresis, was frustrated. A doubling in plasma collection was required if the Canadian plants were going to get enough raw material, but that would entail enormous costs and surpluses of various other blood components that would be either discarded (an insult to volunteer donors) or sold to commercial fractionators (a violation of the non-profit principle). The committee calculated that increased plasma collections would cost as much as $15 million annually, while making up shortfalls by pur-chasing factor concentrate on the open market would cost only $1.5 million.

The committee recommended construction of a second plant for purely political reasons. Just as Ontario demanded that plasma be processed in that province, the Quebec government didn't want the blood donated by its citi-zens creating jobs in Ontario. It didn't seem to matter that the purpose of a single plant was to benefit from economies of scale; politics once again took precedence over common sense.

The health ministers didn't want the public to know just how ugly the politi-cal situation was. In November 1979, Quebec's separatist government, under René Lévesque, had threatened to leave the federal-provincial budget review process and sign a separate contract with the Red Cross for blood collection and distribution. The move would likely have led to the collapse of the blood pro-gram if other provinces followed suit and have caused a good deal of political embarrassment. Because one of its basic principles is political neutrality, the Red Cross would not refuse Quebec's request outright, but it did stall. On February 15, 1980, however, Dr. Denis Lazure, Quebec's Minister of Social Affairs, met with four senior Red Cross officials, including the president, Justice James Wilson, and the national commissioner, retired Lieutenant-General Henri Tellier. According to the minutes of the meeting, Dr. Lazure said that, in return for the Red Cross signing a contract, the Quebec government would build a fractionation plant for the Red Cross at the Institut Armand-Frappier, in suburban Laval. The Quebec cabinet approved construction of a plant with a capacity of up to 250,000 litres, and a contract was drafted and signed between the Red Cross and the Quebec government on June 26 — a deal that lasted for three years — but Quebec still had the bargaining power it needed to get the other provinces to alter the fractionation plan.

Quebec's move got senior health ministry officials in other provinces thinking about who controlled the blood system, and when bureaucrats have a thought it almost inevitably leads their political bosses to appoint a committee. In the summer of 1981 the Inter-Provincial Ad Hoc Committee on a Canadian Authority on Blood Policy became the latest of a long list to investigate Canada's blood program, in particular the blood fractionation issue. The committee, once again headed by Dr. Chapin Key, marked an important turning-point because it recommended the creation of a permanent body to oversee the blood system. (Until then there had been a federal-provincial budget review committee, but Ontario had refused to participate during the battle over fractionation and Quebec had opted out permanently.) The Chapin Key committee was consistent in its inconsistency, with the political interests of the provinces overriding sound business decisions. It too recommended that only non-profit companies be allowed to process volunteer blood, but demanded that the Red Cross sign a long-term contract with the profit-oriented Connaught. The committee also called for the Connaught Laboratories to be modernized so it could process up to 100,000 litres of plasma annually, and for Connaught to be allowed to price its fractionation products in a manner that would allow it to recover 50 per cent of capital costs. (The other 50 per cent would be paid by the province as a job-creation incentive.)

After several more months of back-room bickering, the provinces decided that there should be three regional fractionation plants. Canada being what it is, the west demanded its share of the blood money. But over 40 per cent of the country's blood was collected in Ontario, so it was decided that plasma collected by the Red Cross would be distributed as follows: Connaught Laboratories of Toronto, 50 per cent; and 25 per cent each to the Centre de fractionnement sanguin Armand-Frappier of Montreal, and the Winnipeg Plasma Laboratory. Six years after the Red Cross had started the ball rolling on fractionation, the plants were still nothing but an idea, and no one had budged on the fundamental issue, plasmapheresis, so there was still no adequate supply of plasma for the plants.

Ontario, nevertheless, did get its way. The deal with Cutter was not terminated, although it was watered down considerably; in November 1981 the Red Cross signed a deal agreeing to provide 200,000 litres of fresh-frozen plasma over a three-year period. The Red Cross also signed a three-year contract with Connaught, which was to receive the bulk of the plasma collected in Canada — more than 500,000 litres during the contract period. While Connaught's commercial production capabilities were unproven, hemophiliacs considered its product second-rate and the Red Cross, its prices non-competitive. Ontario insisted that all plasma collected in the province go exclusively to Connaught. Quebec planned a similar demand when its plant got off the ground, and Manitoba figured it should have a claim to all western blood. The health ministers would stop at nothing to land the handful of jobs that would result from the fractionation contracts; even Canada's vaunted volunteer blood system was expendable.

* * *

The Canadian Blood Committee (CBC), composed of thirteen members* — one appointed by each of the federal, provincial and territorial ministers of health — held its first meeting on December 1, 1981. Two months later, the CBC adopted terms of reference that were approved by Canada's health ministers. The Red Cross bitterly opposed the creation of the CBC, arguing that it violated its independence, though the argument seemed to have little credence given that the provinces were paying all the bills. The terms of reference are worth reviewing, if only to underline how utterly the CBC failed in its duties.

> The role of the Canadian Blood Committee is to establish policies with regard to the following:
>
> a. The collection of blood, including plasmapheresis;
> b. the processing of blood;
> c. the distribution of blood products;
> d. the utilization of blood products;
> e. operational research and;
> f. support and maintenance of the four enunciated principles concerning blood and blood products;**
>
> To recommend allocation of resources to meet costs of implementing the above policies;

---

* Quebec, however, did not participate officially until late 1983.
** The four principles were voluntary blood donation; self-sufficiency in supply of blood and blood products; gratuity of blood and blood products; and a non-profit blood system.

To assure adherence to established policies by the Canadian Red Cross, plasma fractionation plants, and others involved in the collection, processing, distribution and utilization of blood and blood products;

To consult with the Department of Industry, Trade and Commerce on appropriate policies for the export and import of human blood and blood products;

To consult with the Bureau of Biologics, Department of National Health and Welfare, on appropriate policies for the regulatory control of the collection, processing and distribution of blood, blood products and their substitutes;

In the short term, to monitor the development of fractionation plants to ensure that their establishment is in accordance with the recommendations of Ministers of Health and allocate resources and priorities for their implementation;

To determine the real costs of producing blood fractions for Canadians and the shareable portion of capital costs to be added to the price of blood fractions;

To ensure that standards for blood, blood products and blood substitutes are developed, and to monitor that such standards are met;

To review and approve the programs and budgets of the Blood Donor Recruitment and Blood Transfusion Services of the Canadian Red Cross Society, subject to the concurrence of all Provinces and Territories;

To report annually to the Ministers of Health on all activities of the Committee;

To be a national forum for the various organizations and associations of the Canadian blood program to discuss issues, and to coordinate the activities related to the management of the Canadian blood system.

The principles appeared to be straightforward, but in practical terms the committee's role was to control costs, keep Red Cross ambitions in check and find means to exploit the burgeoning biotechnological industry. The ministers who endorsed the CBC goals were seemingly oblivious of the fact that blood and blood products were supposed to be used to treat people with life-threatening illnesses, not merely manufactured as a means of job creation. Fifteen years after the first wave of infection of blood products with the hepatitis virus, there was no mention of quality or safety of concentrate, except a vague promise to develop and monitor standards. For Canada's ministers of health, protecting the blood system from the threat of disease wasn't an issue worth exploring, but determining the "shareable portion of capital costs to be added to the price of blood fractions" was a priority. With no legislative authority, no scientific knowledge and no public accountability, the CBC did little more than approve the funds it turned over to the Red Cross each year, and dream up increasingly grandiose schemes for the construction of fractionation plants.

Though the first alarms about blood-borne AIDS were sounded in the summer of 1982, the ministers didn't appoint a committee to study that issue, nor did their Canadian Blood Committee set out to "determine the real costs of producing blood fractions" in social and medical terms. They simply ignored AIDS. In fact, the same week that the U.S. Centers for Disease Control issued its first warning about hemophiliacs being at risk of contracting AIDS, there was a ground-breaking ceremony at the Winnipeg Plasma Laboratory.

In October 1982, Manitoba's Minister of Health, Larry Desjardins, asked that earlier decisions about blood fractionation be reconsidered. He appeared to be worried not about the possible contamination of factor concentrate, but about how much his province stood to benefit from the manufacture of the products. He wanted plasma distributed to each plant in equal amounts, and the pricing structure of concentrates changed so that the host provinces only had to pay 25 per cent of the capital costs of the new plants. The CBC immediately struck another committee. During its first year of existence, the Canadian Blood Committee discussed little else but fractionation.

Extra-Strength Tylenol was taken off the shelves in the U.S. and Canada in October 1982 after someone in the Chicago area tampered with the product and fatally poisoned seven people with cyanide. The manufacturer, Johnson & Johnson Inc., voluntarily withdrew millions of bottles of the pain reliever, a bold move that became a model for responsible corporate reaction to a crisis. Albert Liston, the assistant deputy minister of Health and Welfare, while assuring Canadians that there was no danger of poisoning in this country, said that the department would take preventive measures to reassure the public. It moved swiftly to implement new packaging rules.

At the time of the Tylenol scare, a dozen U.S. hemophiliacs had already died of AIDS and 10 per cent of hemophiliacs were suffering symptoms associated with the disease, not because of the actions of a madman but due to an epidemic that was spreading in the general population. Yet the federal government regulators responsible for ensuring the safety of products, the pharmaceutical companies that manufactured factor concentrates and the Red Cross, which distributed them, took no action.

In December 1982 a group of researchers at the University of Toronto applied to the federal and provincial ministries of health for $100,000 to conduct an in-depth study on the risk to hemophiliacs of AIDS. They were turned down.

Money, however, was available for other purposes. In the two months previous, the federal government had awarded $8.8 million to Connaught to conduct research on recombinant[1] Factor VIII, while Ontario had awarded Connaught $3.35 million to upgrade its much-vaunted but out-of-date fractionation facilities.

The proposed study was needed, according to scientists, because preliminary data from Dr. Christos Tsoukas in Montreal had revealed the alarming statistic that 70 per cent of severe hemophiliacs in Canada were already suffering from cellular immune deficiency consistent with the early signs of AIDS. On January 17, 1983, Dr. Gail Rock, medical director of the Red Cross BTS in Ottawa, wrote to head office expressing the view that blood products for hemophiliacs were not safe. An avid proponent of Canadian self-sufficiency in plasma collection, Dr. Rock felt that importing plasma and blood products like Factor VIII from the U.S. was an unnecessary risk. Her concerns were dismissed.

The scientific advisors to the Canadian Hemophilia Society entered the fray a few weeks later. After meeting with senior members of Health and Welfare Canada on February 7, they expressed the view that "urgent steps" should be taken to reduce the risk of AIDS in the blood supply. The recommendations of that meeting — drafted and distributed by Dr. Hanna Strawczynski, chair of the society's Medical and Scientific Advisory Committee (MSAC) and a physician at the Montreal Children's Hospital — provide a chilling record of what *should have* been done to minimize the infection of hemophiliacs with the deadly new disease.

I — RECOMMENDATIONS TO PHYSICIANS TREATING PATIENTS WITH
   HEMOPHILIA:

a) cryoprecipitate be used to treat patients who have never previously received concentrates; this group includes all newly diagnosed patients, regardless of the severity of the disease;

b) patients who must receive concentrates be treated with Factor VIII manufactured with Canadian source plasma;

c) all new diagnosed and mild cases of Factor IX deficiency should be treated with frozen plasma;

d) while the MSAC recognizes that for most patients, concentrates are the preferred therapy, all healthcare professionals should reinforce the following:

1. therapy should be accompanied by conservative measures such as immobilization and splinting to avoid large doses and prolonged treatment;

2. bleedings should be treated early to avoid severe hemorrhages that require high doses and prolonged treatment;
3. replacement therapy should not be used for arthritic pain;
4. moderate doses are sufficient for most bleeds treated at home.

e) DDAVP [desmopressin] should be used whenever possible for the treatment of Von Willebrand's disease;
f) all elective surgery should be postponed until more information is available about the modes of transmission of AIDS.

II — RECOMMENDATIONS TO THE CANADIAN RED CROSS BLOOD TRANSFUSION SERVICE:

a) serious efforts should be made to exclude blood donors who might transmit AIDS. . . .
b) in reference to I-a and b it is recommended that:

1. plans be made to deal with the possible increase in cryoprecipitate;
2. efforts be made to reinforce the most rational distribution of cryoprecipitate;
3. Factor VIII concentrate made with Canadian-source plasma be distributed proportionally throughout the country.

III — RECOMMENDATIONS TO THE CANADIAN BLOOD COMMITTEE:

Epidemiological evidence from the U.S. suggests that certain groups are at risk both to contract AIDS and transmit it as blood donors. The incidence of AIDS in Canada is three to four times less than in the U.S. In view of this information, it is recommended that urgent steps be taken to expedite the attainment of self-sufficiency in the production of Canadian volunteer donor plasma and fractionation products.

Implicit in the recommendations, even at that early date, was the belief that a good number of hemophiliacs had already been infected with AIDS. The "priority list" of those who should be treated with safer products said as much, by making no mention of those who used large quantities of concentrate. There was nothing comforting in these recommendations for severe hemophiliacs who infused several times a week. Still, implementing even some of the measures would likely have spared children like Serge and Stéphane Landry.

Only some of the recommendations, which were published a month later in the widely read *Canada Diseases Weekly Report*, were followed. The twins' physician, Dr. Rubin, urged their parents to reduce their dosage of concentrate. According to the parents, they weren't offered DDAVP, a safe synthetic product that had been on the market since 1977, nor was it suggested that the boys return to cryoprecipitate. Those recommendations, potential life-savers, were ignored by most treating physicians. Their reluctance was understandable; many had seen patients suffer horribly over the years, and concentrate turned their lives around miraculously. In that context, risking infection with an unknown agent — one that some researchers insisted was fatal only to homosexual men — seemed like an acceptable risk. Besides, the MSAC, the blood experts at the Red Cross, public health officials, federal regulators and the pharmaceutical companies themselves did nothing to reinforce the message of caution. On the contrary, they insisted that bleeds were a greater risk than AIDS.

William Mindell, the Toronto public health official who was proposing that concentrate be made with plasma donated by women, met with members of the Ad Hoc AIDS Group on May 26, 1983, to express his worry about possible contamination of the blood supply. Dr. Derrick, the Red Cross official responsible for AIDS issues, told Mindell that the risk hemophiliacs had of contracting AIDS was one in a thousand — a calculation presumably based on the two confirmed cases among Canada's 2,000 hemophiliacs, and one that ignored the CDC warnings about a lengthy incubation period. Dr. Derrick also balked at the MSAC recommendation that Factor VIII use be curtailed, insisting that factor concentrate, made with the plasma of up to 20,000 donors, were safer than cryoprecipitate, made with the plasma of ten donors, because the AIDS agent would be subject to a "dilution factor" of one in twenty thousand instead of one in five. The theory was ludicrous; scientists had long known that a single unit of blood infected with hepatitis B could contaminate the whole lot of concentrate, and they knew that the AIDS agent resembled the hepatitis B virus. In a memo that same month, Dr. Derrick revealed another concern of the Red Cross: "immense revenues may be lost by the fractionators if the trend to cryo continues."

Also in May, responding to the same scientific research available to the experts in Canada, France banned the importation of U.S. blood products because of the danger of AIDS contamination. Other countries like Belgium and Norway had policies of self-sufficiency that prevented imports, while The Netherlands made it mandatory that all concentrate be heat-treated to kill viruses like hepatitis. (After the AIDS virus was discovered, scientists determined that the hunch had been a good one: heat treatment killed HIV too.[2])

There were no such safety initiatives in Canada, whose proximity to the U.S. and reliance on U.S. factor concentrate left its hemophiliacs much more at risk than those in Europe. Health ministers were busy pursuing their foolhardy dream of a network of Canadian fractionation plants, throwing public health cautions to the wind in the process.

The Canadian Blood Committee working group on plasma fractionation recommended that the 50–25–25 distribution to Ontario, Quebec and Manitoba be maintained. But, in one of the ridiculously bureaucratic compromises that marked the whole fractionation saga, they suggested that plasma collected in excess of 160,000 litres annually should be allocated equally to each regional plant. The decision on costs was similar, with the CBC recommending that the host province pay 50 per cent of plant construction costs but that prices could be adjusted so the provinces would pay only 25 per cent of developmental costs of the new products. While the bureaucrats were splitting hairs to try to make their political bosses happy, little was actually happening that would make Canada self-sufficient in factor concentrate. Despite Quebec's insistence on blood products made in the province, the Armand Frappier fractionation plant remained little more than a concept. Connaught, for its part, decided that it would manufacture the sophisticated blood products of the 1980s with its 1950s technology, modified with government grants. The Winnipeg Plasma Laboratory was the glimmer of hope: the ground-breaking was held in the fall of 1982, and by the winter of 1983 Canada's newest fractionation plant — with a capacity of 75,000 litres annually — was officially open. The fact that it was years away from producing usable concentrate was conveniently overlooked. Worse yet, even this, the newest of the three plants, was installing outdated technology. Manufacturers in the U.S. and Europe had already begun heat-treating their factor concentrate to kill the hepatitis virus, and they were doing research on genetically engineered concentrate. Canadian plants had no plans to manufacture either.

In retrospect, the politically driven decision to build Canadian fractionation plants and rush them into production — dismissing cryoprecipitate as an alternative — is probably the single biggest factor in the infection of hundreds of hemophiliacs with the AIDS virus.

*   *   *

There is little doubt that, in the early days of the AIDS crisis, U.S. plasma from paid donors was far more contaminated than Canadian plasma from volunteers. By the fall of 1983, withdrawals of potentially contaminated Factor VIII were becoming routine in the U.S., even though products were only recalled after a donor actually fell ill with AIDS. In one case, 3 per cent of the U.S. supply — 60,000 vials of Factor VIII — were recalled after a blood banker in Austin saw a story about the city's first AIDS case in the local newspaper and recognized the man as a regular plasma donor. In Canada, where half the Factor VIII was imported from the U.S., withdrawals were also a regular occurrence, but it's worth noting that all of them were voluntary (recalls in the U.S. were mandatory). That spring, though the Bureau of Biologics began testing lots of products, it never ordered a recall.[3] Nevertheless, Dr. Hanna Strawczynski, the MSAC chair, managed to put a positive spin on the troubling withdrawals in an "update on AIDS" mailed to hemophiliacs in September, saying reassuringly that a "recall action is a sign of careful monitoring of blood products and should not cause anxiety or changes in replacement therapy."

The research of Dr. Christos Tsoukas suggests that half of the Canadian hemophiliacs who contracted HIV from blood concentrate may have already been infected by the end of 1983. They were largely the severe hemophiliacs, those who infused on a weekly basis. The others, the mild and moderate hemophiliacs, could have been saved by preventive measures. Researchers and regulators needed only look south to see the horrors that were on the way. By the end of 1983, AIDS was the leading killer of hemophiliacs in the U.S., a fact that should have laid to rest the long-standing argument that bleeds were a greater danger than viral infection.

Instead of investing in plasmapheresis, a means of ensuring long-term safety and security of the raw material needed to manufacture concentrate — instead of switching to cryoprecipitate — the provinces threw away tax dollars on second-rate production facilities. Wastage at Connaught resulted in the loss of at least 50,000 litres of Canadian source plasma during the three-year contract with the Red Cross, the equivalent of pouring more than 200,000 blood donations down the drain. To make up the shortfall, Connaught bought plasma from the U.S., the first time it had been imported since the Second World War. Some of the sources, were, at best, dubious,[4] such as an Arkansas prison. The U.S. blood was often mixed with Canadian donor plasma, contaminating even the safe supplies. Furthermore, the concentrate produced by Connaught was often so therapeutically inefficient (the level of Factor VIII was so far below standard) that they had to be processed anew, cutting the yield of the plasma in half again. All this wastage made it virtually impossible for the Red Cross to meet the contractual obligations it had to provide plasma to Cutter Biologics. In 1983 alone, penalty clauses with Cutter cost the society almost $350,000.[5] The wastage also forced the Red Cross to increase its purchases of factor concentrate made with U.S. plasma — which were already budgeted at 50 per cent of the total concentrate supply — adding even more costs to the bottom line.

The tragic result: Canadian hemophiliacs were infusing U.S. blood concentrate at record levels at the very time that AIDS contamination was peaking in the U.S. blood supply. All told, Connaught's failures required the purchase of 5 million more units of U.S.-source plasma, according to the Red Cross.

Today, the provincial infection statistics tell their own chilling tale. Red Cross policy was to distribute blood products on a proportional basis through-out the country, but Ontario's Connaught-only rule threw a wrench into that system. Already, Nova Scotia had made its own demand: the province would purchase only factor concentrate made from 100 per cent Canadian source plasma. The decision — which dated back to 1978, when all the provinces had agreed to bulk purchases of concentrate to cut costs — was a purely financial one: concentrate made with volunteer Canadian blood was cheaper than that made with imported plasma or purchased on the open market. The result, however, was that the AIDS infection rate among Nova Scotia's hemophiliac community was a fraction of that in other provinces. Canadian source concentrate led to the infection of sixteen hemophiliacs in Nova Scotia; in neighbouring New Brunswick, with a slightly smaller population, fifty-four hemophiliacs, including Serge and Stéphane Landry, contracted AIDS from concentrate imported from the U.S. Moreover, four of the Nova Scotia victims had regularly used products from New Brunswick.

While the Red Cross continued to reassure donors rather than take action to protect recipients, there were doctors who felt they owed it to their patients to adopt a "better safe than sorry" philosophy. Dr. Man-Chiu Poon, a Calgary physician and assistant Red Cross medical director, realized the dangers of AIDS in the blood system and began treating many of his patients with cryoprecipitate or, if they were severe hemophiliacs, reducing their dosage; his colleague Dr. Tom Bowen, director of the Calgary BTS, was convinced by the logic of the measure and did the same. The result, years later, is a dramatically lower rate of infection in Calgary than in Edmonton: twenty-two infected hemophiliacs in Edmonton compared to only eight in Calgary, which has a larger population. Likewise, Dr. Mariette Lépine in Sherbrooke switched all her mild and moderate hemophiliacs to cryo and not a single one was infected with the AIDS virus. Yet just up the highway, at Montreal Children's Hospital, Dr. Strawczynski — chair of the very committee that had made the recommendations — continued using concentrate, most of it American-made, even for her patients with mild hemophilia.* Quebec doctors, the first to use concentrate on a large scale, were also

---

* Dr. Strawczynski later testified that she had a high proportion of severe hemophiliacs at her clinic and virtually no access to safer Canadian-source concentrate.

the most aggressive, treating their patients on a preventive basis, not just as treatment for bleeds. The price for this liberal use of concentrate was high: the Red Cross shipped disproportionate quantities of U.S. source concentrate, about 75 per cent, to Quebec. Sadly, Montreal Children's has the highest infection rate of any treatment centre in the country, and Quebec has the largest per-capita number of hemophiliacs with AIDS.

While the Red Cross initially supported the position of the MSAC that concentrate use should be reduced and that some hemophiliacs should be switched to cryoprecipitate, it soon reversed itself and insisted on doing business as usual. From 1980 to 1983, cryoprecipitate use fell by half. During the first six months of 1983, after the MSAC recommendations, cryoprecipitate use fell another 8 per cent, a trend that changed only after word got out that a hemophiliac had actually died of AIDS. Aside from officialdom's self-interested promotion of concentrate, another problem was the perception that cryoprecipitate was costly (in fact it was cheaper to produce, but required more time and effort by hospital staff). These misplaced concerns over money cost hemophiliacs their lives.

As a mild hemophiliac Chris Taylor rarely required treatment, and when he went to the Cowichan District Hospital in British Columbia in February 1984 for treatment of a pesky bleed on his hand it had been more than five years since he had infused factor concentrate. Despite guidelines published a year earlier that said Chris, as a "virgin hemophiliac", should receive cryoprecipitate, the hospital didn't provide it. (Cryoprecipitate required preparation, freezer space and personnel to administer.) Chris Taylor was returned to cryoprecipitate in early 1985, but it was too late. The 15-year-old boy contracted AIDS from his single use of concentrate. "We were treated as if we were nothing. The life of a child meant nothing," his mother, Darlene Taylor, says.[6]

* * *

With the announcement in April 1984 that Dr. Robert Gallo and his team at the National Institutes of Health had identified the AIDS virus, even U.S. blood bankers couldn't ignore the incontrovertible proof that the disease was blood-borne. The discovery also allowed scientists to determine exactly how many hemophiliacs had been exposed to the deadly virus. Almost three-quarters of U.S. hemophiliacs using Factor VIII concentrate were infected; among those who infused concentrate more than once a month, the infection rate was 90 per cent. Before long, research in Canada would reveal similar rates of infection.

The news was shocking, even to those who had predicted the worst. But still there was no sense of urgency. Concentrate continued to be distributed, with the federal regulator's seal of approval. Unlike the makers of Tylenol, manufacturers of blood products that had infected thousands of people with a deadly disease didn't bother to change a thing. In fact, months before, a Red Cross official specifically ordered Cutter not to include a warning about AIDS on the product insert.

In the summer of 1984 researchers confirmed the assumption that heat treatment could kill the AIDS virus, but the Canadian Red Cross continued to doubt the efficacy of the process. Besides, Connaught was incapable of producing heat-treated concentrate, and it was getting difficult to buy heat-treated products from the U.S.; most manufacturers there were switching to heat treatment to stay competitive, and large quantities of non-heat-treated concentrate were being destroyed as unsafe. Because of the lag between collection of plasma and delivery of vials of factor concentrate — about six months — supplies were tight. On October 11, 1984, CHS representatives met with Red Cross officials to express their concern about recent shortages of Factor VIII concentrate. The Red Cross had only a two-week inventory of the product, down from its normal two-month supply.

Strangely, the solution proposed was not to do the same as in the U.S. — dump the unsafe product and move immediately to heat-treated — or to step up the production of cryoprecipitate, but to increase collections of Canadian source plasma. The fervent belief that volunteer blood donations couldn't carry the disease, an increasingly naive excuse for inaction, once again prevailed.

On October 13, two days after the CHS-CRC meeting, the scientific advisory committee of the U.S. National Hemophilia Foundation recommended an immediate switch to heat-treated products. When the CHS reiterated its demand for the safer, heat-treated product, the Red Cross countered with three arguments: Canadian fractionators were not licensed (meaning they couldn't sell heat-treated products even if they were able to manufacture them); national self-sufficiency would be compromised by switching to heat-treated; all users would want heat-treated products even though evidence that they were safer was inconclusive.

The first two points were clearly monetary ones, and spurious at best. Any company with a licence from the U.S. Food and Drug Administration — and there were already seven — could get temporary licence approval in Canada virtually overnight. The reality was that the Red Cross had to buy from Connaught for political reasons, and that the archaic laboratories were barely able to produce non-heat-treated concentrate, let alone heat-treated. A change in policy would mean 100 per cent of Factor VIII concentrate would have to be imported, which would embarrass the Ontario government, the principal funder of the Red Cross blood program. In addition, the lower yields of heat-treated products (in the early days as much as 25 per cent was lost in the treatment process) would require more imports of U.S. plasma, further undermining the much-vaunted but non-existent state of self-sufficiency. The net result was that a move to heat-treated products would cost millions of dollars.

Finally, a bureaucrat in Ottawa inadvertently called the politicians' bluff. On November 13, 1984, Cutter Biologics was granted a licence to manufacture heat-treated concentrate in Canada. Three days later, David Pope, assistant director of the Bureau of Biologics, issued a directive to all manufacturers of Factor VIII and Factor IX (the next most common deficiency) requiring that they provide heat-treated products. In a telex to the Red Cross and the producers, Pope wrote that, because heat treatment of concentrate "has shown to inactivate some viral agents that may cause serious disease, further reliance on AHF products that have not been heat-treated cannot be justified." The federal regulator ruled that untreated coagulation products be replaced with heat-treated products as soon as possible, a process it predicted would take two to three months.

Just as it had fallen silent after expressing its initial concern about AIDS in blood concentrate in mid-1982, Health and Welfare again disappeared from the picture. Senior officials in the federal health department had known for four months that more than half of Canada's hemophiliacs were infected with AIDS before they recommended change. The Canadian Blood Committee itself had no emergency response mechanisms, so it took almost a month to call an emergency meeting — in response to a directive that had been a long time coming.

7

CONSENSUS FOR INACTION
HEAT-TREATED CONCENTRATE

> A great man does not think beforehand of his words that they may be
> sincere, nor his actions that they may be resolute — he simply speaks
> and does what is right.
>
> Mencius
> *The Works of Mencius*

James Kreppner, Toronto

*A hemophiliac who was infected with AIDS by contaminated factor concentrate,
James is angry at the buck-passing and denial that has surfaced since the public
inquiry into tainted blood started its hearings.*

"We should put a wash basin up here because all the agencies come up here and
essentially wash their hands of their own responsibility for what occurred."

(*March 21, 1994*)

Antonia Swann, Toronto

*The common-law spouse of James Kreppner, Antonia says the official response to the
tainted blood tragedy is so academic and bureaucratic that it is adding insult to
the injury already suffered by the victims and their families.*

"AIDS is ruining our lives. The blood system players can sit back and forget what
they didn't do to minimize risk but, when we walk out of here, we carry AIDS with
us every minute, every day and wait for its final, bleak culmination. This is not an
academic exercise for us. It is the day-to-day reality and horror of tainted blood.

I say this regarding James: What a waste of a kind, intelligent, articulate, gentle man. The risk could have been lowered. The risk should have been lowered."

(March 21, 1994)

NO SINGLE EVENT OFFERS BETTER INSIGHT into the root causes of Canada's tainted-blood tragedy than the December 10, 1984, Consensus Conference on Heat-Treated Factor VIII — a meeting that brought together every major player in the Canadian blood system, and some of the country's top AIDS experts, after the Bureau of Biologics sent out its telex. Gathered at Ottawa's Congress Centre, just blocks from Parliament Hill, were representatives of the users, the manufacturers and the regulators of blood products. They were faced with a serious problem, the fact that blood concentrate — more specifically, Factor VIII — used in large quantities by hemophiliacs were contaminated with the AIDS virus. But they had an easy solution, because recently published scientific studies demonstrated beyond the shadow of a doubt that the AIDS virus could be killed by a simple process of heat treatment. The manufacturers also had a clear mandate from the users, represented by the Canadian Hemophilia Society, and the regulator, the Bureau of Biologics of Health and Welfare, to make the switch to safer products as soon as possible. While there was a sense of concern as the thirty-eight delegates strolled from the table of coffee and Danishes into the main meeting room, there was no sense of urgency.

Ambrose Hearn, Newfoundland's deputy minister of health and the chairman of the CBC, called the conference to order. Significantly, his first and last act was to turn the chair over to Dr. Perrault, director of the BTS. From that point on, not a single representative of the provinces contributed to the meeting. Members of the Canadian Blood Committee sat silently as the conference proceeded. The CBC, a glorified budget review committee, wasn't prone to taking the initiative, and on the key question of safety its record was even more lamentable than that of the Bureau of Biologics.

Dr. Perrault opened the conference by summing up the events leading to the meeting. On October 30 the scientific advisory subcommittee of the CBC had met to discuss the concerns of the Canadian Hemophilia Society regarding the availability and quality of Factor VIII concentrate. On the one hand, hemophiliacs were being denied the large quantities of Factor VIII they required for prophylactic treatment and surgery because concentrate was considered unsafe. But on the other hand, nothing was being done to minimize the contamination.

Ken Poyser, past president of the CHS, pointed out to the subcommittee that four U.S. fractionators were already heat-treating concentrates to kill viruses, while in Europe heat-treated products had been available since 1980. Behringwerke AG, a German manufacturer, had developed and marketed the first pasteurized Factor VIII; other manufacturers had the technology; but making more profitable products, not safer ones, was the priority.[1] Australia and West Germany had ordered a switch to heat-treated products in previous months, while in The Netherlands it had been policy since early 1983.

Dr. Wark Boucher, head of the blood products division of the Bureau of Biologics, responded that due to the "inconclusiveness of evidence that heat treatment was effective" and to the "significant loss of Factor VIII activity" (the ability of the enzyme to do its job — in the case of Factor VIII, clotting blood), the Canadian regulator had not recommended a switch. Neither of these arguments was valid. In September *The Lancet*, a respected and widely read British medical journal, had reported that heat treatment could kill a mouse retrovirus used to contaminate blood. While that research was being conducted the AIDS virus had been discovered, and scientists at the U.S. Centers for Disease Control, replicating the research using the HIV, had found heat treatment was highly effective for killing it as well. Moreover, the heat treatment method employed by CDC scientists was the one used by Cutter Laboratories, the major supplier of blood concentrate to the Canadian Red Cross. In October 1984 Dr. Man-Chiu Poon, an assistant medical director of the Red Cross and a member of MSAC, had even travelled to Washington to witness heat treatment tests at the CDC laboratories, and had urged his superiors to make the switch immediately. (At the time, the Red Cross was still purchasing non-heat-treated concentrate.) As for the loss of Factor VIII's ability to aid clotting, it was reduced only marginally by heat treatment — less than 10 per cent. What was lost in the heating process was not efficacy but yield, the quantity of the Factor VIII that could be derived from plasma and used to manufacture concentrate. And Dr. Gail Rock of the Red Cross in Ottawa had already suggested two methods to dramatically improve yield: priming collection bags with heparin instead of dextrose, and giving plasmapheresis donors DDAVP to increase the Factor VIII in their blood.

All that came out of the advisory subcommittee meeting was a recommendation for yet another meeting "at the earliest opportunity". Six weeks later, in the same Ottawa meeting room, Dr. Perrault reminded the delegates that they were fulfilling that obligation. One important fact he didn't repeat was an observation he had made to the subcommittee: the Red Cross inventory of Factor VIII was equivalent to a two-month supply, and there was enough plasma "already in the pipeline" to produce about eight million units of Factor

VIII, about three more months' worth of products. Those inventory and turnover figures would help explain the delays later on.

After his introduction to the consensus conference participants, Dr. Perrault turned the floor over to Dr. Norbert Gilmore, a doctor at Montreal's Royal Victoria Hospital and chairman of the National Advisory Committee on AIDS, a blue-ribbon panel that reported directly to the Minister of Health. Dr. Gilmore summarized the AIDS situation in Canada and compared it favourably to other countries. According to the quarterly "Update on AIDS", published by the federal Laboratory Centre for Disease Control, there had been 177 adult cases of AIDS in Canada to date, and 93 of those had died. The means of infection, Dr. Gilmore told the delegates, were varied: homosexual or bisexual practice, 127 cases; intravenous drug use, one case; clotting factors for hemophiliacs, 2 cases; in 15 other cases, the means of transmission was unknown.

In Western Europe the number of AIDS cases had tripled to 762 cases in fourteen nations in 1984. While not all countries kept detailed statistics, West Germany reported that two-thirds of its hemophiliacs carried antibodies to the virus, which had prompted the government to order a switch to heat-treated concentrate. Around the time of the consensus conference, a wave of panic was spreading across Britain, after authorities reported that at least 55 surgery patients had been treated with a batch of coagulation products that was later found to be contaminated. In December 1984 the U.S. CDC reported that 7,699 Americans were dead or dying of the disease, among them 49 hemophiliacs and 90 transfusion patients.

After Dr. Gilmore wrapped up his brief presentation, Dr. John Furesz of the Bureau of Biologics explained the rationale behind its decision that use of non-heat-treated concentrate "cannot be justified". He said the bureau had issued its November 16 telex because of "increasing scientific evidence that a human retrovirus, HTLV-III [now HIV], is the agent or one of the agents implicated as the cause of AIDS." That was typical of the federal government's understatement; U.S. researchers had announced the discovery of the AIDS virus a full seven months earlier, and the French had done the same in May 1983.

Dr. Furesz went on to say that U.S. research showed the virus was almost certainly transmitted by blood and blood products. He cited a study in *Mortality and Morbidity* of October 26, 1984 stating that 74 per cent of Factor VIII users and 39 per cent of Factor IX users in the U.S. were infected. In Canada, he noted, there was a "significant number" of infections. But he didn't mention an important revelation in his notes. They read: "Preliminary data from Canadian studies indicate that 55 per cent of hemophilia patients who have received Factor VIII have antibodies to the virus." Senior officials at Health and Welfare and the Red Cross had been aware of that troubling information since July 1984, when Dr. Michael O'Shaughnessy, director of laboratory research at the Federal Centre for AIDS, had presented the findings to his superiors. Around that time, Red Cross and government health officials had stopped arguing that there was no proof that AIDS could be transmitted by blood. Instead, they had started behaving as though there was no use acting now because most hemophiliacs were already infected.

Health and Welfare had considered Dr. O'Shaughnessy's research[2] significant enough to send its scientists to present the results at the International Symposium on Medical Virology in San Francisco and at a meeting of the Canadian Association of Clinical Microbiology and Infectious Diseases in Vancouver in previous months. Dr. O'Shaughnessy had even presented his findings to the NACAIDS meeting on October 9, 1984; by coincidence, it was the same week the Centers for Disease Control said that heat treatment of factor concentrate was no longer just a wise precaution but an "absolute necessity". Inexplicably, Dr. Furesz did not share the news of the 55 per cent infection rate with the consensus conference.

He did set the record straight on a couple of other issues. He contradicted what Dr. Boucher had told the CBC scientific advisory subcommittee just a month earlier: heat treatment did kill the AIDS virus, with very little loss of Factor VIII potency. He said submissions for licensing of heat-treated products would be given high priority, so that products manufactured in Canada could be on the market within two months. In addition, he promised that approval of lots of heat-treated Factor VIII from the U.S. would be expedited, so they could be available within a couple of weeks.

The problem with rushing heat-treated products to market was that it would cause certain difficulties for the Red Cross, and no small amount of embarrassment for the provinces and their fractionation plants. For the next hour, senior Red Cross officials outlined those problems. First, Dr. Ray Matthews, an advisor to the Blood Transfusion Service, explained the background. The Red Cross not only collected the raw plasma that was sent for fractionation, it was also responsible for buying factor concentrate on the open market, and for distribution of the products to hemophiliacs. Dr. Matthews too kept some of his views to himself; just weeks earlier, at a meeting of the consultative committee of the Red Cross BTS, he had expressed concern that the agency wasn't respecting the Food and Drug Act and that that could result in some "legal and financial risks". The consensus conference was deemed a good venue for sharing those risks.

Dr. Martin Davey, assistant national director of the BTS, explained the financial and logistical impact of switching to heat-treated concentrate. Heat-treating would require a 10 per cent increase in plasma collection, due to loss of yield. As well, because there were already insufficient quantities of plasma, more concentrate would have to be purchased from the U.S., imposing additional costs. Heat-treated Factor VIII cost about two cents more per unit — the Red Cross was paying 8.7 cents a unit for non-heat-treated products — which added up because annual use of Factor VIII exceeded 43 million units. Heat treatment of Factor IX, he noted in passing, resulted in no loss of yield and no cost increase, but that was the last mention of Factor IX, a concentrate used by almost 400 hemophiliacs. Dr. Davey didn't mention to those gathered at the consensus conference that, ten days after the bureau telex calling for a switch to heat-treated products, he had sent a letter to the president of Connaught Laboratories saying the Red Cross would continue to accept non-heat-treated products until March 31, 1985.

Dr. Derek Naylor, director of Blood Products Services at the Red Cross, was essentially the shopkeeper for the nation's supply of blood products. As the next delegate to address the meeting, he explained the modifications required to existing programs in order to make the switch to heat-treated products, chief among them that Red Cross contracts for the purchase of Factor VIII with Connaught in Canada and Cutter in the U.S. would have to be renegotiated. Because it was time to finalize contracts for 1985, a decision needed to be made immediately, he added. What Dr. Naylor didn't tell the consensus conference was that, just five days earlier, he had received from Travenol, a U.S. manufacturer, preliminary results of research it was conducting on heat-treated concentrate; not a single hemophiliac who had been treated exclusively with heat-treated concentrate was infected, while 75 per cent of those who had used non-heat-treated products tested positive for AIDS antibodies.* The lead time for manufacturing, Dr. Naylor told the conference, was about five months, meaning that heat-treated products made with Canadian donor plasma could be available by May 1, though an eight-week "transition period" would be required. Deciding which patients would get heat-treated products in the interim would be difficult, he said, but they would likely go to children and newly diagnosed hemophiliacs. There was a significant assumption in his statement that, in retrospect, seems particularly egregious: as prior users were likely already infected, it was acceptable to continue supplying them with non-heat-treated products rather than discarding these products. Contaminated blood, apparently, was preferable to no blood

* The full results of the research, conducted by Dr. Luc Montagnier, were essentially the same numbers, and were published in *The Lancet* in February 1985.

at all. The July 1 target for transition was easily arrived at: two months' inventory plus five months' lead time meant that if distribution of the heat-treated product was kept to a minimum, by Canada Day all the non-heat-treated concentrate would be gone.

Dr. Naylor was not challenged. A decision was made to use up stocks of blood products, and it was tacitly endorsed by the conference.

* * *

In the days before and after the December 1984 consensus conference, a jury sat in a Toronto office tower listening to testimony about a different kind of problem with a blood product. The Ontario coroner's inquest was investigating the death of Evelyn Lee, a 73-year-old leukemia patient who had died after receiving a transfusion of platelets at Toronto General Hospital on October 6, 1983. The very day the Thornhill woman died, Dr. Andrew Kaegi, assistant medical director of the Red Cross BTS centre in Toronto, withdrew all the blood products that had been packaged in a kind of bag known as the PL1240, made by Baxter Travenol Laboratories Inc., as a precautionary measure. There had been about ten other, milder reactions, ranging from nosebleeds to fever, reported in patients who had received platelets from the PL1240 bag, and it was discovered later that another leukemia patient had died five days earlier. "I felt at the time that I had discontinued the use of the bag on some pretty thin evidence," Dr. Kaegi testified at the inquest. But, he added, it was better to withdraw the product and conduct studies than risk giving a dangerous product to patients. The Red Cross distributed about 300 bags of platelets daily in the Toronto area, and the blood product was used mainly by cancer and heart-surgery patients. (Hemophiliacs in the Toronto area, by comparison, were using about 50,000 units daily of factor concentrate.)

Immediately after Lee's death, the disease and epidemiology division of the Ontario Ministry of Health launched an investigation into the bag's safety and asked that its use be discontinued after discovering traces of a noxious chemical that seemed to have been created in the manufacturing process. (Patients receiving platelets are usually suffering from immune suppression, and are particularly susceptible to poisoning.) Baxter withdrew the product world-wide, recalling and destroying more than 600,000 PL1240 bags. The coroner's jury, disturbed by the fact that medical devices weren't subject to the same scrutiny as prescription drugs, had some harsh words for Health and Welfare Canada. "The federal government should take a leadership role in ensuring the safety of medical devices by amending the present laws to require testing for the safety of a device before it is sold," the jury said in its recommendations. Dr. Kaegi said he welcomed the suggestion. "If stronger regulations aren't enacted, I think we will have a repetition of this kind of tragedy," he said.

The tragic irony for hemophiliacs is that, had the blood concentrate they injected at a rate of 3.5 million units a month been packaged unsafely, they probably would have been recalled. Yet public health officials knew that the powder in the vials of Factor VIII and Factor IX was likely infected with the AIDS virus, and the company wasn't forced to make a precautionary withdrawal; provincial epidemiologists conducted no studies, and Health and Welfare regulators even gave the potentially tainted concentrate their stamp of approval; they did nothing but monitor them. The AIDS virus killed slowly, not quickly like the chemical in the PL1240 bag. But it did kill. The PL1240 bag was implicated in two deaths, and ten cases of illness; prior to the consensus conference, two hemophiliacs had died of AIDS and hundreds more were known to have been infected. A coroner's jury had also investigated the March 1983 AIDS death of Artibano Milito in the months prior to the consensus conference, but, while they had harsh words for the regulators, no changes had been made.

Why was action so swift after the leukemia patient died, and so sluggish after the hemophiliac died? It was the politics of disease. The stigma and homophobia that were pervasive in the reaction to AIDS ensured that victims would keep a low profile; on the other hand, leukemia and cancer patients would never stand for their rights being violated, and the public would be outraged if they were. Above all, the motivation was money. Ending the poisoning of leukemia patients was cheap. Ending the poisoning of hemophiliacs would cost a couple of million dollars. While the rhetoric of the conference focused on a smooth transition to heat-treated concentrate, it came down to a cost-benefit analysis: how much should be spent on the protection of people who, in large part, were already infected?

The hard numbers had been presented to the consensus conference by yet another Red Cross official. Craig Anhorn, manager of Blood Products Services, told the assembled delegates that the switch to heat-treated products would cost the provinces $1.1 million annually, about 20 per cent more. His calculations, prepared specifically for the meeting that was supposed to determine the details of the phase-in, were based on a single option: switching to the heat-treated products no earlier than May 1985 and, afterwards, purchasing all heat-treated concentrate from Cutter Biologics. Anhorn didn't calculate the cost of destroying the inventory and replacing it with heat-treated products, but the calculation is easy to make with the figures he provides. Spot purchases of heat-treated

Factor VIII (buying off the shelf from a manufacturer instead of at a contracted price) cost 18.6 cents per unit, about 10 cents a unit more than non-heat-treated. Given that a one-month supply of Factor VIII for all of Canada was about 3.5 million units, five months of spot purchases would have added $1.75 million to the bottom line. The two-month inventory of non-heat-treated concentrate the Red Cross kept on hand was worth another $550,000, so responding to the emergency and destroying the AIDS-contaminated products would have cost, at most, $2.3 million. Proceeding at a leisurely pace and using up the inventory before switching to safer products cost only $770,000. To save $1.5 million — the cost of treating a dozen AIDS patients — some 2,000 Canadian hemophiliacs were exposed to blood products that were increasingly contaminated with AIDS for another six months.*

William Rudd, then president of the Canadian Hemophilia Society, was an accountant from New Westminster, British Columbia. He could have done the calculations on the scratch pad in front of him. As a boy, Rudd had been the first hemophiliac in Canada to be treated with Connaught factor concentrate. Without the miracle product he wouldn't have been able to attend university, marry, hold a good job and be a father to two beautiful girls. For months Rudd, who was all too aware of the potential impact of AIDS-contaminated concentrate, had lobbied to get heat-treated products, yet he was not prepared to accept either personally or on behalf of his members the loss of freedom that would come with a return to cryoprecipitate. At a meeting with senior Red Cross officials on October 19, 1984, he had bluntly stated that hemophiliacs didn't care about national self-sufficiency; they wanted the safest products available, regardless of where they were manufactured. But he was always told that the alternative to the potentially contaminated products was no concentrate at all, and he knew the suffering that would cause. Just a couple of months earlier, Rudd had attended the coroner's inquest into Milito's death — an inquest that recommended immediate measures to minimize the risk of AIDS contamination of Factor VIII concentrate. Rudd didn't speak at the consensus conference. We will never know why. What we do know is that, like most Canadians, he trusted the system. No one told Rudd that 55 per cent of hemophiliacs were already infected. As it turned out, he was one of them.

The only consumer representative who spoke at the conference was Ken Poyser, past president of the CHS and a member of the CBC advisory subcommittee. Like Rudd, he was accorded observer status and wasn't on the formal list of speakers, but after the cold-hearted financial analysis he felt

---

* At least six babies at Toronto's Hospital for Sick Children were infected during the "transition" period.

compelled to speak out. As an accountant from Edmonton, Poyser could do the number-crunching, but he reminded the medical experts that the issue was not dollars and cents but safety. He had been pushing for almost two years for the introduction of heat-treated products to cut the risk of contracting hepatitis, and firmly believed that the process would kill AIDS too. Surely, Poyser asked the delegates, spending a couple of pennies more per unit of Factor VIII was worthwhile if it could prevent infections? His intervention wasn't even recorded in the minutes. Hemophiliacs had come to expect that kind of response; their opinions on treatment and safety were never actively sought, and when they expressed their concerns they tended to be dismissed as hysterical.

Another person who remained silent at the crucial meeting was Dr. Derrick. Back on August 4, 1982, he had been contacted by Dr. Furesz of the Bureau of Biologics to discuss what should be done about the possible transmissibility of AIDS via blood and blood products. Until late 1984 Dr. Derrick had believed that the proof that AIDS was transmissible by blood was inconclusive, and that, even if the pathogen was blood-borne, the Canadian voluntary system would minimize the risk of contamination. He was the leading proponent of the wait-and-see approach. In the month before the consensus conference, however, he changed his view. In a background paper prepared for presentation at the meeting, dated November 15, 1984, he wrote that there were "compelling reasons" to switch to heat-treated products, notably new research that showed the process killed both the AIDS virus and the as-yet-undiscovered virus that caused non-A-non-B hepatitis (hepatitis C), a potentially debilitating liver disease that is many times more common than AIDS. Dr. Derrick noted that failure to provide the safer product "would undoubtedly lead to strong protests from hemophilia treaters and patients country-wide and could also heighten the vulnerability of the Canadian Red Cross Blood Transfusion Service to legal action in the event that hemophilia patients developed AIDS subsequent to the time that it became apparent that additional, apparently well-based precautions against contracting it were feasible." By his calculation the transition would cost about $300,000, substantially less than Anhorn's estimate. Yet, at the same time, Dr. Derrick argued that the switch would make little difference because so many hemophiliacs were already infected. In a memo to Dr. Roger Perrault just a couple of weeks earlier, Dr. Derrick had presented this argument against switching to heat-treated products. "There can be no assurance. . . that use of heat-treated Factor VIII concentrate will lower the incidence of AIDS in this high-risk group," he wrote, since "all but virgin hemophiliacs [those who had never been treated with concentrate] have almost certainly been exposed to the putative AIDS agent." Dr. Derrick was not called upon by his superior to speak at the meeting, and in the hierarchical Red Cross that meant he was to remain silent.

The next person to take the floor after Anhorn was Dr. Robert Card, chairman of the Canadian Hemophilia Society's MSAC. He spoke of the great advances in hemophilia treatment over the years, and the concerns of hemophiliacs and their physicians about the contamination of coagulation products with the AIDS virus. Echoing the recommendation made by the scientific advisors of the U.S. National Hemophilia Foundation in October 1984, he said the switch to heat-treated products should be made even if the scientific proof wasn't incontrovertible, and that, for added safety, children, newly diagnosed hemophiliacs and those with mild clotting disorders who rarely needed treatment should be treated with cryoprecipitate, not concentrate. The MSAC had requested back in August 1983 that the Red Cross switch to heat-treated concentrate, which had been approved by the U.S. Food and Drug Administration with some fanfare in previous months. Edward Brandt, the assistant U.S. health secretary, had said that since heat treatment killed the hepatitis virus, researchers were confident it would prevent the spread of AIDS too. The MSAC request, however, was refused by the Red Cross; Dr. Naylor, director of Blood Products Services, said "use of this product in Canada would further compromise goals of national self-sufficiency." Dr. Card was certainly aware of the infection rate among hemophiliacs, but he accepted the view of the Red Cross that the heat-treated products couldn't be made available before May 1. He also endorsed the Red Cross suggestion that the MSAC draw up a priority list of who should receive the limited supplies of the safer product.

The final three speakers at the consensus conference stood to lose the most from a rapid transition to heat-treated products. They were the fractionators, the manufacturers of the concentrate, and none of them had the ability to produce heat-treated products. Gilles Cossette was vice-president of marketing at Connaught Laboratories Ltd.[3] and a member of the advisory committee to the CBC. He told of Connaught's long history of involvement in the blood program, and of its being the sole Canadian producer of fractionation products. (The Winnipeg and Montreal plants were not yet functional.) Cossette didn't mention that the company's manufacturing facilities were archaic, and that hemophiliacs complained about the poor quality of Connaught Factor VIII.*

---

* The lone hemophiliac employee of Connaught refused to use the company's product, opting for cryoprecipitate. He felt conditions that included frozen plasma bags being opened by carpet knives were not sanitary.

Cossette focused on the economic arguments, and on the bloody-minded obsession of the Canadian Blood Committee with attaining self-sufficiency. Without a long-term contractual commitment from the Red Cross and CBC, Connaught couldn't rationalize the retooling of its facilities, which would cost upwards of $10 million. In their internal briefing notes, officials at the Bureau of Biologics estimated that if Connaught purchased the heat treatment process from Cutter Biologics it could start production in three months, but that if it developed its own procedure it could take six to twelve months. Dr. Furesz had told the executive committee of the CBC earlier that heat treatment was the least of Connaught's worries; it had long failed to fulfill its contractual obligations on the quality and yield of Factor VIII.

Dr. Albert Friesen, executive director of the Rh Institute, was the next to speak. The non-profit Rh Institute, affiliated with the University of Winnipeg, produced the world-renowned blood product WinRho, a vaccine that corrects Rh-incompatibility between a pregnant woman and her fetus. The institute was now setting up the Winnipeg Plasma Laboratory, which was slated to begin production of factor concentrate in July 1985 but was experiencing all sorts of problems that had put it behind schedule. Because heat-treated products had not yet been approved, making the process mandatory would further delay the start-up date because new equipment would have to be purchased. Yet in background papers prepared for the meeting Dr. Friesen had argued that "the use of heat-treated Factor VIII should begin as soon as possible." Dr. Jacques Gélinas, a member of the CBC advisory committee and president of the Armand Frappier fractionation plant, joked that his was probably the only organization that wouldn't be affected by a switch to heat treatment. Its facilities were little more than blueprints, and construction wasn't set to begin before late 1985.

What happened next at the conference is a bit of a mystery. Dr. Perrault, the nine members of the CBC and the four members of the CBC secretariat absented themselves from the conference room. The remaining twenty-four delegates — including seven employees of Canadian fractionation companies, six senior Red Cross blood program administrators, three senior officials of Health and Welfare and a single hemophiliac — drafted a series of recommendations, under the guidance of Dr. Gilmore of NACAIDS. There are no minutes from those proceedings; those who were present only remember that much of what was said at the main meeting was repeated, and that there was very little disagreement when recommendations were proposed. The CHS representatives felt that, despite all the negative talk, they had won — that hemophiliacs would start getting heat-treated products in the very near future.

The full group reconvened and, after a brief discussion, the conference settled on the following recommendations:

That this Conference:

1. Endorses the introduction of heat-treated Factor VIII concentrates in Canada as soon as is feasible before May 1985, with a transition period not exceeding eight weeks thereafter when both heat and non-heat-treated will be transfused to Canadian hemophiliacs;
2. Asks the Canadian Bureau of Biologics to expedite licensing of further heat-treated Factor VIII in Canada, including approval of heat treatment procedures for material in process in Canada;
3. Recommends that all Factor VIII products currently in the plasma or cryoprecipitate stages should be heat-treated;
4. Recognizes that the CRC will continue to direct all FFP [fresh frozen plasma] to facilities currently licensed to produce heat-treated Factor VIII until Canadian fractionators are licensed to produce heat-treated concentrates, when the CRC will redirect plasma to licensed Canadian facilities;
5. Recommends that the CBC recognize costs of development of heat-treated Factor VIII concentrates as legitimate costs to be met through sales of fractions by the CRC to the provinces;
6. Recommends that the CBC continue surveillance of and promote and support further research by primary and secondary producers towards the development of safer Factor VIII concentrates;
7. Recognizes that it is most important that the CBC continue to support the development of self-sufficiency in fractionation products in Canada;
8. Recommends that the criteria for the use of heat-treated and non-heat-treated concentrate during the transition period be agreed upon by the hemophilia treaters who are members of the Medical Scientific Advisory Committee of the CHS, using existing national representation;
9. Recommends that the CBC encourage national efforts to continue surveillance, serological investigations and other research in an effort to understand the effects of retrovirus infections on hemophiliacs.

The next day, the executive committee of the CBC held an extraordinary meeting to approve the recommendations. Although all seven provincial representatives had attended the meeting the day before, they were not in on the drafting of the recommendations, and had some "uncertainties" about the timing of the transition as stated in the first recommendation. To clear up the confusion, they called not the person who had chaired the portion of the meeting that drafted the suggestions, but someone who had been absent from the discussions, Dr. Perrault of the Red Cross. The switch from non-heat-treated to heat-treated concentrate, he said, would start May 1, 1985, and would take eight weeks. The delay was necessary, he said, to "deal with the inventory", because neither the consensus conference nor the CBC had requested that it be written off.

The executive committee of the Canadian Blood Committee approved the decision. They decided at the same meeting that the matter should remain quiet "to avoid the creation of concerns in hemophiliacs' minds". It was an odd approach to public health: people were going to be infusing AIDS-contaminated blood concentrate, and the principal concern of the deputy ministers of health was that they not worry about it.

The senior bureaucrats did not keep the decisions secret from everyone, however; they reported to their political bosses. Briefing notes prepared for federal health minister Jake Epp included a summary of the deliberations of the consensus conference and a quick analysis of the impact on hemophiliacs. According to the bureaucrats, the decision to delay implementation could "create anxiety. . . regarding who will receive the heat-treated products." The impact on the blood program, Epp was told, would be an additional cost of $1.5 to $2 million, "although the present inventory of non-heat-treated products will not be destroyed." The switch to heat-treated products, the minister learned, would result in temporary diversion of plasma to U.S. fractionators until Canadian plants could produce the new product. Self-sufficiency "will be partially achieved by the end of 1985."

It was, in the end, consensus for inaction.

*   *   *

The same day that Jake Epp received his briefing notes about heat-treated Factor VIII, Heather Coulter-Bowen, a spokesperson for Consumer and Corporate Affairs, announced that a number of fake Cabbage Patch dolls were being banned from sale in Canada.

The dolls were excellent imitations of the popular toy but smelled of kerosene, and in a handful of cases were believed to have provoked rashes.

Consumers were urged to return the products immediately; the federal govern-ment wanted to ensure that little girls had a happy, safe Christmas.

The Lancet noted in a December 22, 1984, editorial, "It would be indefensi-ble to allow prescription and home use of material known to be at risk of HTLV-III [HIV] when safer preparations are available." But it was too late for Canada's hemophiliacs.

Two weeks after Christmas, Connaught Laboratories was informed that three donors whose plasma was included in lots purchased from Irwin Memorial Blood Bank had been diagnosed with AIDS. The 3,000 vials of Factor VIII concentrate manufactured with that plasma were set to expire in January 1985. Connaught informed the distributor, the Red Cross, which in turn contacted the regulator, the Bureau of Biologics. John Weber, director of Quality Control and Regulatory Affairs, wrote back to say, in essence, that all the contaminated products had likely been used up so "no further action has to be taken on these lots".

*　　*　　*

Although Connaught didn't have the facilities to produce heat-treated concen-trates, it was allowed to continue manufacturing non-heat-treated products with plasma "already in the pipeline". As a result of the consensus conference, however, the Red Cross nixed plans to continue that policy until the end of March. Beginning December 12, all of Canada's plasma was diverted to Cutter, which was contracted to produce 12 million units of heat-treated Factor VIII concentrate for delivery on April 15, 1985.* Within days, however, Cutter said that yields on heat-treated concentrate were lower than expected and that there might be additional delays in production. Nevertheless, on December 17 the Cutter order was increased to 30 million units, and another 10 million units were ordered from Armour, a pharmaceutical company (subject to licence approval); in total, it was a full year's supply.

Today the Red Cross contends that it was impossible to provide hemophiliacs with heat-treated concentrate any faster than it did. Yet at the CBC executive com-mittee meeting on November 22, 1984, Dr. Peter Glynn, the assistant deputy minister of Health and Welfare, had asked if Cutter was in a position to supply heat-treated products. He had been told yes, at any time. In fact, prior to the con-sensus conference seven pharmaceutical companies were already producing heat-treated products, at a rate of about 300 million units per company annually. The

---

* Connaught delivered non-heat-treated concentrate from Canadian-source plasma until March 8, 1985, and from U.S. source plasma until April 12, 1985.

entire U.S. blood system was switching to heat-treated concentrate, as were a number of other countries, yet there is no evidence that any company ever refused an order. They couldn't afford to in such a competitive and lucrative field. Besides, Canada's annual needs amounted to just over one per cent of total U.S. production. "The production capacity of manufacturers greatly exceeded demand; there were plenty of products available for export," said Jack Reasor of the Market Research Bureau in Laguna Beach, California, which has tracked the inventory of blood products for the past twenty years. Further proof that fractionators were eager to do business can be found in a December 21 letter[4] from Travenol to the Red Cross in which the company offered a five-year royalty-free licence to manufacture and sell heat-treated factor concentrate in Canada, in hopes that corporate generosity would result in some sales. The Red Cross refused that offer and, while there are no records of efforts to purchase safer Factor VIII immediately on the open market, Dr. Martin Davey wrote to the CBC that "conversations with various U.S. contacts had indicated there is no ready availability of heat-treated Factor VIII for spot purchases."

On April 19, 1985, the Medical and Scientific Advisory Committee of the Canadian Hemophilia Society formally drafted a "priority list" for distribution of heat-treated products, as promised by Dr. Card at the consensus conference. During the transition period, the physicians decided, heat-treated products would be distributed in the following order of priority:

1) Previously untreated or rarely treated patients who require concentrate therapy during the conversion period.
2) Previously treated patients known to be sero-negative for HTLV-III antibodies.
3) Young children who require concentrate during this period.
4) Those regularly treated with cryoprecipitates who require factor concentrate for isolated indications, including major surgery or travel.
5) The distribution across the country to be equitable.
6) The decision of priorities to be done by Hemophilia Clinic Directors in consultation with CRC BTS Centre Directors.

Just days later, on April 20, 1985, the board of directors of the Canadian Hemophilia Society unanimously endorsed what came to be known as "Schindler's List", an ironic reference to the German manufacturer who saved Jews from Nazi concentration camps. Many CHS members would later see this endorsement by a group that was the sole representative of users as the ultimate

betrayal.* The reality was that board members were convinced triage was necessary for a few months due to severe shortages. The situation was painted as
one in which a ship was sinking and there were only enough lifeboats for the
children. They decided to sacrifice themselves to save the next generation.
More than half of the twenty-four board members who made that fateful decision would themselves die of AIDS, and none of them would be unaffected by
the overwhelming number of deaths in the community.

Had the Bureau of Biologics done its job and ordered the unsafe products
destroyed, had the consensus conference emphasized safety, had the Red Cross
resisted the temptation to use up existing stocks, heat-treated products would
have been distributed to everyone months earlier, and no priority list would
have been required.

The Cutter products were late and some of the Armour products failed to
pass Bureau of Biologics inspection, but shipments started trickling in: 1.63
million units from Armour on April 25, 2.5 million from Cutter on April 29.
By May 1 the Red Cross had 7.8 million units of heat-treated products in
inventory, but during that month it delivered only 343,795 of those units to
hemophilia treatment centres. Despite a healthy inventory and assurances that
two large orders would arrive early in June, the priority lists were rigidly obeyed
and the stock was held back so the unheated products could be used.

On May 30, as he had done in March, Dr. Naylor wrote to BTS medical directors to remind them to distribute untreated products. While a two-week supply of
heat-treated products would be sent out on June 10, he noted, "routine requests"
should be filled with untreated products until July 1. True to its word, the Red
Cross continued to stockpile, accumulating 15 million units of heat-treated concentrate, a four-month supply. Only a fraction of the Factor VIII shipped out during
the "transition period", one million units, was heat-treated.[5]

As if that weren't enough, in several instances untreated products that
were returned by one hemophiliac were redistributed to another to ensure
that they were used. Products considered unsafe in Regina were returned to
the Red Cross warehouse in Ottawa and were immediately sent out to
Montreal. On June 29, 1985, just seventy-two hours before the end of the
transition period, Serge and Stéphane Landry, then age eight, were given
non-heat-treated products that had been returned to a Moncton hospital the

---

* Some of the treatment centres and hospitals that provided factor concentrate had priority
lists that actually listed the names of people eligible for the safer products. These lucky few,
about 3 per cent of the hemophilia population, were nicknamed PUPs, for previously
untreated patients.

day before, even though the hospital had ample stock to provide them with heat-treated products.

That the Red Cross expected all non-heat-treated concentrate to be used up was also explicitly confirmed in a September 27 memo from Craig Anhorn, the manager of Blood Products Services. The Red Cross head office was bickering with its regional Blood Transfusion Service centres and with hemophilia clinics about credits for products returned to be destroyed. Anhorn wrote that no credit should be given for non-heat-treated products received before June 1 because "all BTS centres and hemophilia treatment centre directors were notified with sufficient time to ensure that no stockpiles of product were in place at the time of transition." In other words, centres and hospitals that didn't use up the non-heat-treated products suffered a financial penalty.

More than 11 million units of untreated Factor VIII were distributed to hemophiliacs after the Bureau of Biologics ordered a switch to heat-treated products. In the end, after an excessively long phase-in period, 1.8 million units[6], worth less than $250,000, were destroyed — not even less than a two-week supply. Fully one-third of the non-heat-treated units remaining in hemophilia treatment centres and hospitals had been shipped to them during the phase-in period, further proof of efforts to exhaust inventory. And the recall process was so slipshod that non-heat-treated products remained in patients' fridges for many more months.

"It angers me that people actually let this happen," Normand Landry, the father of Serge and Stéphane, told the Commission of Inquiry on the Blood System in Canada when it visited New Brunswick in July 1994. "The more I look at the facts, the more I realize it was basically all about money — money, not medicine. They had us give a product to our children that they knew was contaminated by telling us there was not enough heat-treated product to go around. 'Your kids are already infected, so give them the contaminated product,' is what they were really saying. To me, it is inconceivable that they did this."

Equally inconceivable is that many hemophiliacs were tested for AIDS without their knowledge, and a good number weren't told of the diagnosis. Much more effort was put into documenting the ravages of the disease than in to preventing its spread. In January 1987, Normand and Anne-Marie Landry attended a hemophilia conference in Montreal. There, for the first time, they heard news of an ongoing study of hemophiliacs. The research of Dr. Christos Tsoukas showed that 90 per cent of severe hemophiliacs were infected with AIDS, while 85 per cent of hemophiliacs who had received only heat-treated products were free of infection; overall, the rate of infection was close to 50 per cent. The parents knew immediately that the twins were in danger. When they returned to

Moncton, they learned that Serge and Stéphane had been tested for AIDS in June 1985, and two more times since. All the results had been positive.

Normand and Anne-Marie Landry were as angry as they were frightened. They felt betrayed not only because they hadn't been informed that the products they injected into their sons' arms were contaminated, but by the secrecy surrounding the diagnosis. Still, there were virtually no treatment options at the time, so they kept the news from the boys for another year. After all, you needed to look no further than the daily newspaper to see the plague of hatred and discrimination that followed on the heels of the AIDS epidemic. In the most highly publicized case, in Arcadia, Florida, the Ray brothers — Ricky, ten, Robert, nine, and Randy, eight — had been physically driven out of church and barred from school, and their family home had been fire-bombed, all because they were hemophiliacs with AIDS. The same thing had happened, on a lesser scale, to young hemophiliacs and their families in Montreal, Winnipeg and Vancouver.

One day in June 1987, Normand and Anne-Marie Landry sat down at the kitchen table with the twins and told them they were infected with the AIDS virus. They had information pamphlets and reassuring hugs, but they couldn't answer the question that sprang from childhood curiosity: why? "It was the hardest thing we ever had to do in our lives," said Mrs. Landry. "Imagine having to tell your children that they're going to die." Serge and Stéphane were not yet eleven years old — the same age as the AIDS epidemic.

*   *   *

In June 1985 Connaught Laboratories decided that it would build a new fractionation plant, but it faced two major roadblocks — an inability to get liability insurance and a seeming lack of the government largesse it had depended on for decades. In the spring of 1987 Connaught gave the Canadian Blood Committee an ultimatum: the provinces must guarantee financing of the new plant, or it wouldn't be built. The CBC went one better; despite Connaught's abysmal record, the provinces guaranteed the Canadian fractionator that it would get all Canadian donor plasma once it was licensed to produce concentrate. The CBC had already, surreptitiously, paid for the private companies to switch to heat treatment, to stifle their objections that the move to the safer products was unwarranted. From May 1, 1985, to March 31, 1986, the Red Cross had provided Connaught with financial assistance of $124,000 a month to quiet the company's complaints that the switch to heat treatment was "premature", and had paid for implementation of heat treatment equipment as well as providing donor plasma for testing. But the insurance problem could not be resolved, so in June 1987 Connaught withdrew from the factor concentrate business. In total it had received $1.75 million for the manufacturing changes, the latest of indirect and direct subsidies it received for the failed experiment that was the fractionation plant — more than it would have cost to make the switch to heat-treated products back in December 1984. The Winnipeg Plasma Laboratory, which had operated since February 1986, shut down its fractionation facilities within weeks; it had managed to swallow up a whopping $28 million in government subsidies — $6 million from the Manitoba government and the rest from the Canadian Blood Agency — without ever producing saleable concentrate.[7] The Centre de fractionnement sanguin Armand-Frappier had never produced any usable concentrate either, but it managed to gobble up another $10-million in government grants. The self-sufficiency project, a débâcle from beginning to end, was dead.

But the tainted-blood scandal wasn't over. In 1987 Canada experienced a second wave of transfusion AIDS, and new warnings about the dangers of hepatitis — aspects of the story that are rarely discussed, but that demonstrate just how little was learned from the errors made at the outset of the AIDS epidemic. While blood products were now being heat-treated to kill HIV, there were still unresolved problems. Some of the Factor VIII on the shelves of hospitals and in the fridges of Canadian hemophiliacs was manufactured with plasma that hadn't been tested for HIV. In a February 1987 memorandum, Stephen Vick, acting director of Blood Products Services for the Red Cross, wrote that "it has come to our attention that some hospitals are still holding stocks of unscreened, heat-treated Factor VIII concentrate and Factor IX complex," and he urged them to return them for safer products. At least one hemophiliac in Manitoba is known to have been infected with HIV after receiving heat-treated product made with untested plasma, which he injected between September 1986 and July 1987.

The problem was that, while these products had been heat-treated, the process used by Cutter and Armour, the two companies the Red Cross was buying from, was far from an unqualified success. An article in *The Lancet* in mid-1986 warned that the dry-heat process didn't guarantee viral inactivation; the wet-heat process, or vapour treatment, had a much better success rate at killing HIV. Both The Netherlands and the U.K. banned the import of Armour products in October 1986 after some hemophiliacs contracted the AIDS virus from the product. That same month, the Canadian Hemophilia Society demanded the withdrawal of all Armour products and an immediate switch to wet-heat-treated concentrate. Both the Red Cross and the Bureau of Biologics rejected the demand, still insisting that the volunteer blood donor system would guarantee safety.

Hoechst AG was the only company licensed in Canada to produce wet-heat-treated concentrate, but the Red Cross didn't buy from it. In late 1986 and early 1987 there were hundreds of lots of Factor VIII concentrate recalled[8] after hemophiliacs contracted AIDS from the heat-treated product, while other lots failed to pass Bureau of Biologics inspection. (Federal inspectors didn't test every unit, but samples were taken from each lot for testing.)

In early November 1987, it was revealed that seven hemophiliacs — six in British Columbia and one in Alberta — all of whom had been free of infection in January of that year, had contracted AIDS from dry-heat-treated concentrate. In response to the infections, the Bureau of Biologics asked the manufacturers, Armour and Cutter, to withdraw sixty-seven lots of their products, about 15 per cent of the national supply. The move sparked panic because almost 1,500 hemophiliacs were using the product. In the preceding months, most of the users had become acutely aware of the devastation caused by tainted blood prior to the introduction of heat treatment, despite the official statistics that listed only twenty-three AIDS deaths among hemophiliacs. On December 9, 1987 — the same day the U.S. Food and Drug Administration ordered a switch to wet-heat treatment — the Bureau of Biologics issued this opinion: "The process of wet-heat treatment appears to be superior to dry-heat treatment in the inactivation of the HIV virus." Once again, there was no order from the federal regulator to get the unsafe products off the market.

It would be February 1988 before the next meeting of the Canadian Blood Committee, where the switch to wet-heat treatment had to be approved. The safer product would cost $1.675 million more that year. In the interim, the source of infection of the seven hemophiliacs was narrowed down to three lots of Armour concentrate, so the other sixty-four lots were released to the Red Cross. While they were waiting for the safer products, the hemophilia treatment centres fell back on the trusty "priority list", and once again stocks were virtually depleted by the time the new product arrived.

Even before heat treatment of concentrate and testing of blood donations for AIDS were instituted, hemophiliacs had begun to worry about another blood-borne disease, non-A-non-B hepatitis, which causes fatal liver disease in about 15 per cent of cases. While the virus had yet to be identified, there was growing evidence of the public health risk, so on August 26, 1986, the American Association of Blood Banks adopted two surrogate tests to screen out potential carriers: anti-HBc, the hepatitis-B core test, and ALT, a test that measures the level of the liver enzyme aminotransferase. The Canadian Blood Committee was well aware of "market pressure to adopt this testing", but when its advisory subcommittee debated the issue at a meeting on June 19, 1986, Dr. Perrault warned that the initiative could cost a lot, at least $10-million annually — not because of the cost of testing alone, but due to the loss of thousands of units of blood that would be screened out. For the next four years the issue was debated regularly, but no decision was taken until the virus, renamed HCV or hepatitis C, was identified in late 1989 — at which time it was decided to wait until an antibodies test was available. In the short-term, the delays saved the blood program $30-million. The Canadian Hemophilia Society estimates that 12,000 Canadians were infected by HCV-tainted blood during that four years of foot-dragging, and that could translate into another 1,800 deaths by tainted blood.

Wait-and-see, lack of regulatory initiative, concerns about money rather than safety, another Schindler's List, more hollow reassurance. Despite the horror, the administrators of Canada's blood system had learned absolutely nothing from their mistakes.

8

ONE IN A MILLION
AIDS TESTING BEGINS

So the people said something would have to be done,
But their projects did not at all tally.
Some said, "Put a fence round the edge of the cliff."
Some: "An ambulance down in the valley."

Joseph Malines
"Prevention and Cure"

Sherry Lencucha, Edmonton

A relationship Sherry had with a hemophiliac in the fall of 1982 came back to haunt her a decade later. In the interim, she married another man and had two children. Sherry's first child, Megan, was born with AIDS but never properly diagnosed. Her son Kyle was born in 1991 and neither he nor his father is infected. Sherry, the founder of the Alberta Society for Positive Women, was one of the first Canadian women with AIDS to go public.

"My daughter Megan was born in August 1987 and died in March 1988. My daughter had recurring bacterial pneumonias, unexplained body rashes, failure to thrive. She did not grow the way normal babies do. When she died at seven months, she had never sat up, she had never cooed or babbled, she had never eaten from a spoon. At the end of her life, she was blind, she did not recognize me or my husband, except by touch. . . .

I went public because women deserve a voice. There are a lot of people out there *who are silent, who are living in fear, who are afraid of the stigmatization that comes with this disease."*

(April 22, 1994)

BLACKSPOT RESTAURANT WAS OFF THE BEATEN PATH, tucked away in Alberta cattle country, two miles off Highway 2, but Tony Zucchelli made the search worth the effort. The owner-chef was known far and wide for his succulent veal cutlets, but it was Zucchelli's friendliness that had customers repeating the forty-mile trip south from Calgary. He tried to slip out of the kitchen long enough to greet visitors as they came into the popular eating-spot, and on occasion, late at night, he would serenade the customers with his violin. When 18-year-old Kirk Stratychuk sat down at the counter of the Blackspot just after one p.m. on February 13, 1985, Tony strolled from the restaurant kitchen at the back to offer a cheery hello. The response from the teenager, who was depressed at being unable to find work, was to raise a .22 calibre rifle and say, "This is it, Tony. Goodbye." Then he pulled the trigger.

Tony Zucchelli lost a lot of blood in the shooting, more during the ambulance ride to Calgary and still more when doctors at Holy Cross Hospital removed the bullet in his abdomen, then opened him up again to cut out twenty-two inches of his damaged colon. He was transfused with five units of blood during the emergency surgery on Valentine's Day, and received another five units five weeks later, when surgeons performed a colostomy. (Ten units is the equivalent of 4.5 litres of whole blood; the average man has 5.5 litres of blood in his body.)[1] Though he had been close to death on the floor of the Blackspot, doctors were predicting that the burly Italian immigrant would be back on his feet in no time.

More than 300,000 Canadians a year undergo surgical procedures, and many of them receive blood both during surgery, to prevent shocks, and after, to speed up recovery. In Canada a unit of blood, in its myriad forms, is transfused every twenty seconds. What few patients realize is that any major surgery, requiring five units or more, can be likened to an organ transplant and, as such, carries risks. About one-third of surgery patients suffer from hemolytic reaction, a sort of allergy to the blood itself.* Others are infected by blood-borne

---

* Hemolytic reaction usually results in fever, chills, nausea and vomiting, but can be fatal. It was the main reason blood transfusions were risky before the discovery of blood groups. The reaction is not caused by allergy per se, but by the accumulation of cytokines, a chemical released by white cells. The longer the blood has been stored, the more serious the reaction tends to be.

viruses and bacteria, even when screening measures are in place. Massive blood replacement also depletes the immune system, making a patient more susceptible to disease. Still, since the Second World War, Canadian doctors had been taught to use blood liberally.

The surgeons skilfully removed the bullet fragments from Tony Zucchelli's abdomen, but they left behind a far more insidious killer. One of the units of blood he received was infected with HIV. A month after the operation, the restaurateur began suffering from the flu-like symptoms that are the first indicator of AIDS.

The catchphrase at the time was that the risk of contracting AIDS from a transfusion was one in a million.* In early 1985 doctors didn't even mention the risk to surgery patients; they seem to have had a far greater chance of dying from the anesthetic than from tainted blood. According to federal government statistics, there had been only one AIDS death attributed directly to blood — that of the baby girl who was transfused in Montreal in October 1982. (The same statistics told of only two AIDS deaths in the hemophilia community. But the figures that seemed so reassuring were in fact testimony to the lengthy incubation period of AIDS.)

In January 1984, however, *The New England Journal of Medicine* had published a paper about twenty-eight people with AIDS whose only risk factor was having received a blood transfusion. "The current number of cases of transfusion AIDS is small, representing about one per cent of reported cases in the United States," the researchers wrote. "These 28 cases were diagnosed during approximately 12 months, a period when over three million persons in the United States received transfusions. However, most of these patients received their transfusions between 1979 and 1982, a time when the prevalence of AIDS — and presumably of donors affected by the putative AIDS agent — was much lower than during 1982 and early 1983." In other words, they were the tip of the iceberg. Epidemiology 101 taught that, if an epidemic disease was left unchecked, the number of people infected increased exponentially. The risks of transfusion AIDS might at one point have been one in a million, but now they were growing rapidly. But the administrators of Canada's blood system, taking comfort in the apparently tiny infection rate, contented themselves with staying the course, blind to what lurked ahead, below the surface.

---

* The one-in-a-million risk, often cited over the years, seems to have come from a July 19, 1983, press conference where Dr. Roslyn Herst said, in response to a question, that the risk to transfusion recipients was one in a million. That figure was based on U.S. statistics that showed fourteen cases of transfusion AIDS over a three-year period during which there had been ten million transfusions.

The official announcement of the discovery of the AIDS virus, in April 1984, had made it possible to confirm what epidemiologists had predicted. In the U.S. the infection rates among high-risk groups were staggering: almost 90 per cent of intravenous drug users, three-quarters of hemophiliacs who regularly infused factor concentrate, and two-thirds of sexually active homosexual men. The CDC had generously provided the Laboratory Centre for Disease Control in Ottawa with 20,000 test kits, and its testing on high-risk groups was giving similar results. By September 1984, American blood banks had started large-scale clinical trials with the ELISA (enzyme-linked immunosorbent assay) test. Five of the world's largest pharmaceutical companies[2] were vying to produce the first commercial blood test for AIDS; the competition in the $100-million-a-year sweepstakes was furious, so tests were everywhere.

On October 5, 1984, members of the Canadian Red Cross working group on AIDS discussed the implementation of testing donations for AIDS. The society had been approached by several companies who wanted to conduct clinical trials in Canada. With its centralized buying, the Red Cross was a much bigger market than most U.S. blood banks but the humanitarian agency didn't jump at the chance to introduce a new safeguard. Instead, it concluded that the need for testing was unproven and worried that there were "very serious psycho-social implications to instituting such testing prematurely". What it was really worried about was the implications for its blood program; the sting of criticism from its ban on gay and Haitian donors a year and a half earlier was still fresh, and the same groups were concerned that testing would bring more discrimination. Two days later, the Red Cross reiterated its position at a meeting of the National Advisory Committee on AIDS. Despite the fact that, back in February 1983, the Medical and Scientific Advisory Committee of the Canadian Hemophilia Society had called for testing to be implemented as soon as it was available, and despite the fact that clinical tests had been under way for months in the U.S., NACAIDS had never examined the issue. So it appointed a subcommittee, the Task Force on AIDS-Associated Retrovirus Testing. At its first meeting, on November 2, 1984, the task force did little more than endorse "in principle" the idea of testing blood for AIDS.

By December 10, 1984, when the consensus conference gathered all the main players in the blood system to formulate a response to the problem of contaminated factor concentrate, it had been obvious for several years that Factor VIII and Factor IX concentrate were likely contaminated with the AIDS virus. Yet the experts limited themselves to discussing heat treatment of Factor VIII. They ignored the fact that two dozen other blood products were derived from volunteer blood donations and transfused into hundreds of thousands of Canadians, and they certainly didn't discuss tackling the problem at its root, with preventive action like testing.

The next day, December 11, at an extraordinary meeting of the executive committee of the Canadian Blood Committee executive director Dr. Denise Leclerc-Chevalier, who had said nothing at the consensus conference, told provincial representatives that they might "be requested to approve testing of blood for HTLV-III antibodies at a cost of $5 million, or $10 million if two tests are conducted."* Dr. Roger Perrault informed the executive committee that three conferences on testing were planned for early 1985, hosted by the U.S. National Institutes of Health and the Centers for Disease Control. While the Red Cross was skeptical about the need for testing — it still viewed volunteer donor blood as risk-free — officials would attend those information sessions, he said. The CBC executive left it at that.

At its next meeting, on January 15, 1985, the CBC resolved a matter that had been long outstanding: the relocation of Red Cross headquarters from Toronto to Ottawa. The charitable organization had decided to relocate in October 1982, around the time federal health officials first urged it to begin investigating the problem of transfusion AIDS. Building the new head office would cost $27 million and would take just over two years. The agency had lobbied hard for funding, most recently in a private meeting with health minister Jake Epp, and the federal government had agreed to pay $10 million, which the provinces jointly matched; the same health ministry bureaucrats who dithered and fretted about spending a couple of million dollars to make the blood supply free of AIDS had no trouble approving $20 million for a new building. AIDS was not even on the agenda at the CBC meeting that day; the 1985 budget for the blood program was approved without any provision for testing.

Meanwhile, after months of trials, the U.S. Food and Drug Administration (FDA) was gearing up to release the first commercial AIDS test on February 15 — the day after Tony Zucchelli received his fatal transfusion. Ten days earlier the Red Cross had received its first test kits, and it was conducting clinical trials at a rate of 375 tests daily. As it turned out, the first commercial test wasn't licensed in the U.S. until a couple of weeks later, on March 2, 1985; the financial stakes were so high that the FDA wanted to make sure the quality of the test was beyond reproach, and that it was available in large quantities. That the licence was granted on a Saturday morning indicates the sense of urgency that

---

* This was a reference to the initial ELISA test and the confirmatory Western Blot, and an indication that U.S. blood banks were already considering a sophisticated two-step testing procedure.

was prevalent in the U.S. Within hours of official approval, Abbott Laboratories — the company that had been selected — was delivering its test kits to more than 2,300 U.S. blood banks. The first recipient was the Irwin Memorial Blood Bank in San Francisco, which had the dubious distinction of dispensing more AIDS-tainted blood than any other blood bank in the world. But at least the Irwin management was willing to talk about the problem of transfusion AIDS — which infuriated other blood bankers, who still insisted that the risk of contracting AIDS was the mythical one in a million.

The day after the U.S. approved the commercial AIDS test, the AIDS Committee of Toronto urged Canada not to implement testing because it would foster hysteria and fear among those who tested positive. "These people are really clutching at straws . . . and people don't realize this test is not diagnostic. It's just not worth it in terms of the fear it will spread," said spokesman Phillip Shaw. Dr. Perrault still gave credence to that view. He questioned the accuracy of the ELISA test — despite the international reputation of the FDA — and stated that the Red Cross wouldn't implement testing if it was too expensive. "When you have more questions than answers, you have to be careful," Dr. Perrault said; in any case he saw no need to rush to test blood because there were "no confirmed cases" of transfusion AIDS in Canada.

On March 7, 1985, the NACAIDS task force finally got down to discussing the testing issue seriously. It recommended that country-wide testing be in place by April 30 and asked the Red Cross to submit, as quickly as possible, an analysis of the costs. The Red Cross drafted an implementation plan and estimated that Canada-wide screening would cost $2.6 million for the remaining six months of 1985, and $5.5 million for 1986. With the necessary funds, the Red Cross could begin work on May 1 and could be testing all blood donations in the seventeen regional BTS centres by August 1, twelve weeks later. As it turned out, there was not another NACAIDS meeting until May 15. By the end of March, 99 per cent of blood banks in the U.S. (all but three small facilities) were screening blood for AIDS antibodies; implementation had taken two to three weeks. In Canada, it took that long to get people to a meeting.

On April 1 the Bureau of Biologics approved the sale of the Abbott test kit in Canada, and two weeks later it gave its stamp of approval to a second kit. Hospitals and provincial laboratories were buying kits to test patients for the virus, but plans to test blood that would be transfused into surgery patients had still not been formalized.

In mid-April the Irwin Memorial Blood Bank published the results of its first month of testing. A dozen of the 5,300 units of its volunteer blood donations were infected with AIDS, even after rigorous screening. That meant the chances of receiving an AIDS-tainted blood transfusion in San Francisco were a staggering 1 in 440. The statistic was discarded as meaningless in Canada because of the city's large gay population. Yet the American Red Cross reported nation-wide results that were not much different: 1 in 500 volunteer donors tested positive for the AIDS virus. As the numbers trickled in, Canadian healthcare officials clung, rather pathetically, to the notion that the border provided some kind of miraculous shield from the pandemic — despite the fact that clinical trials of the Abbott test being conducted at the Red Cross showed an infection rate of 3.7 per 1,000 — even higher than the U.S. rate. On April 25 Dr. Robert Card, chairman of the Medical and Scientific Advisory Committee of the Canadian Hemophilia Society, wrote a letter to the Red Cross demanding immediate institution of AIDS testing. In his mind, testing blood was even more urgent than heat-treating concentrate, because it tackled the problem at the source. Instead the Red Cross continued clinical trade of various test kits, not even discarding the units of blood that tested positive.[3]

On May 9, 1985, five days after 70-year-old Vic Drew died at Vancouver's Royal Jubilee Hospital, the Red Cross admitted publicly for the first time that someone had died of AIDS contracted during a blood transfusion. "We have taken all the precautions that we could," Dr. Derrick said that day. "It certainly appears the inevitable has happened." Yet what had made Drew's death (and many more to come) inevitable was the flagrant lack of precautions. The risk of transfusion AIDS had been recognized three years earlier, after the Montreal baby died. Yet it had taken until April 1985 for the symptoms of AIDS to be mentioned in the "Important Message to Our Blood Donors" pamphlet, and not even the deaths had convinced Red Cross and public health officials to speed up testing. The day after the announcement of the transfusion AIDS case, the first National AIDS Conference was held at the Université du Québec à Montréal. Dr. Alistair Clayton, director-general of the Laboratory Centre for Disease Control, told delegates that AIDS was bloodborne but again downplayed the risk as negligible. Dr. Clayton, the country's top AIDS official, did not mention that AIDS tests were readily available to determine the cause of death of hospital patients, but not to test blood products for those whose lives could be saved.

Tony Zucchelli's case provides the perfect example of the failure of the blood system. A bullet to the stomach constitutes an emergency, and no expense is spared to save the victim; yet the knowledge that the transfusion may kill the recipient can be dismissed. Leaving Zucchelli to bleed to death on the floor of the restaurant was unthinkable; refusing to move rapidly to institute AIDS testing should have been equally unthinkable.

To be considered a public health emergency, however, an event had not only to be visible but pay political dividends. In the spring and summer of 1985, Dr. David Korn, Ontario's Chief Medical Officer of Health, was dispatched to deal with a PCB spill on the Trans-Canada Highway near Kenora, to a hydrogen spill from a tanker car in Smiths Falls and to a London nursing home where there was a flu outbreak. But — despite his experience with the World Health Organization containing a smallpox outbreak in Ethiopia, and his desire to tackle AIDS as a public health priority — Dr. Korn was told by senior provincial bureaucrats that the disease was not within his mandate. AIDS was still seen as a disease of those on the fringes of society, and as such it was a second-rate problem — one that paled in comparison with the need to keep holiday traffic flowing on the Trans-Canada.

On May 15 the NACAIDS task force met again to discuss the testing issue. Dr. Perrault was coy about the results of the clinical trials. About one in every 220 blood donations in the sample had tested positive, but he did not reveal what percentage of blood donors were actually carriers of the AIDS virus.* Dr. Perrault said the society was concerned it would lose its insurance if news of the infection rate got out. The Laboratory Centre for Disease Control in Ottawa was more forthcoming; it had tested 9,000 samples from members of high-risk groups — gay men, hemophiliacs, intravenous drug users and prostitutes — and found 3,000 of them to be infected with AIDS. That day, the NACAIDS task force formally recommended that testing proceed according to the Red Cross implementation plan. Because it involved spending money, however, the plan had to be submitted to the Canadian Blood Committee meeting on June 4, 1985. The CBC decided that it could only approve testing "in principle" because there were a number of "sociological, ethical, legal and medical concerns . . . beyond its mandate".

It was true that issues like alternate testing sites — to ensure that people didn't go to blood donor clinics as a way of being tested for AIDS — and contact tracing — contacting the sexual partners and previous recipients of blood from donors who tested positive — had implications beyond the blood system. But these issues fell within the mandate of the CBC members, who were all senior health ministry officials. Besides, the argument that Canadians might flock to blood donor clinics to get AIDS tests was a spurious excuse for inaction; had there been a genuine fear, the Red Cross could have told donors that they wouldn't be informed of their test results, or had them sign a form confirming

---

* However, positive responses to the ELISA test do not necessarily mean that blood is infected with AIDS. The confirmatory Western Blot test is required.

that positive test results, and their names, would be passed on to public health authorities. If people went to blood donor clinics for AIDS tests, as they did for a decade after testing was instituted, it is a reflection of the lack of AIDS education, and the lack of knowledge, on the part of both doctors and patients, about the availability of anonymous testing.

The real reason for the delay was that the bureaucrats were reluctant to approve any spending outside budgetary periods. Just months before, for example, the CBC had refused to let the Red Cross hire a part-time janitor. Such decisions, regardless of how small the amount, had to go right to the top. Dr. Leclerc-Chevalier, executive director of the CBC, told the Red Cross it could expect a definite answer by June 30. In the meantime, the Red Cross decided that, because it didn't have the money up front, it would do no preparatory work to speed up implementation. While the Red Cross sat idly by, CBC members passed the buck to their political bosses, who bounced it back to other health ministry bureaucrats.

On June 11, 1985, British Columbia's health minister, Jim Nielsen, had finally had enough. Transfusion-AIDS was a political embarrassment, so the province decided to act alone: it granted $550,000 to the Red Cross for testing and $450,000 to St. Paul's Hospital in Vancouver to establish an alternate test site. The plan was to buy the test kits in nearby Seattle for $5 each. The next day, David Kirkwood, the federal deputy minister of Health and Welfare, invited his provincial and territorial counterparts to a consensus meeting on July 4. This time, they didn't even make the pretence of inviting interested groups. The deputy ministers of ten provinces, two territories and the federal government agreed that testing blood for the AIDS virus should go ahead, and that each province should designate one or more laboratories to do AIDS testing for the public (the so-called alternative test sites). But the guardians of a $60-billion-a-year healthcare system couldn't agree to spend $5.5 million to make Canada's blood system free of the deadly virus. That, they decided, was up to the Canadian Blood Committee — a committee of their subordinates.

So, on July 17, the CBC members met again. They approved the testing budget, except for Ontario, a province consumed by political turmoil, and Manitoba, a province still miffed about fractionation. In the first six months of 1985 Ontario had had four different health ministers[4] as the province went from a majority Conservative government to a minority Conservative government and then to a minority Liberal government. Stephen Dreezer, the Ontario representative on the CBC at the time, still insists the go-slow approach was not due to politics. "You can do things in a week and screw them up. We had to decide what was best for Canada. There's a big danger in looking south of the border and totally accepting whatever they do down there. We were concerned about the accuracy of the testing, the number of false negatives and what to tell people if their blood was infected," he recalls.

It's not clear how those issues were resolved over the next couple of weeks, but Manitoba quickly came aboard and, on August 1, five months after the test kit went on sale in the U.S., Ontario finally agreed to pay its share of testing — $1 million of the $2.5 million start-up costs. (Each month of foot-dragging had reduced the testing budget by about $500,000.) But the wait wasn't over. Only then did the Red Cross start training staff and upgrading its laboratory facilities; only then did the provinces start setting up alternate test sites. In Toronto, testing was in place within six weeks. But nation-wide testing of blood donated to the Red Cross wouldn't be in place until twelve long weeks later, on November 4, 1985.

At least two hospitals refused to brook such a delay. In July 1985 the Royal Victoria Hospital in Montreal — where Dr. Norbert Gilmore, chairman of the NACAIDS, was on staff — bought test kits directly from the United States and tested each unit of blood provided by the Red Cross before using it in surgery. The secret testing led to delays in almost 500 elective surgeries and cost $40,000, but it also saved lives. (The procedure was kept hush-hush to avoid a rush of patients who wanted safe transfusions.) In three months, laboratory technicians at the Royal Victoria tested 3,800 units of blood and discovered that 8 of them were contaminated with AIDS (an infection rate of 2 per 1,000). The Victoria General Hospital in Halifax took a similar initiative, inventing its own simple test using a bit of AIDS virus replicated in a petri dish.

In September 1985 the "tainted tuna" affair dominated the news. Fisheries minister John Fraser, who had overruled federal inspectors and allowed a million cans of foul-smelling tuna to go to market, was forced to resign amidst the furor, and the senior bureaucrat in Fisheries, deputy minister Art May, was fired even though he had advised his political boss not to let the product be sold. Within weeks the government had implemented a six-point plan to restore Canadians' faith in tuna. No one had died, no one had even gotten sick, but the government had been embarrassed.

In that same year almost a million units of untested blood were used for transfusion and the manufacture of blood concentrate, even though officials knew there was contamination in the system, and even though a test was available. By September three men had died of transfusion AIDS, and hundreds of others had contracted the deadly disease. Unlike the "tainted tuna", the tainted blood was not recalled. None of Canada's thirteen ministers of health lost their jobs, nor were any departmental officials fired, despite their inability to make a decision. It would be years before the tainted blood would embarrass the politicians. So far, it was merely killing people.

*   *   *

Back in January 1983, Dr. Donald Francis of the U.S. Centers for Disease Control had pounded his fist on the table and demanded to know at what point officialdom would be willing to act against the epidemic. By the time testing for AIDS was fully implemented in Canada in November 1985, his question about the "threshold of death" resonated loudly. At least 300 Canadians had been infected with AIDS during surgery before universal testing of blood, in addition to about 750 hemophiliacs. Many if not most of the deaths were preventable.

Yet the infections that are most difficult to accept are those that occurred in the eight months after the test kit was approved for sale. Dr. Man-Chiu Poon had been in the audience on the day of the outburst by Dr. Francis. Many years later, he and Jack McDonald, a professor in the Faculty of Social Work at the University of Calgary, conducted a study that revealed that fifty-five Canadians were infected with AIDS by transfusions administered between the time the test kit was approved in the U.S. in March 1985 and the full implementation of testing in Canada in November. The foot-dragging had cost seven lives a month. No single statistic more graphically illustrates the human costs of bureaucratic dithering in the tainted-blood tragedy. In itself, Ontario's indecision about testing probably cost two dozen Canadians their lives. The tests cost $5 each. Yet there was no shortage of money; Canada's blood program was $4 million under budget in 1985.[5]

As with factor concentrate, blood that was already in the pipeline was not discarded. Dr. Martin Davey, assistant national director of the Red Cross BTS, had told medical directors to test their stocks "if resources allow". Red cells, for example, have a shelf life of thirty-five days, and some Red Cross directors didn't want to lose a month's inventory at a time when there were shortages. So when Mr. C.*, a 67-year-old Montreal-area man, went in for heart surgery on November 7, 1985, he received untested blood. Because of delays and shortages caused by the new screening procedure, Mr. C.'s family had been asked by the doctor to give blood; twelve family members did so before he went into the operating room. The family was under the impression that their blood would go directly to Mr. C.; the Red Cross, however, does not allow directed donations because it says administering the system would be costly and

---

* Mr. C's family have asked that he not be identified, to ensure the privacy of his widow.

would not ensure a safer supply.[6] Their fresh, tested blood would go to some-one else. Mr. C. received blood that had been collected at the height of infec-tion, in a city with a rate far worse than anywhere else in the country. Though he received only three units of blood, one of them was infected with AIDS. Mr. C. not only died of AIDS, but infected his wife as well.

One of the mysteries of the tainted-blood tragedy is exactly how many transfusion patients actually contracted AIDS. Blood is the most efficient AIDS transmission route; more than 90 per cent of people exposed to conta-minated blood are infected. Yet, as research has shown, between 40 and 60 per cent of major-surgery patients die of their original condition within a year of transfusion. As well, because transfusion recipients were not considered a high-risk group, AIDS often went undiagnosed. The true number of transfu-sion infections is likely much higher than the 300 cases reported; some epi-demiologists suggest three to four times the number.

What is known is that the risks grew tremendously as time passed. One study conducted for the Quebec Ministry of Health found that the risk of a patient being exposed to AIDS-contaminated blood during surgery was sixty times higher in 1985 than in 1980, the year of the first known transfusion infection in Canada. In 1985 alone, when screening was poor and AIDS testing was delayed, the risk doubled. Dr. Robert Rémis, the Montreal epidemiologist who conducted the research, estimated that one in every 2,000 units of donated blood was infected with HIV in 1985. For multiple transfusions — an average of five units during surgery — the "risk was six per 1,000, or one infected per-son out of every 166 who received transfusions." By comparison, the risk of getting tainted blood during multiple transfusions in 1980 had been about one in 10,000. The Toronto Hospital for Sick Children found that fully half of its patients who contracted AIDS had received tainted blood in 1985, a clear indi-cation that aggressive screening would have saved lives.

The only other comparative statistics come from the period immediately after screening was implemented. In the first three months of testing, one in every 3,300 donations to the Red Cross was contaminated, and that was after donors were screened with a questionnaire asking about high-risk activities. Within the year the rate fell markedly, largely because the infected repeat donors were finally weeded out. Among them were Mr. E., a Toronto man who had had hundreds of homosexual partners yet had given blood thirty-two times, and the wife of a hemophiliac in Saskatchewan who had given blood every three months for all of her adult life — people who never should have gotten through the screening procedure, and who should have been targeted by education campaigns.

While there were tremendous variations in the infection rate from region to region, the province of Quebec had more than half the AIDS-infected blood donors in the country. Of 117 HIV-positive units in the province in the first year of testing, 114 were in Montreal, and more than half of those had been collected at three clinics in the downtown area. In a memo Dr. Perrault speculated that the disproportionately high infection rate might mean that French Canadians were genetically predisposed to get AIDS, the way scientists years earlier had thought homosexual men were, but in fact the high rates were attributed to the placing of donor clinics in high-risk areas. To make matters worse, Quebec didn't open any alternate test sites until four months after the Red Cross began testing. Some doctors actually referred patients to blood clinics to be tested, and some people continued to go to the Red Cross on their own initiative because the alternate sites weren't advertised. This was a nation-wide problem. In early 1986, the student council sponsoring a blood clinic at the University of Saskatchewan posted a big sign that read "Free AIDS Test".

Accepting blood from people who were at high risk of being AIDS carriers was risky for a couple of reasons: 1) there is a "window" after exposure during which antibodies to the virus do not yet show up in the blood, and 2) the Red Cross was having technical problems introducing the new test. There were interruptions in supply, a number of defective test lots and human errors. Pat Humphreys, director of laboratory services at the Red Cross, sent a June 1986 memo to technicians that told of a man who had been hospitalized with AIDS symptoms just days after giving blood. He had twice donated since testing had been introduced, and all his tests had been negative — a problem the lab manager said was due to "mislabelling". Suffice it to say that infections did not end with the introduction of testing.

Despite a significantly large infection rate during clinical trials, there were still efforts to cut corners. At the time, units of blood that tested positive in the ELISA test but negative in the Western Blot were transfused. The Red Cross also continued to use untested blood for the manufacture of factor concentrate until December 1985, on the premise that the virus would be killed during heat treatment. The heat treatment process used was soon shown to be less than 100 per cent effective, but some concentrate made with untested plasma was still in use as late as 1987.

In 1986, growing numbers of transfusion patients learned that they had been infected with the AIDS virus. Those who had contracted the disease early were getting sick, and others began to worry when they read the stories that were popping up in newspapers. What few people realized was that evidence of a parallel tragedy was beginning to emerge, the widespread infection of transfusion recipients with non-A-non-B hepatitis, a virus so mysterious it was defined by what it was not. Testing blood for AIDS was now routine and blood-borne HIV infections had been virtually eliminated, but there was still no test to detect the type of hepatitis that could cause debilitating liver disease. In 1985, Dr. Harvey Alter, chief immunologist at the U.S. Institutes of Health, published research that calculated more than 100,000 people a year in the U.S. were contracting non-A-non-B hepatitis* — that translates to about 10,000 in Canada — and in April of the next year, he proposed a simple method of eliminating about half of those infections using surrogate tests. The Red Cross did preliminary testing with the surrogate tests — in fact, the Montreal Blood Transfusion Centre was prepared to institute the procedure in early 1987 — but the Red Cross, as it had done with AIDS, decided that more evidence was required before it acted. This despite a study published in 1987 that showed 9.2 per cent of transfusion recipients at Mount Sinai and Toronto General Hospital were contracting non-A-non-B hepatitis.** So flagrant was the inaction that Dr. Alter proposed using Canada as a control group to judge the efficiency of U.S. surrogate tests. By comparing Canadian and U.S. data, scientists were able to determine that the tests screened out about 40 per cent of hepatitis C cases.

*　　*　　*

Tony Zucchelli began to wonder about the blood he had received in surgery; he was back operating the restaurant, but he was always tired. In 1987 his doctor in High River, who had never been contacted by the Red Cross or public health officials about the risk of blood-borne AIDS, told him that receiving tainted blood was as likely as having a star fall out of the sky and hit him on the head. That summer the Red Cross received its final payment from the federal government, and in August it officially opened its new Ottawa headquarters, marking the fortieth anniversary of the peacetime blood program.

In 1988 Helen Zucchelli was found to be infected with a parasite that's common in people with AIDS. Tony's doctor had always discouraged him from getting an HIV test, arguing that his own wife had been transfused the same month and she was in good health. But Tony, because he didn't want to harm his wife, insisted on a test. The results were positive. He broke the news to

---

* The virus was named hepatitis C when it was finally discovered in 1989.
** About half of the people who contract hepatitis C don't get sick, while about 40 per cent develop chronic illness, with symptoms like fatigue and jaundice. About 10 per cent of victims develop cirrhosis of the liver or cancer, though it can take up to 30 years after infection for symptoms to appear.

Helen on New Year's Day, as they were returning from a ski trip. To Tony's great relief, Helen tested negative. Zucchelli told a couple of family members, but they reacted badly so he was determined to keep his status secret. When he went to the hospital in High River for tests, however, the nurses recognized him from the restaurant. Soon there were rumours, and the locals stopped coming to the restaurant; then the cars stopped turning off Highway 2. Tony would hide in the kitchen, hoping the customers would return.

In 1990 the couple sold the Blackspot and gave up their dream. The chef never accepted his fate; having AIDS was like taking a bullet to the gut every day. He was so terrified of transmitting AIDS that he would barely touch his wife and grandchildren. Without the restaurant, without the cooking, with his own body an enemy, Tony Zucchelli's sole remaining pleasure was the violin. He took refuge in music until the disease caused him to lose feeling in his fingers. Another victim had been silenced, dead before his fifty-fifth birthday.

9

THROUGH THE LOOKING-GLASS
LOOK-BACK AND TRACE-BACK

Too late is the medicine prepared,
when the disease has gained strength
by long delay.

Ovid

James Hackett, Aurora, Ontario

Watching his wife Florence die, at age 59, a gruesome death from a mysterious illness doctors could not pin down, James is angry that serious efforts were never made to track down former recipients of blood. Florence received a transfusion in late 1984 and died seven years later, just days after being tested for the virus.

"I watched my wife go from a healthy, vibrant woman to skin and bones. All she had left at the end was her fighting spirit.

During all those years after the transfusion, nobody ever advised me she might have received tainted blood. I keep thinking if treatment had started earlier, she might still be alive . . . I just can't forgive and forget."

(*February 21, 1994*)

Linda Collins, Aurora, Ontario

A registered nurse, and the daughter of James and Florence Hackett, she says her mother was treated with less compassion than an animal. Linda says that, during a recent scare about infectious canine affliction, she was telephoned by her veterinarian and told to have her dog tested.

"We're talking about a dog here, and I got phoned. But no one ever phoned about Mom. Why do we treat animals better than we do ourselves? The authorities seemed to believe that ignorance is bliss. Well, we're paying for that bliss with the lives of our loved ones."

(February 21, 1994)

THEY CALLED IT OPERATION 300.

After the deaths of Vic Drew and "Mr. F." in early 1985 — the first publicly acknowledged cases of transfusion AIDS in Canada — Colonel Neville Robinson, administrator of the Vancouver Blood Transfusion Service of the Red Cross, set out to pinpoint the source of the tainted blood that had killed them. The former paratrooper had seen active duty in North Africa, Sicily and Korea, but nothing in his military training could have prepared him for being parachuted into the minefield of AIDS at the height of public hysteria.

Vic Drew, a former soldier, had died of AIDS at Victoria's Royal Jubilee Hospital on May 4, 1985, two years after successful heart surgery. Mr. F. was a 52-year-old Vancouver man who had been seriously burned in a house fire in July 1981, and had died of AIDS on April 22, 1985. Colonel Robinson's task, on the surface, was straightforward: to contact the donors of the blood products the two had received and bring them in for AIDS testing. Yet the exercise to determine where the fatal transfusions had come from was rife with legal, ethical, medical and practical issues. Did the donor have a legal obligation to be tested? Did public health authorities have to be notified? What purpose did it serve to find the infected donor if there was no treatment for the disease? What about the donor's right to privacy? What if there were other recipients of an infected donor's blood? And then there was the sheer number of donors involved; Mr. F. alone had received donations from 301 donors,* hence the codename "Operation 300".

The goal of Robinson's search, in fact, was to limit the legal liability of the Red Cross. The admission that two recipients of blood products had died of AIDS had had an unexpected, double-barrelled result: the threat of lawsuits,

---

* The 301 blood products included 107 units of plasma, 76 units of whole blood, 41 units of platelets, 40 units of concentrated red cells and 37 units of frozen plasma. Mr. F. had also been transfused with 20 vials of albumin, but donors of plasma used in fractionation products like albumin were not traced because each vial contained portions of thousands of donations.

coupled with a threat by the Red Cross's insurance company to cut off coverage. A couple of lawsuits could not only destroy the credibility of the humanitarian agency, but could bankrupt it. For almost a week after the public admission by Dr. Derrick that two recipients were infected with AIDS, Robinson spent his days huddled with lawyers. Dr. Perrault, director of the Blood Transfusion Service, flew in from Toronto. The lawyers advised doing everything possible to track down the donors, up to and including hiring private detectives, and testing them promptly to avoid new cases. Unlike the switch to heat-treated concentrate and the institution of testing, both of which had taken eight months to get off the ground, the "trace-back" program began within a week. At first, when the Red Cross itself felt threatened, the problem was considered an emergency; then the agency decided this was another issue best left to the bureaucracy.

The approach to finding the donors and recipients of the tainted blood was virtually identical to the process of introducing heat-treated products. On May 15 Dr. Perrault was in Ottawa for a meeting of the National Advisory Committee on AIDS, where he recommended that a consensus conference be called to discuss the medical, legal, sociological and ethical issues involved. He said the Red Cross would eventually notify donors if it was given the mandate and the funding to do so, but that the agency had no interest in tracking recipients, a matter he argued should be "handled separately". Randy Starkman, a lawyer for the federal Department of Justice, backed that division of responsibilities, as well as a go-slow approach because of the legal repercussions. According to the minutes of the meeting, he "indicated that, from a legal point of view, major concerns may be related to donors but there was a growing swell of additional concerns on the part of recipients." NACAIDS decided to strike a task force to examine these issues. Dr. Richard Mathias, a professor of epidemiology at the University of British Columbia and chairman of the Task Force on HTLV-III Testing in Canada, was outraged by this position, which he felt was an unacceptable response to a blood-borne epidemic disease. But his was the lone vote of dissent. Dr. Perrault didn't even tell the NACAIDS members about Operation 300.

On May 16, 1985, Colonel Robinson began phoning the seventeen people — eleven men and six women — whose blood had been transfused into Mr. Drew. He started with the men because they were far more likely to be infected. It took less than two hours to contact the first six, but it would take two more weeks before everyone agreed to be tested. During the calls, Robinson read from a lawyer-prepared script that the donors had been chosen as "part of a research process" that required an additional blood test, but he reported to his superiors that "90 per cent of them knew right away it was about AIDS." The plan was to have the local donors come into the Vancouver BTS centre, and to fly a nurse to outlying regions. When a shift worker in Dawson Creek insisted that his own doctor take the sample, the procedure was changed. A woman who lived in Prince George, over 400 miles away, offered to fly her own plane to Vancouver to be tested that very day, a move typical of both the donors' fear and their eagerness to help. A couple of the donors mentioned that they had had multiple sexual partners, or bisexual partners; the Red Cross was still screening out only members of high-risk groups, not people who engaged in high-risk activities. Another woman, whom Robinson had been unable to contact, turned up by chance at a clinic; she became the first donor whose blood was tested without specific consent. But one of the worst fears of the Red Cross was confirmed when one donor contacted his lawyer before agreeing to be tested, because he feared being sued by the recipient.*

While various committees hemmed and hawed over the need for testing, only the Laboratory Centre for Disease Control in Ottawa had the facilities to do AIDS tests. Both Air Canada and Canadian Pacific Airlines refused to fly blood samples that might be contaminated with AIDS, so they had to be shipped overland from Vancouver to Ottawa. By June 20 the results from Mr. Drew's donors were in. It turned out that not one but two of the men were HIV-positive — yet back in 1983, when their donations had been made, the risk of transfusion AIDS had been considered relatively low.

From the initial test case, Colonel Robinson drafted a set of standard operating procedures for the trace-back of donors, and a nurse, Marlene Coulthard, was enlisted to help. By the end of July 1985, Operation 300 had ballooned; two new AIDS cases — both of them young women from remote British Columbia communities who had received blood components due to complications during childbirth — involved blood from forty-eight donors. All the cases dated from 1981 to 1983, and the biggest problem was that donor records were outdated. About 15 per cent of people had moved — some couldn't be found, while others had to be tested by doctors in other provinces — and a few had died. The Red Cross, following legal advice, told donors the bare minimum about the implications of testing, and worried that outside doctors would tell all. There were also bugs in the system. A couple of donors were called to attend clinics while their blood was off being tested for AIDS. In one case the registrar forgot to enter the "L" code in the computer that indicated that the donor had tested positive for the AIDS virus, and the person, whom they

---

* There have been hundreds of lawsuits against doctors, hospitals, the Red Cross, the provinces. Though many of the donors have been traced, no donor has ever been sued in Canada.

hadn't been able to track down, gave blood again. Because of the absence of the computer code, the contaminated blood was collected; because of the lack of testing, it was transfused into another patient.

Operation 300 ended on December 31, 1985. After 150 days of searching, the Red Cross had located and tested 304 of 366 donors, an 83 per cent success rate, Colonel Robinson reported. Only two people had refused outright to be tested, but a good number simply couldn't be found. Yet the mission could be considered only "partially successful" because contaminated donations had been located in only three of the four cases, Robinson concluded. The exercise had cost the Red Cross just over $35,000, or about $100 per donor. His final recommendation — in keeping with his military background — was to keep Operation 300 confidential and to destroy all documents in five years.

*　*　*

As with many aspects of the tainted-blood tragedy, what wasn't done was as significant as what was. Colonel Robinson carried out a "trace-back" to find donors, but there is no indication that he conducted a "look-back" — tracking their prior blood donations to ensure that other recipients of their blood were tested. Aside from a briefing to British Columbia's assistant deputy minister of health, the details of the exercise were kept confidential by the Red Cross, a policy that does not appear to have been challenged by public health officials. An epidemiologist reading the report on Operation 300 would have immediately raised some red flags: 1) only one of the four donors who tested positive was sick and only two of the four were gay men, meaning that the majority of infected donors would not have been detected by screening measures; 2) given what was known about the incubation period of the virus at the time — it was believed to be about six years — those early infected recipients were an indication of many more to come; 3) the sexual partners and children of former transfusion patients and donors were also at risk.

There should have been a determined effort to track down and test recipients of potentially tainted blood — at least back to 1981 — to limit the spread of the disease. People with AIDS should have been asked systematically if they had been blood donors, and recipients of their donations contacted. And, given that 300,000 people a year receive blood, doctors across the country should have been alerted to the possibility of transfusion AIDS. There were a number of ways to limit the spread of AIDS: a general public announcement by the Red Cross, regional campaigns by the provincial medical officers of health, a letter to physicians by groups like the Canadian Medical Association and advertising in medical journals. Instead, the wait-and-see approach ruled: waiting for the provinces to make up their minds on testing, and waiting for transfusion patients to die before looking for the source of their AIDS. From the Red Cross's point of view, Operation 300 had alarmed a number of donors, cost a good deal of money and monopolized the time of senior workers. The society wasn't challenged to act differently by public health officials, who still behaved as if they believed AIDS was a disease of the marginal, of the 4-H club, and therefore not a priority. In fact, unofficial policy in both federal and provincial ministries of health was to downplay the risks of blood-borne AIDS, to avoid the reality that AIDS had moved out of the gay community.

Yet there was every reason to worry. In the latter part of 1985 there were ten new cases of transfusion AIDS* in Canada, and that was before testing began formally on November 4. There would soon be more. In mid-November, for example, Mr. L., the Chrysler worker, returned to the blood donor clinic at the Legion Hall in Ajax. Once again he breezed through the screening, but this time his blood was tested. By then the trace-back procedures had been modified. The Red Cross wasn't calling donors individually but sending them a carefully worded form letter. A few weeks after his donation, Mr. L. received a letter, and on January 12, 1986, he and his girlfriend were tested for the AIDS virus: he was positive, she was negative. The recipients of his donation, including Kenneth Pittman, would not have the benefit of early diagnosis.

On January 20, 1986, Dr. Guévin, medical director of the Montreal BTS Centre, wrote a memo to Dr. Davey, assistant director of the Blood Transfusion Service, asking if all centres had to repeat Operation 300. Montreal, like Vancouver, had a rash of transfusion AIDS cases in late 1985. There was a two-year-old girl, and two middle-aged men who had undergone surgery during the last three years, all three of whom died of AIDS in November. (Of the first twenty transfusion AIDS cases, twelve were due to blood provided by the Vancouver and Montreal centres.) It was Dr. Guévin, not Colonel Robinson, who had conducted the first trace-back, way back in 1983, after a six-month-old infant had died of AIDS at Ste-Justine Hospital. He had had a fairly easy time of it; the girl had received only five units of blood, and he easily found the five donors. In the days before there was an AIDS test, all he could do was ascertain whether the donors were members of high-risk groups or had any AIDS symptoms; the medical director found four "straight-forward young healthy males" and was left with "some doubt as to the sexual habits of the fifth blood donor", a sexually active homosexual man who had given blood before there were any screening measures in place.

---

* Then, as now, the federal government kept track of AIDS cases only, not the number of HIV infections, which greatly skews the statistics of a disease with a long incubation period.

In his memo to Dr. Davey, Dr. Guévin made a key point: the Red Cross computer wasn't adapted to doing trace-back and look-back procedures. Each BTS centre had some form of computer for donor records, but the machines weren't very sophisticated and, more important, weren't linked to hospitals or other BTS centres. The lack of an electronic data base had been a long-standing problem. Way back in 1972, the Canadian Hematology Society had identified as the number-one priority in the country's blood system the need to computerize donor records. The problem then was inventory control — thousands of units of blood were unaccounted for each year — but the advent of fractionation products and infectious diseases like hepatitis made the issue more urgent. A study conducted by the Hospital Systems Study Group of Saskatoon led to the creation of a regionally decentralized computer system. By 1976 the Blood Information System (BLIS) project was under way, with the Red Cross switching from a manual, file-card system to electronic data processing of donor records. But when the Hematology Society did a follow-up report a year later, topping the list of deficiencies once again was the state of computerization — more specifically the fact that computers weren't used in the laboratories, or to keep track of hepatitis tests. Almost a decade later, in 1986, Dr. Guévin had the same complaint: BLIS was strictly a donor records system, designed to help the Blood Donor Recruitment division get donors coming back. It still didn't address blood product inventory or general laboratory requirements. In the era of AIDS, with a million blood donations a year being tested for the deadly virus, testing and trace-back records were still being done manually.

The response to Dr. Guévin's concern was a non-answer that the long-time employee understood all too well. In the Red Cross, as in the army, you spoke only when spoken to, and didn't take initiative. In a memo to medical directors soon after Dr. Guévin's query, Dr. Davey explained that donors who tested positive for the AIDS virus would be notified according to a strict procedure. There were three basic principles underlying the approach, which had been cleared by the society's lawyers*:

a) while donors must be informed of tests, specific consent is not required for testing itself;

b) the Blood Transfusion Service must not establish a doctor-patient relationship with any donor;

c) BTS centres should keep donor records confidential as far as the law allows; test results should only be provided to a physician if agreed to by the donor.

---

* He identified the honorary counsel of the Red Cross, P.H.H. (Peter) Ridout, Q.C.

Dr. Davey made no mention of recipients of tainted blood because the Red Cross felt it had no particular legal responsibility towards them, a notion that would finally be dispelled in later lawsuits. Two years earlier, U.S. blood bank administrators — including the American Red Cross — had expressed an "urgent need" to establish a system to trace recipients of contaminated blood for "epidemiological purposes", but the Canadian blood banker felt then that it was too early to act because there wasn't yet a commercial test available. In the months various committees had taken to consider the issue of testing — supposedly to resolve all the related issues — testing had barely come up, and there was certainly no policy in place once AIDS testing was implemented. In October and November of 1985, when testing was still only being phased in, 45 of 180,000 blood donations in Canada tested positive for AIDS; the donors promptly received a letter urging them to be tested, but there was still no formal plan in place to notify recipients of previous donations. (This is particularly important because 85 per cent of Canadians who give blood to the Red Cross in any given year are repeat donors.)

At a March 1986 meeting, four months after the implementation of nationwide AIDS testing of blood, Red Cross medical directors discussed the tracing of recipients, but decided to wash their hands of the matter. They behaved as if Operation 300 had never been conducted. Policy decisions, they decided, should be left to NACAIDS. In June 1986, U.S. blood bank administrators said trace-back was necessary to prevent the further spread of AIDS among the sexual partners and newborn children of transfusion recipients. The Canadian Red Cross, however, issued its own statement, saying that transfusion-associated AIDS wasn't a major problem in this country: of 604 cases of AIDS that had been identified at that time, only 23 had been "linked positively" to blood transfusion. The idea of look-back needed to be studied further, the agency said, to determine "whether and how such a system could be implemented in Canada, if it proves feasible and cost effective."

By March 1986, when a 12-year-old girl in North Bay, Ontario, was found to have been infected with AIDS by blood she had received a couple of years earlier during surgery, each one of the seventeen Red Cross Blood Transfusion Service centres had reported a case of transfusion AIDS. Despite the fact that public health authorities made no effort to find recipients of tainted blood, two dozen more transfusion AIDS cases were reported in 1986. The diagnosis usually came just days before, or after, death. At a meeting of a subcommittee of the Canadian Blood Committee on June 19, 1986, Dr. Perrault estimated that "450 recipients might be involved annually in any look-back procedure." As the number of cases climbed — just as epidemiologists had predicted — logic dictated that some kind of action was necessary. Provincial and federal officials did nothing, so the Red Cross took some initiative, though half-heartedly.

In January 1987, for the first time, the humanitarian agency urged in a public statement that former transfusion patients who were concerned about AIDS consult a physician about the need to be tested. Yet Dr. Derrick went out of his way to downplay the risk. "It's obvious that there was a very small chance of acquiring AIDS. An educated guess is that a person would have a chance of about one in 200,000 of acquiring the virus prior to the tests being done now," he said. But there was nothing "educated" in his statement; it was pure sophistry. Dr. Derrick knew very well that, although the one in 200,000 figure might apply to the seven-year period prior to testing, it was as meaningless as the often bandied about "one in a million". The fact was that, in the first year of testing, one in every 5,750 donations was contaminated — and that was after a much tougher questionnaire had been introduced to eliminate high-risk donors. The point that should have been made was that transfusions were a small risk compared to other means of contracting the disease but that the risk was significant from 1984 to 1985, and not negligible in the years prior.

On March 17 the U.S. Public Health Service urged blood transfusion recipients, particularly those from 1983 to 1985, to get tested for AIDS. It estimated that there were about 12,000 transfusion-AIDS cases in the U.S., though only a fraction of them had been detected. Health Canada remained silent, and the Red Cross again had reassuring words. Kenneth Mews, technical information officer with the society, urged former transfusion patients to speak to their doctors but said it "would be in no one's interest" for all transfusion recipients to get an AIDS test. The problem was that the physicians were getting the same information from the Red Cross as was the general public, so they had no reason to believe tainted blood was any more of a risk than falling stars.

The result of the absence of trace-back and look-back programs was that although Tony Zucchelli and Ken Pittman and many other recipients of multiple transfusions should have been listed as members of a high-risk group, their doctors never thought to have them tested for AIDS, or even actively discouraged the idea. The person who donated the blood that infected Zucchelli was never located. As unbelievable as it seems today, the blood that Mr. L. donated had killed two people, but no one ever told Pittman, the third recipient. The Red Cross didn't even get around to telling the Toronto Hospital that one of its patients had received a contaminated donation until June 12, 1987.

The principal reason why the Red Cross took eighteen long months after Mr. L.'s blood donation tested positive for the AIDS virus to contact the hospital was that it wasn't a priority. The first step of the look-back, connecting the donation to the donor, was relatively easy and paid immediate dividends for the Red Cross, because it eliminated a contaminated donor from the pool. The next step, finding previous donations and the blood components that had resulted, was a far more time-consuming and expensive process, while the final stage of look-back, tracing the unit numbers within hospitals and back to the recipients, was more complicated still. In February 1987 the Toronto branch of the Red Cross conducted a "peek-back", an informal tracing of HIV-positive blood from four donors including Mr. L., to determine how difficult it would be to trace recipients. Dr. Roslyn Herst, medical director of the Toronto BTS — like Colonel Robinson before her — was enlisted to come up with a methodology. The paperwork and the headaches were formidable.

Tracing a current donor was simple: you looked up the name in the computer and sent a letter. A blood donation, on the other hand, was divided into a minimum of three parts — plasma, red cells and platelets — and each part might be shipped to a different institution. Plasma sent for fractionation was a whole different matter, for it was pooled with up to 20,000 other donations, and all it took was one infected unit to contaminate the lot. Many of the records were still kept manually, and, until 1984, those that were on computer were often purged after a year. But the bottom line was that, with enough investment of time and money, many recipients could be found. For the next four months, Red Cross and Ontario public health officials dickered about who should be responsible for notifying the recipients of potentially tainted blood.

During a lawsuit many years later, the Red Cross would argue that it had no legal duty to contact recipients because it had no access to patient records to make the contact. Technically that was true. But in the bizarre regulatory netherworld in which the Red Cross operated, it was the agency, not public health officials, that was responsible for accrediting hospitals to receive blood products. On paper, the Red Cross required that "records must be kept that provide details of the receipt and disposition of all blood products provided to patients." In practice, however, the rule was not enforced, and the only sanction available to the Red Cross — cutting the flow of blood to a hospital — would have violated its most fundamental principle.

In reality, the debate about who would contact recipients was moot. Determining which patients had received what blood components would be a far greater obstacle. The Red Cross records were in impeccable condition compared to those in the blood banks of Canadian hospitals, and most hospitals had given virtually no thought to the implications of blood-borne AIDS.

After it was finally alerted to Mr. L.'s contaminated donation, in June 1987, the Toronto Hospital — the largest user of blood and blood products in the country — had no idea what to do with the information. The hospital was still relying on a manual filing system in which blood records were attached to individual patient files, which were filed by year. Without a cross-listing for the date of operation and the unit number of the blood product, tracing a potentially infected unit of blood was a logistical nightmare; stacks and stacks of files had to be searched for the six-digit bag number, and a single patient could have received up to three hundred units. The hospital resolved to correct the error, but there was no sense of urgency, no sense that the units of blood in question were a poison that had been tranfused into patients and that, as a result, the lives of their spouses, lovers and children could also be in danger. Instead of being a race to save lives, the tracing of tainted-blood recipients was a tedious, low-priority exercise in accounting.

Eventually the hospital decided to set up a computer system from scratch to figure out which of its patients had received the infected unit. It began the process in February 1988, more than two years after Mr. L. had been notified of his infection. Because the budget was tight, a single clerk was hired, and it took her five months to enter just one year of blood records into the computer. Later, as the cases piled up and the absurdity of the time required to find a recipient could no longer escape hospital officials, a "quick and dirty" system was put in place, and three years of records were inputed in a mere five weeks. Shortly thereafter — on February 24, 1989 — Kenneth Pittman's name was linked to cryoprecipitate unit number A96490, donated by Mr. L. forty months earlier. The information was passed to Pittman's family doctor, Stanley Bain. After all that effort, Doctor Bain chose to keep that knowledge to himself — another example of the lack of education in the medical community.

*   *   *

In 1988, NACAIDS finally recommended that former transfusion patients should be tested for the AIDS virus — a full three years after it had recommended testing of blood. While the call wasn't widely advertised, some doctors paid heed. Soon after the NACAIDS recommendation, in September, Lena Mary Dadd had her 11-year-old son, Bobby Mathieson, who was suffering from a strange skin ailment, tested for AIDS. He had received multiple transfusions back in 1980, during open-heart surgery as a toddler, and it turned out that he was infected with the virus. Across the country, former transfusion patients were learning they too were infected.

While little effort was made to find the victims of tainted blood, even less thought went into the counselling and education of those who had learned they were infected. The exception was in Calgary, where social worker Jack

McDonald set up the HIV-T Group, a self-help group that was founded in February 1988. Elsewhere in Canada, transfusion patients, unlike hemophilia patients, had no support network. Dadd's family physician in St. Catharines, Ontario, refused to treat the boy because she didn't want to take the disease home to her own children. When the family moved to nearby Niagara Falls, parents circulated a petition to have Bobby banned from school. Children threw smoke bombs at him in the schoolyard, and slashed his mother's tires. When Bobby went for treatment at the Hospital for Sick Children in Toronto, the nurses dressed up in gowns, goggles and masks before approaching him, and he had to go to the door of his hospital room to pick up his meals because staff refused to approach him.

In March 1989 the Canadian Blood Committee endorsed development of a nation-wide computer system, and provided $1.5 million over three years for start-up costs. The Computerized Information System for Centre Operations (CISCO) was going to link blood records from both the recruitment centres and the laboratories and, ultimately, allow the Red Cross to know the history of any unit of blood with a few keystrokes. The pilot project began in Tony Zucchelli's province, Alberta. CISCO would, however, become another in a long line of expensive failures. The earlier Blood Information System (BLIS) had clearly been inadequate, so in early 1987 the Red Cross had spent $1.6 million to purchase new hardware and software. In early 1988 the CBC had approved spending almost the same amount again to further upgrade the BTS centres' minicomputers, as an interim measure pending the establishment of a Blood Programme Management Information System (BPMIS). "The cost of upgrading such equipment was covered by savings realized in overall lower equipment maintenance costs," Dr. Perrault wrote in a report to the Canadian Hematology Society. By the time work began on developing CISCO, an integrated computer system, in 1989, the Red Cross had already spent more than $7 million on computerization — yet laboratory tests of blood were still being recorded by hand.

The computer system took on particular importance because, in 1989, blood was classified as a drug and became subject to the terms of the Food and Drug Act (it would be several more years before the regulations pertaining to blood were drafted, so blood remained unregulated into the 1990s). Under the proposed regulations, the computer system was supposed to include a national deferral registry, monitoring of laboratory testing records, and trace-back and look-back functions. Another little-noted but significant development in 1989 was a technical ruling in a civil suit against the Red Cross by the estate of Bud Sharpe, one of the first recipients of tainted blood to sue. The court ruled that the Red Cross must take all means possible to locate the donors of tainted blood because their testimony could be relevant. As a result, the Red Cross hired a private detective agency, Albright Investigators Ltd. of Unionville, Ontario, to locate errant donors — an approach it had rejected years earlier during Operation 300. It also provided the donors with free legal counsel.

In December 1989, when the federal government announced its Extraordinary Assistance Plan (EAP) to provide compensation to victims of tainted blood, the importance of record-keeping again escalated. To prove they were eligible for the EAP, hemophiliacs and transfusion patients needed records from the Red Cross, but victims and the Blue Cross, which had been contracted to administer the EAP, found the humanitarian agency uncooperative when asked to conduct trace-back procedures. The problem was that the Red Cross's insurance policy contained a standard clause that prohibited it from providing evidence to a potential claimant in a lawsuit. "This puts the Society in the position of providing evidence in support of a potential lawsuit against itself while Government funds potentially assist in the pursuit of such action," Red Cross president H. Robert Hemming wrote to health minister Perrin Beatty on January 12, 1990.

In December 1990 the Red Cross signed a contract with Etcom Inc. of Edmonton to develop software for CISCO, the much-vaunted computer system that would link all seventeen BTS centres. By early 1992 it was obvious that the project, budgeted to cost $11 million, was in big trouble. "The CISCO project is floundering, with no indication of significant improvement in the near future. Maintaining CISCO on its present course is not a viable alternative," the management and systems consulting company G. Gargarella & Associates Inc. wrote in a 1992 report to the Canadian Blood Agency. The consultant recommended capping expenditures at $12.5 million, but by the time its report was presented costs had already exceeded $18 million, with no end in sight.

*   *   *

The intense and long-overdue media coverage of the tainted-blood tragedy finally began in late 1992, and brought a good number of former transfusion patients to their doctors for AIDS testing, while the growing number of lawsuits prompted a whole new round of look-back and trace-back procedures. The watershed event, however, came in 1993, when Dr. Susan King, head of the infectious diseases division at the Hospital for Sick Children, conducted a seven-month research project to determine if contacting former transfusion patients was a worthwhile exercise. The HIV Information Project chose a target group, former pediatric cardiac patients who had received multiple transfusions between 1978 and 1985, and opted to contact them via their family physicians instead of by letter. (A highly publicized 1987 study in San Francisco found that only 12 per cent of former transfusion patients responded to letters.) The results of the research, that 17 of the 1,783 children were infected with the AIDS virus,* or 1 per cent, made headlines around the world.

A decade after the transfusions, one-third of the children still had no symptoms of AIDS. The data also provided some disturbing facts about public understanding of the risks of transfusion AIDS: fully two-thirds of the patients, even though they had huge scars to remind them of surgery, were unaware that blood had been used in their treatment; while knowledge of the risk of AIDS was high, few connected the risk to themselves until they were approached directly; 70 per cent of former patients only went for testing due to media coverage, demonstrating that, in addition to enlisting general practitioners, it was important to publicize the trace-back campaign. The publicity surrounding the study led directly to the discovery of six other transfusion AIDS cases in Ontario alone. With those kinds of results, the hospital decided that it should contact all 17,000 of its transfusion patients during the high-risk period, an approach that would be copied by most pediatric hospitals in the country. Yet the response remained more emotional than scientific; hospitals still balked at tracing former adult transfusion patients even though they were more likely to be sexually active, and thus a much greater public health threat.

One of the most troubling aspects of the research, Dr. King said, was that a group of doctors in Alberta initially refused to tell forty former pediatric patients that they were at high risk of infection and should be tested for AIDS. The physicians refused to co-operate because they feared legal action, but eventually they changed their minds. Lawyers at Sick Kids had warned the HIV Information Project that their efforts to find patients could provoke lawsuits. "We were aware that by finding cases of infection we might incur litigation . . . but it was our medical and ethical duty to proceed," Dr. King says. Her view was that contacting former transfusion recipients should be considered part of the "continuing care" provided to patients by physicians and hospitals.

The Sick Kids study finally led public officials to change their minds about the need for testing — or at least embarrassed them into action — and prompted the publication of epidemiological studies about the number of Canadians with transfusion AIDS. Jack McDonald, Dr. Man-Chiu Poon and Gerald Devins had estimated in their research commissioned by Health Canada

---

* Six patients were actually identified as infected during the research; the other eleven had been identified as seropositive earlier, which prompted the hospital to conduct more in-depth research.

that there could be 50 new cases annually through to 1997, bringing the total number to over 500. (In early 1993 there were 261 cases enlisted in the federal compensation program, and 419 transfusion AIDS cases had been identified by various surveillance programs.) Dr. Robert Rémis, the epidemiologist at Montreal General Hospital, and his colleague Robert Palmer estimated that between 942 and 1,441 patients had been infected with AIDS by transfusion, and that about half of them were still alive. (As noted, between 40 and 60 per cent of major surgery patients — five units or more — die of their underlying illness or injury within a year of transfusion.) Epidemiologists at the Laboratory Centre for Disease Control confirmed those numbers, and extrapolated that as many as 245 former transfusion patients could be infected and still unaware of their status. The Commons Sub-Committee on Health Issues also keyed in on the startling fact that, a decade after testing of blood became routine, hundreds of Canadians could still be unaware that they were infected with a deadly virus.

By the end of 1993, virtually every provincial public health department had made a public call for former transfusion patients to be tested. As always, the speed of action varied. Most notable for its slow reaction was Manitoba, where political priorities once again overrode public health concerns. Dr. John Guilfoyle, Chief Medical Officer of Health in the province, wanted to issue a bulletin on the testing of transfusion patients in July 1993, around the time Ontario made its very public announcement, but he wasn't allowed to do so until October 18. The delay was due to the fact that five by-elections were planned for September 21 and, while tainted blood wasn't an issue *per se* during the campaign, the Conservative government of Premier Gary Filmon was highly sensitive to criticisms in the area of healthcare reform and cuts to health spending.

The Ontario Hospital Association joined the calls for former transfusion recipients to be tested in June 1994, and followed that up with an advertising campaign and media blitz led by its executive director, Dennis Timbrell, who years earlier had been the provincial health minister touting Connaught. The general warnings about transfusion AIDS were necessary because the sorry state of hospital records ensured that the majority of recipients of tainted blood would not be tracked down.

Even at Sick Kids, one of the first hospitals to computerize its blood bank records, look-back procedures were still ineffective. Of the thirty-one look-back requests Sick Kids had received from the Red Cross — meaning that the donor of a unit of blood was infected and the hospital should find the recipient — it had been unable to complete sixteen. The problem was particularly acute at children's hospitals because blood is often shared; for example, one unit of blood at Sick Kids left four children infected with AIDS. "Computerization of blood bank systems is really still fairly new. Of all laboratory systems, the blood bank has been the last to computerize," said Dr. Annette Poon, director of the hospital's blood bank.

The paper trail was so rife with dead ends that technicians at the Red Cross resorted to poring over the names on an AIDS memorial in downtown Toronto, writing down the inscriptions and trying to match the names of the dead with the names of blood donors who couldn't be located. They managed to close at least eight trace-back cases using that rather macabre method. One of the names on the memorial was eerily familiar: Dr. Derek Naylor, director of Blood Products Services at the Red Cross. That the person responsible for purchasing blood products for Canadian hemophiliacs had been a gay man infected with the AIDS virus was a tragic reminder of the lack of co-operation between the agency and gay groups at a time when concerted efforts could have saved a lot of lives.

The vast majority of recipients of tainted blood were never contacted by public health authorities. The Toronto-based HIV-T Group (Blood Transfused), in a survey of its members, found that only 5 out of 41 people (12 per cent) had been contacted as the result of a trace-back or look-back. Earlier research by Jack McDonald found that 26 of 97 infected persons (27 per cent) had been identified by official means. Just as important, half the cases had been discovered since 1990. Most had found out due to poor health, after blood tests for insurance purposes or because a spouse or child had died of the disease. Many were diagnosed only after their own deaths, and many more — an estimated 627 in the study by Dr. Rémis and Dr. Palmer — had likely been infected with HIV but had died of other causes.

Lynn Kampf, a nurse from Pickering, Ontario, was one of the people who finally got tested in July 1993. She had been transfused with two units of blood after an ectopic pregnancy more than twelve years earlier, and in recent years had suffered persistent flu-like symptoms. Married with three teenage children, she was not classified as a member of a high-risk group and never considered herself a person at risk of AIDS. Kampf can't understand why public warnings were issued promptly in numerous *causes célèbres* such as the Tylenol scare, and action taken promptly in others like the tainted-tuna scandal, but so little was done for transfusion patients. The veteran healthcare worker notes wryly that, for years after her transfusion, St. Michael's Hospital managed to contact her to ask for donations to their building fund, but they made no attempt to urge that she be tested for AIDS.

"Why? Why did things happen the way they did?" asks her husband, high school teacher Gabriel Kampf. "Where were the public advocates, the watchdogs of the public health system?

"It appears that everyone with a vested interest in the blood system didn't address the issues that were staring them in the face. They have obviously not acted in the best interests of the public. We believe there has been a breach of faith."

Gabe Kampf is particularly angry at the state of the trace-back and look-back system because, as a sexual partner, he was continually at risk, though he managed to escape infection. "We've lost eight or nine years of possible care, and I've lived my life in jeopardy. I would like to know who made the decision that my life was expendable."

10

MONEY CAN'T BUY ME LIFE
THE FIGHT FOR COMPENSATION

> Look to your health; and if you have it,
> praise God, and value it next to a good
> conscience; for health is the second
> blessing that we mortals are capable of;
> a blessing that money cannot buy.
>
> Isaak Walton
> *The Compleat Angler*

Garry Colley, Vancouver

As the only hemophiliac living on Vancouver Island for many years, Garry kept himself healthy by learning a lot about treatment, but says the authorities never provided any warning about factor concentrate being infected with the AIDS virus.

"*Forty-seven years of being in and out of hospitals, I know enough medicine to make a first-year resident blush. What I want to know before I die is how this was allowed to happen. . . .*

My future right now is pretty bleak. I expect my life will soon be terminated, but I'm going out kicking and scratching all the way. . . .

I want to make one last comment. I don't think we're going to solve the problem that caused tainted blood until we decide if our priority is people or money.

If budgets are going to rule our lives, then we're fodder. If caring for people is going to rule our lives, then budgets had better go out the window. We had better do something that is correct. If there is another infection, not just AIDS, but any other infection, it must be jumped on. We must think about the people who will be affected, jump on it promptly, and to hell with the cost."

(March 31, 1994)

THE FULL MOON HAD PASSED a couple of weeks earlier so the ward at Montreal Children's Hospital was no longer packed to bursting. The nurses remarked, only half in jest, that there was something in the moonbeams that made the bleeders bleed. It was worse in the fall, when the dampness gnawed at their joints and made them howl with pain. The nurses also knew that the last few days of hospitalization were the toughest time; a sure sign that the boys were recovering was when they became restless. On this day, September 8, 1964, the kids were particularly rambunctious, singing loudly and racing up and down the halls in their wheelchairs. Behind the stern words and scoldings, the nurses were secretly happy to see the young hemophiliacs getting a taste of childhood. They knew that the snippets of freedom were rare, that many of their charges wouldn't live to adulthood. Besides, the younger nurses shared the excitement. They knew it wasn't just full moon fever or relative good health that was at the root of the hyperactivity. It was Beatlemania.

No one was more excited by the news that the Beatles were coming to town than Randy Conners, the son of a soldier from the nearby military base at Longueuil. The 8-year-old, like many other hemophiliacs, often turned to music to help pass the countless days he spent confined to bed. Randy, who already knew all the words to the Fab Four's hits, had his ear glued to the transistor radio. In just a few hours John, Paul, George and Ringo would be right across the street at The Forum for their afternoon show. He would be able to climb up on a chair and peer out the window, across the park, when the limousine pulled up, just as he and his friends did when Jean Béliveau and his fellow Montreal Canadiens came to play.

The problem was that Randy wasn't recovering as well as many of his ward mates. He was a severe hemophiliac treated with transfusions of whole blood or plasma, and a spontaneous joint bleed could take weeks to heal sufficiently, so he was often excluded from the fun and games. As older boys like David Page fooled around, Randy watched the rain and lightning and played with his toy soldiers. Still, when all the pyjama-clad kids huddled around the big window, pointing excitedly at the crowd and crowing each time a big car was spotted, Randy fully expected to be part of the gang. But the nurses would have none of it. Despite his bitter protestations, Randy Conners was strapped to the bed. The technique was often used to hold children still during painful transfusions and aspirations (when fluid was removed with an oversized needle), or to immobilize them if they had particularly bad hemorrhages in their joints. But this day the leather straps seemed like an advanced form of torture inflicted on a boy whose only crime was a longing to fit in. As the tears streamed down Randy's face, the Beatles pulled up to the stage door of The Forum, then took to the stage. From across the street Randy could only hear the screams, and the distant din of music mingling with thunder. In his dreams that night he danced recklessly in the rain as they sang "Can't Buy Me Love".

Thirty years later, almost to the day, Randal Duane Conners was freed from the nightmare of AIDS through death. His loving wife, Janet, was at his side. During their short time in the public spotlight, this couple from Dartmouth, Nova Scotia, had changed the face of AIDS in Canada. Their plight had driven home the message that, left unchecked, the deadly disease spared no one. Randy Conners had been infected with HIV when he was transfused with blood products. Janet Conners, thirty-eight years old, had contracted the virus by making love with her husband, despite the fact that they practised "safe sex". That was something to which just about anyone, single or married, could relate. That they were a middle-class Maritime couple with a teenage son, concerned with the impact their illness would have on meeting their mortgage payments, made their story all the more poignant.

Shortly before his death, Randy Conners spoke of the Beatles incident as an event that had marked his life. While he repeatedly apologized for his faltering memory — a result of the dementia that is one of the most devastating symptoms of AIDS — he remembered the day in 1964 as if it were only yesterday. Like many hemophiliacs, he had spent a lifetime striving to escape being tied down by the disease. Cryoprecipitate freed him of the emergency room tether. He dropped out of high school to hitch-hike across Canada. Later he returned to school and became a computer programmer, landing a job with the federal government in Halifax. But his quest for a normal life, for a long, fruitful life like that of his colourful grandfather, the Reverend Hollis Kimball,[1] was cut short by AIDS.

*   *   *

The hemophiliacs' fight for compensation began quietly in the fall of 1985. There was much grumbling at the time about delays in testing blood donations for HIV, but the consequences of the foot-dragging really hit home in late October 1985, when a group of almost a hundred Canadian hemophiliacs attended a joint conference of the Canadian Hemophilia Society and the U.S. National Hemophilia Foundation in Houston. The Canadians were shocked by the ravages that AIDS had wrought on the U.S. hemophilia community. In the angry rap sessions they heard stories that left them stunned: the fact that medical journals had begun warning of the dangers of transfusion AIDS in 1982; the refusal of blood bankers to take preventive action despite warnings from U.S. public health officials that thousands could be infected; the rumours that pharmaceutical companies had imported contaminated blood from Haiti and Africa and used it to manufacture the concentrate they injected into their veins every day; the revelation that half of all hemophiliacs in North America were infected with AIDS and were going to die. Though many of the members of the delegation were infected, they had been led to believe that AIDS only killed homosexual men.

The Houston meeting not only frightened the Canadians, it also got some individuals talking openly about the disease they thought was their private shame, and galvanized their anger. Over the next two years a handful of activists resolved to find out what had really happened. They scoured the files and followed the detailed activities of blood system administrators over the years. The information, gathered into a single volume that stretched out to hundreds of pages, documented a scandal of staggering proportions. The volumes didn't originally have a title, but it became known as the Archival Study. [2] Members of the group realized that the procrastination over AIDS testing was not an isolated phenomenon; it was part of a pattern of inaction and neglect that had lasted for years and had caused them to be infected in large numbers. In fact, they estimated that as many as 1,500 hemophiliacs and transfusion recipients had contracted the AIDS virus.

The Archival Study, and the dozens of boxes of material from which it was culled, implicated public health officials in every province and territory, and pointed to stunning indifference among the country's ministers of health. That it remained on a shelf, collecting dust, for a number of years is an unsettling testament to the stigma of AIDS. Many hemophiliacs didn't want a public link made between the blood disorder and the "gay plague". Already, U.S. hemophiliacs were being barred from school and thrown out of Sunday school. Life was getting difficult for bleeders in Canada too; in Montreal, Niagara Falls, Winnipeg and Vancouver, parents were demanding that children infected with the AIDS virus be removed from schools; adult hemophiliacs found co-workers keeping their distance.

Besides, most hemophiliacs were forgiving to a fault. The Red Cross blood program, after all, was a lifeline to them. Virtually all had had their lives saved by blood transfusions, and their way of life transformed by new products like cryoprecipitate and factor concentrate. Many would say they could no more blame the Red Cross for giving them AIDS than they could blame their mothers for giving them a hereditary disease. The doctors and nurses who treated them were often like a second family.

Like most Canadians, hemophiliacs trusted their healthcare system implicitly. Accessible, free and state-controlled, it was universally admired. The volunteer blood system and the provision of drugs to people with hereditary diseases were examples of what made the medicare system so special.* The absence of the profit motive eliminated, in many people's minds, the risk of scandal, just as the lack of paid blood donors was said to prevent donations of contaminated blood. It was a comfort that federal and provincial health authorities accepted at face value the Red Cross argument that the contamination of blood products with the AIDS virus had been unavoidable. It was reassuring when the humanitarian agency said that Canada's blood system, already one of the best in the world, was even safer since the switch to heat-treated concentrate in July 1985 and the introduction of AIDS testing in November 1985. But now a vocal minority told a tale of betrayal at the highest levels — a possibility that many hemophiliacs simply refused to entertain.

Yet by 1987 everybody had friends who were getting sick. For many it was becoming impossible to work, just as it had been in the bad old days before home treatment. Some hemophiliacs were dying, and others were realizing that the talk of hemophiliacs simply being carriers of the virus was nothing more than wishful thinking. Users of factor concentrate wondered why they hadn't been more leery of the miracle product in the fridge, but they kept using it, clinging to the hope that the problem had been resolved. Then came news that seven hemophiliacs in western Canada had contracted the AIDS virus. All of them had been using Armour concentrate that was heat-treated to kill HIV. That meant no one was safe.

An unprecedented wave of panic swept through the hemophiliac community. Stories began popping up in the mainstream media, featuring familiar words of reassurance that seemed increasingly inappropriate alongside the facts. News that seven "virgin" hemophiliacs had joined the ranks of the infected cast all the claims about the inevitability of infections prior to the switch to heat treatment in a different light. Tough questions were asked.

It's important to note that the CHS, in its first thirty-five years of existence, had rarely behaved like a consumer group. Its primary focus was education. The group tried to inform doctors outside the three big cities about modern

---

* In the U.S., by contrast, it costs hemophiliacs about $25,000 to $500,000 a year to purchase factor concentrate, and most aren't eligible for insurance. A unit of blood transfused during surgery in a U.S. hospital costs about $125.

treatments for hemophiliacs, and politely lobbied government for practical improvements like comprehensive care centres. This was not a wasted effort; after all, as late as the 1980s some hospitals were still treating hemophiliacs with intravenous drips of fresh-frozen plasma instead of using cryoprecipitate and concentrate, not for the sake of safety, but out of ignorance. Major cities were still without hemophilia clinics more than three decades after the first opened in Montreal. Still, while the CHS continued to douse these brush fires, the AIDS epidemic was raging out of control. The CHS was a volunteer group; its leaders never railed and never denounced, and they always trusted the advice provided by medical professionals. More often than not, the group's newsletters were a conduit for conservative medical opinion and their own modest goals.

As AIDS moved unchecked through the community, the CHS made polite representations to the Red Cross and government regulators, but little else. When it asked for changes to blood policy, they inevitably mirrored the demands of its U.S. counterpart, the National Hemophilia Foundation — a group that was shamelessly aligned with major pharmaceutical companies. With no history of activism, and few resources in terms of money or scientific personnel, the CHS was at best a tame advocate.

When it became apparent that almost half of Canada's hemophiliacs were infected with the AIDS virus, and that many were already dying, the CHS had two major projects: the Million Dollar Club, aimed at creating a million-dollar fund to promote hemophilia research; and the computerization of comprehensive care clinics to better track the use of factor concentrate. (At the time, the Red Cross was lobbying governments to provide more money for research and development, and attempting to create its own nation-wide computer system.) Some hemophiliacs rebelled against this business-as-usual approach. At a meeting in Toronto during the first weekend in May 1987, a dozen or so hemophiliacs (half of them infected with HIV) who were in town for a board meeting got talking over dinner on Friday night.

The discussion was emotional and angry. The wine, and the tears, flowed freely. After hours of talking, the people found themselves holding hands and saying a silent prayer together. They formed a compensation committee to press governments to ease their suffering, with, as its main weapon, the Archival Study. Their determination was galvanized by the news the next day that Frank Schnabel, the man known as "Mr. Hemophilia", had died. David Page, who announced the news to the board, recalled how Schnabel, when people expressed surprise at the way he was wasting away, would say only, "Welcome to my nightmare." Until that weekend the word AIDS was almost never uttered by hemophiliacs. That would soon change. The organization Schnabel had founded was reborn; an era of activism began.

* * *

In November 1987, Robert O'Neill — chairman of the CHS task force on HIV and AIDS, and one of the authors of the Archival Study — made the first formal call for compensation. He did so after the founding meeting of the CHS committee, in Dartmouth, a stone's throw from Randy Conners's home. It was as good a place as any to begin a consultation with the membership, in order to determine their priorities in dealing with the AIDS crisis. The CHS also hired an accounting firm to put together a detailed actuarial study of the potential monetary losses incurred by AIDS sufferers. In February 1988 the Canadian Hemophilia Society put its request for compensation in writing to the Canadian Blood Committee. It fell flat, but two months later the Royal Society of Canada, a national academy whose object is to promote scientific learning and research, made the first public call for compensation, saying that the government had a legal obligation to aid recipients of tainted blood. The co-chairman of the Royal Society panel was Mr. Justice Horace Krever, who five years later would head the Commission of Inquiry on the Blood System in Canada; the project director for the Royal Society investigation was Dr. Maung Aye, who would later become director of the Red Cross Blood Transfusion Service.

In August 1988 the CHS sent a document entitled "Hemophilia Catastrophe Relief: An Urgent Request to the Government of Canada" to Jake Epp, the Minister of Health and Welfare. The executive summary read as follows:

> One thousand Canadians with hemophilia have been infected with the human immunodeficiency virus (HIV) from the use of government approved medical treatment. Their lives and the lives of their families have been totally thrown into disarray even though most of them have not yet felt the full impact of this terrible virus.
>
> This is a horrendous medical catastrophe, a colossal failure of the country's blood system. The system failed in four ways:
>
> 1) there was no national blood policy, and on several occasions when products were at risk, there was no national agency willing to take emergency action;

2) there was substantial wastage of Factor VIII from Canadian plasma, resulting in increased dependence on American blood products during the critical years of HIV transmission;

3) there were delays in implementing measures to protect the Canadian blood supply against the transmission of HIV;

4) there were inadequate and incomplete efforts to recall potentially harmful blood products from distribution.

The Canadian Hemophilia Society now seeks the support and compassion of the Government in order to help the 1,000 infected families maintain the quality of their lives to the extent that this is possible in the face of this tragedy. We believe the Government has the moral responsibility to do that, and for that reason: We respectfully urge the Government of Canada to act now to counteract the financial consequences of this catastrophe on hemophilia families:

1) by reimbursing HIV-infected hemophiliacs for the loss of their earnings while disabled and for out-of-pocket costs of their medical care;

2) by providing the families with adequate financial security upon the death of the infected person;

3) by providing all HIV-infected hemophiliacs with an adequate cash payment as relief for the pain and suffering they have endured and for the loss of enjoyment of life.

We ask that the Government respond swiftly and compassionately to help these people before they succumb to the disease. HIV-related illness has already devastated the lives of many of these people.

HIV-positive hemophiliacs are a clearly-defined and finite group. Scientific knowledge suggests that their numbers will not increase since the blood products used by hemophiliacs are considered safe. They deserve sympathy and compassion and must be entitled to financial support from the Government.

At the time the CHS forwarded its request to the minister, seven other countries had already established compensation plans for recipients of tainted blood. The actuarial study commissioned by the group put the total price tag on a Canadian "catastrophe relief" package at about $340 million. The initial request, however, did not call for lump-sum or equal payments. Rather, a complex formula was proposed covering three distinct areas:

1) Relief for loss of earnings due to infection with the AIDS virus.

First, a disability pension, geared to income, was requested, according to the following scale:

> 100 per cent of the first $5,000 annual income
> 75 per cent of the next $25,000
> 60 per cent of the next $30,000.

For infected people earning in excess of $60,000, a pension of 55 per cent was recommended, to a maximum of $5,000 monthly. For young people, it was suggested they become eligible for the benefits, based on the average wage in their age group, after their 18th birthday.

There was also a three-tiered request for medical costs not covered by medicare, such as nursing care at home and AIDS medications. The annual costs incurred by a person infected with AIDS were pegged at $34,000, compared to $11,000 for someone suffering from ARC [AIDS Related Complex], and $3,000 for a mildly symptomatic individual.

2) Financial security for the family after the death of the HIV-infected hemophiliac.

As survivor benefits, the CHS recommended spouses receive the disability pension for one year after the infected person's death, then a lifetime annuity equivalent to two-thirds of the pension. Children would receive five per cent of the pension until age 18.

Further, the government was asked to pay a $10,000 lump sum for funeral and related death expenses.

3) Compensation for pain and suffering, and loss of enjoyment of life.

The CHS asked for a $110,000 lump sum payment for all individuals infected by blood and blood products. This was proposed as a sort of life insurance equivalent because virtually no hemophiliacs had insurance due to the prohibitive cost of premiums.

For Randy Conners, who was thirty-two at that time and had a $38,000 annual salary, the proposed package would have resulted in a pension of $28,550 a year, plus $3,000 because he was mildly symptomatic at the time, and the $110,000 lump-sum payment. After his death, Janet Conners would have received a pension of $18,850 a year, and their son Gus would have had a meagre $1,425 annually to compensate for growing up without his dad. Notably, the initial package contained no provision for the compensation of spouses who had been infected, and none for children infected at birth. While the proposed benefits were modest, the total cost was high because the infected hemophiliacs were so young; almost 85 per cent of them were under age forty. Still, according to the CHS actuarial study, it would have cost the province $401,550 to provide financial relief for Randy Conners and his family, and less than half that amount in initial payments.

The request for compensation didn't get very far with the bureaucracy. The CHS couldn't even get a meeting with the minister to discuss the matter. Soon there was a federal election campaign; then, in November 1988, a new minister. The process had to start all over again.

On March 22, 1989, a 48-year-old Montreal hemophiliac held a press conference at the offices of the Quebec Civil Liberties Union. Claude Varin, looking gaunt and frail, told the assembled journalists that he was launching two lawsuits for more than $2 million in damages because he was infected with AIDS by Factor VIII blood concentrate. In one suit, filed in the Quebec Superior Court, he claimed that the manufacturer, Cutter Biological, and the distributor, the Canadian Red Cross Society, had been negligent in not providing sufficient warning about the dangers of the blood product. In the second lawsuit, filed in the Federal Court of Canada, he alleged that Health and Welfare Canada was negligent in approving the product for use in Canada, and for failing to order its withdrawal when the risks became evident. The lawsuits provided a summarized version of the explosive information in the Archival Study. David Page, the once-frequent hospital mate of Randy Conners who had grown up to become a teacher and vice-president of the Canadian Hemophilia Society, revealed that as many as 950 Canadian hemophiliacs were infected, and stressed the fact that the government refused to provide compensation. Varin said he would gladly drop his lawsuit if the authorities would apologize and provide him with a modest disability pension, a refrain that would be heard for many years to come. He also suggested that an inquiry would be a good idea, to find out how he and so many others had been infected with AIDS. "I'm not doing this for the money, but for other guys like me. You know, so it won't happen any more," Varin said, conscious that he would probably not live long enough to see the lawsuit settled.

By coincidence, the morning Varin's story appeared in the newspapers, health minister Perrin Beatty was scheduled to meet representatives of the CHS. He spent ninety minutes with the delegation, and almost immediately accepted the principle of financial assistance to recipients of tainted blood. But over the next few months government accountants and lawyers whittled away at the initial request. A lump-sum payment for "pain and suffering" was out of the question because it implied wrongdoing. The income replacement approach was also rejected; all the payments had to be equal, the bureaucrats decided, to avoid legal challenges under the Charter of Rights and Freedoms.

On December 14, 1989, Beatty announced a "humanitarian assistance" package for people infected with AIDS by blood or blood products. The government offered $120,000 tax free, over four years, to the victims. In return, they had to waive their right to sue the federal government. A fixed payment was preferred because it was much easier to administer, while the four-year term reflected the widely held view that the victims would all be dead soon, or so sick that they would be receiving some form of welfare or disability payment. The CHS had acknowledged as much in its actuarial study, which estimated that, by 1993, 500 hemophiliacs would be dead and 400 others afflicted with ARC. It was subsequently decided, again in response to lawsuits, that persons who had been infected during blood transfusions would also be included in the package. Health and Welfare Canada estimated that, in total, there were about 1,250 Canadians infected by AIDS-tainted blood. It was estimated that the Extraordinary Assistance Plan would cost Ottawa approximately $150 million. The program administrator was Greg Smith, a civil servant who had been involved in AIDS issues since the beginning. In fact, he had attended a meeting of the Ad Hoc AIDS Group, at the Red Cross, way back in December 1982, when the threat of blood-borne AIDS was first discussed, and he had been Health and Welfare's representative on the Royal Society panel on AIDS.

Beatty summarized the EAP as follows: "Our goal is two-fold: to ensure that public confidence in our blood supply remains high, and to provide a form of disaster relief to Canadians who are facing extraordinary hardship. With the assistance announced today, I believe we are responding in a way that expresses the fairness and compassion Canadians expect from their government, while recognizing the overall objective of fiscal responsibility."

Despite the soothing words, the minister was irked. The provinces, he knew, were largely responsible for the administration of the blood system, and they should be paying their share of compensation. Beatty had written to his provincial counterparts on August 25 and again on November 10. Just days before the announcement he met a delegation of health ministers to make one last pitch for a joint assistance package, but the provinces refused to join in. This was typical of what was wrong with Canada's blood system: thirteen governments could never agree on anything, so initiatives were half-completed, no matter how urgent or humanitarian. In a letter to the president of the CHS, Beatty wrote, "I have invited the provinces to do their part in responding to those needs in view of their role in the national blood supply system and I support the society's efforts for obtaining additional assistance from the provinces." In fact, Ottawa's plan had been to provide $120,000, the equivalent of the lump-sum payment for pain and suffering, while the provinces and territories would provide $260,000, a combination of a modest disability pension and a life-insurance payment to the victims.

Beatty refused to include the Red Cross in the waiver because it would absolve the provinces, who paid for the blood program, of financial responsibility. But the Red Cross had only $5 million in liability insurance, making its financial situation precarious. Worse yet, it was supposed to provide EAP claimants with information on the tainted blood they had received — information that could be used in lawsuits against the Red Cross itself, a violation of the agency's insurance policy. In the early months of 1990 senior officials at Health and Welfare tried to get the Canadian Hemophilia Society to include the Red Cross in the waiver, but it refused to do so unless the provinces came through with additional compensation.

On the surface, it seems unusual that a cash-strapped government would so readily agree to a $150-million payment, particularly as the story of the infection of hemophiliacs had hardly caused a ripple. There were a number of extenuating circumstances that contributed to the decision. The overriding concern, however, was financial. The Canadian Blood Committee, the federal-provincial body that was supposed to oversee blood policy, was an unincorporated and uninsured body, which meant that its legal liability was virtually unlimited. Faye E. Campbell, senior counsel in the legal services office of Health and Welfare, estimated that each lawsuit by a victim of tainted blood would cost $150,000 to defend, and that the average settlement would likely be $3 million. If the Department were to lose in litigation, the cost could be around $1 billion, she had warned months earlier.*

Apart from the money, the government couldn't afford the political consequences of a spate of lawsuits by hemophiliacs and transfusion patients who were dying of AIDS. The federal government had just hosted the Fifth International Conference on AIDS in Montreal, and it had been stung by criticism of its do-nothing approach. Furthermore, the Red Cross saved the state hundreds of millions of dollars a year by collecting blood on a volunteer, non-profit basis, and a Conservative minister wasn't going to suggest that it be

---

* February 3, 1989, memo from Greg Smith reporting on discussions with Campbell.

replaced by a government agency. Perrin Beatty's emphasis on maintaining confidence in the blood system reflected this concern. The Canadian blood system, as the CHS stated in its brief, was leaderless, so nothing prevented an ambitious new minister from taking charge and leaving his mark. Yet the deciding factor was Beatty himself. AIDS was a hot social-policy topic, and he was an ambitious minister. A genuinely compassionate individual, he was also convinced by the CHS that compensation was the right thing to do. It would take several more years before a provincial health minister would show the same concern.

Beatty's leadership role, as laudable as it was, served to underline an important but often overlooked aspect of the tainted-blood scandal. When a minister decided to act, the impact was almost immediate. But over the years countless persons in positions of power had failed to take action. Usually the most politically expedient approach to the problem of AIDS, and AIDS-contaminated blood in particular, was to do nothing. Luckily for the victims of tainted blood, the international AIDS conference had focused the world's attention not only on the disease but on Canada.

Prime Minister Brian Mulroney made his first public statement on the disease at the Montreal conference, on June 4, 1989, more than a decade after the epidemic hit Canada. "Having this illness neither diminishes people's humanity nor limits their rights. People with AIDS are entitled to our respect as well as to our compassion. Shunning people with AIDS or attaching stigmas to the illness obscures the existence of AIDS when precisely the opposite is required," he told more than 10,000 delegates at the opening ceremonies in the Palais des Congrès. "It is morally offensive, at the very least, to make persons with AIDS the outcasts of the twentieth century. It is also inhuman, the sort of blind ignorance which should make us thoroughly ashamed."

Throughout the speech, a small group of protesters from the activist group AIDS Coalition To Unleash Power (ACT-UP) stood in front of the stage where Mr. Mulroney was speaking, with their backs turned to him and their mouths gagged. At the end they booed loudly and chanted, "The whole world's watching, Mulroney, you've left us to die." They carried signs and wore T-shirts featuring the group's slogan: Silence=Death.

Less than three months after Mulroney's speech, the health ministers of Canada's provinces and territories met in St. John's. On the compensation issue, they decided to let Ottawa foot the bill and do nothing themselves. In fact, they struck a pact of silent solidarity. The idea was that, if no province bowed to the demands of the victims of tainted blood, none would have to offer apologies or compensation. The ministers and their advisors were convinced that there would be no political fallout. They were betting that the stigma of AIDS would keep the victims from making much of a fuss. Indeed, people like Randy Conners were disappointed with the compensation package, but they didn't want to be singled out in their communities as carriers of AIDS. Conners would take to calling his $30,000 annual cheques from Ottawa "shut-up-and-die" money.

*   *   *

Just two weeks after Mulroney spoke of the "blind ignorance which should make us thoroughly ashamed", and just weeks before the provincial health ministers would display it with their pact of silence, a baby girl was born at Ottawa's Civic Hospital. She was already infected with HIV.

The birth of Billie Jo Decarie, not too far from Parliament Hill, on June 19, 1989, marked the beginning of the second generation of Canada's tainted-blood scandal.

Billie Jo's mother, Johanne Guindon, had been infected by a transfusion of AIDS-contaminated blood just after the premature birth of her twins four years earlier, in August 1985. She had suffered a stroke and liver problems that required surgery; her treatment included 125 units of blood — concentrated red cells, fresh-frozen plasma, platelets, cryoprecipitate and twenty-nine units of Factor IX concentrate — over the next ten days. While virtually all blood banks in the U.S. had been testing donations for the AIDS virus since early April, Canada had decided that testing would not be fully implemented until November 1 — a decision that will ultimately cost Johanne and Billie Jo their lives.

One of the units of red cells Guindon received was infected with HIV, but the Red Cross didn't learn this until the donor returned to give blood again and tested positive. It would be eight months after surgery before Guindon learned that she had received tainted blood. Six months into her pregnancy with the twins, her first husband had left her. The recovery from the stroke had taken months, and hadn't been helped by the fact that she was now a single mother with two babies. But her life was turning around. She was still only twenty-six, and she had married a wonderful man, building contractor Bill Decarie; they were getting along famously. Joanna's biggest fear after her diagnosis was not her own health, but that Bill would leave her. Instead, they decided to face the formidable adversary, AIDS, together. Bill won custody of his three children from a previous marriage, and the family of eight settled in Rockland, Ontario.

After the diagnosis Johanne and Bill practised safe sex, but on occasion "we got carried away," she says. Sometimes a condom broke. They never worried about it too much because they were both healthy. Then, in the fall of 1988,

Johanne learned she was pregnant. After much soul-searching the couple, both Roman Catholic, decided against an abortion. Doctors told them the chance of the baby being infected was 50–50.* Because a baby shares the mother's anti-bodies for the first weeks of life, diagnosis of a newborn can be difficult. But at the age of six months Billie Jo contracted PCP, a sure sign of infection with HIV, and an illness that is often fatal.

Bill didn't get tested. With a wife and child at home infected with the AIDS virus, he just didn't want to know his status. In September 1992 the couple attended a retreat sponsored by the Canadian Hemophilia Society in Geneva Park, Ontario. More than three hundred people attended the seminar entitled "Coping As Couples". They talked a lot about their financial situation, the colossal drug bills and the fact that the federal compensation money was about to run out. Many had filed lawsuits against the province, the Red Cross and pharmaceutical companies. After the conference, where his new friends talked about the need for healthy living and early treatment, Bill decided to get tested for the HIV. The test came back pos-itive. He wasn't eligible for the federal EAP, nor was Billie Jo, because they were considered "secondarily infected". He and his wife decided to sue.

In October 1992, more than a decade after the Bureau of Biologics had first shown a passing interest in blood-borne AIDS, tainted blood became front-page news in Canada. A series of coincidences led to the media interest. Four senior members of France's blood system, including Dr. Michel Garretta, the head of the National Blood Transfusion Centre, were facing criminal charges for distributing AIDS-tainted blood products to hemophiliacs. U.S. tennis star Arthur Ashe announced that he was HIV-positive, the result of a transfusion a decade earlier. The Ontario College of Physicians and Surgeons found Dr. Stanley Bain guilty of professional misconduct in failing to tell Kenneth Pittman that he was dying of AIDS. In Calgary, Jack McDonald published his research revealing that fifty-five transfusion patients — including Johanne Decarie — had been infected with HIV during the eight-month delay in intro-ducing AIDS testing. He also estimated that there were more than 250 transfu-sion patients who were infected with HIV but didn't know it. Then *La Presse*, a Montreal newspaper, looking for a local angle on the French scandal, published some of the details of the Archival Study. Officials at the Canadian Hemophilia Society said matter-of-factly that Canada's tainted-blood scandal was just as bad as that in France.

---

* More recent research has found that about one child in three born of HIV-positive moth-ers contracts the virus. Seropositive women who take the drug AZT during pregnancy can reduce the risk of transmission to about 8 per cent.

The suggestion that hundreds of Canadians were infected with AIDS due to criminal malfeasance — a conclusion reached by a journalist, not the CHS — sparked a media frenzy. On November 5 the CHS called a press conference at its Montreal headquarters to clarify its position. "We have no indication, like in France, that some people knowingly distributed contaminated blood products, we have no such evidence," David Page, the vice-president, said that day. "We maintain that the crime was not one of commission, but a crime of omission. Governments failed to put in place safety procedures, and no one assumed leadership and exercised their responsibility of ensuring public health." Page said the group didn't particularly want a criminal investigation or public inquiry into the tragedy, it simply wanted the provinces to honour their initial promise of compensation, as Ottawa had done. "Our position is to demand compensation for those affected, and that we put this whole thing behind us. These people have lived years of difficulty and misery, and they want to live out the rest of their lives in peace and security."

*   *   *

In the fall of 1992, Randy Conners was in a severe depression, moping around the house and convinced he was going to die. Janet was angry, and the media coverage made her angrier. She walked into the bedroom and told Randy she was tired of his self-pity: "I don't believe you're as sick as everyone says you are. You're just wasting your life away. You're wasting our life. Get out of that bed and do something." Across the country, HIV-infected hemophiliacs had started telling their stories, demanding a public inquiry to shed light on the tragedy and emphasizing the fact that they had been abandoned by the government. Randy and Janet Conners decided to tell their story in a bid to draw attention to the compensation issue. They appeared on CBC Television in Halifax, in silhouette, calling themselves Jack and Jill. The story of how their ordinary life had gone tumbling out of control, broadcast on November 30, captured the public's imagination. The next day — World AIDS Day — the couple joined a group of activists who met with Nova Scotia's Minister of Health, George Moody. "I said to myself, this is my one chance, so I launched into it," Janet Conners says. "I told him: Mr. Minister, you may want to believe it's only homosexuals, but hemophiliacs and anyone who has ever had a blood transfusion could have AIDS." At a press conference after the meeting, the couple went public.

Randy and Janet Conners maintained a high public profile, and they had two more meetings with Moody in early 1993. At the third meeting they had their most intimate discussion, and Mrs. Conners wept as she told of their "ordinary fears" of being incapable of work, unable to afford drugs to ease their suffering, and losing their home. Moody asked for six weeks to come up with a solution, and he immediately wrote his provincial and territorial counterparts asking them to "revisit the issue of compensation to see if there can be a consensus." The other ministers were less than enthusiastic. But George Moody, like Perrin Beatty before him, was a man of his word. He decided that politics would not stand in the way of compassion.

During the six-week period, there were two important developments. On April 1, 1993, most infected hemophiliacs and transfusion recipients received their final cheques from the Extraordinary Assistance Plan. The majority had not, as expected, died during those four years. In fact, 321 had died; 655 were still alive. Randy Conners was among the living, but he was ill with PCP. With a provincial election imminent, the Conservatives couldn't afford to have a high-profile activist die while the government was paralysed by indecision. On April 14, George Moody, Janet Conners and Randy Conners summoned the press to Victoria General Hospital to announce that a settlement had been reached. Mr. Conners had to be wheeled to the press conference in a wheelchair. Moody said that the pact of inaction between the provincial and territorial ministers of health was untenable. "I think we all have to follow our conscience. I did this because I felt it was right. This isn't an issue of legal liability, it's an issue of compassion. These people should be able to live without having to beg to survive." The couple agreed to one special request by Moody, that the terms not be revealed until after the election.

The CHS had urged the couple not to accept an individual compensation offer, but instead to use their renown to push for a deal for all the victims. In fact, Nova Scotia's willingness to settle the matter put tremendous pressure on the other provinces and territories. Then, in May, the Commons Sub-Committee on Health Issues released the report of its investigation of the tainted-blood tragedy. It not only called for the provinces to reconsider their decision not to compensate, but recommended that the federal government extend the EAP beyond four years. A week after that report, federal health minister Benoît Bouchard bowed to pressure and agreed to call a full-scale public inquiry.

That announcement, more than anything else, made the provinces eager to resolve the outstanding claims. That summer the provincial health ministers began saying, one by one, that compensation was overdue: first Quebec, then Ontario, British Columbia and finally Alberta, which recommended that a deal be hashed out at the scheduled health ministers' conference in September. Everyone agreed to that except Quebec health minister Marc-Yvan Côté, who wanted to settle the issue quickly and cheaply. The Quebec chapter of the

CHS, like all other provincial chapters, approached the government with an updated version of the original 1988 request. They asked for $56 million for disability pensions, drug costs and funeral expenses; Côté offered a $10 million package that came with a means test and skewed payments towards children whose two parents died of transfusion AIDS (children with one parent secondarily infected received less). The association flatly rejected the offer.

Meanwhile, Randy and Janet Conners signed their contract with the province. It was Moody's last act as minister of health; his government was defeated. The deal, which was offered and accepted by all sixteen tainted-blood recipients in Nova Scotia, provided $30,000 a year for life, tax free, along with free prescription drugs. Children of the victims were entitled to four years of post-secondary education, all expenses paid. The province also agreed to provide a death benefit of $50,000, and $5,000 in funeral expenses. Recipients had to sign a waiver agreeing not to sue the province, and to share any awards against other parties, such as doctors, the Red Cross or pharmaceutical companies with the province.

Eligibility for provincial assistance was based on the victims having been accepted by the federal EAP. The order-in-council[3] that was passed soon after Beatty's announcement was straightforward: "HIV-infected blood or blood products recipient means a person who, in the opinion of the Minister on the basis of an independent medical review, received blood or blood products in Canada between 1978 and 1989 and became infected with the human immunodeficiency virus as a consequence." Over the years, bureaucrats administering the humanitarian assistance program had rejected sixty-nine applicants, most on the grounds that based "on the balance of probabilities" they had most likely contracted the AIDS virus in other ways. Some people who had received blood or blood products were refused compensation because they were homosexual (having tattoos or pierced ears was also considered to indicate ineligible risk), while others were turned down because they had also received blood products in the U.S. Only one case was appealed to federal court, and the claimant, Mario Landry of Montreal, died before his appeal was heard. What was sadly ironic was that, while blood system administrators had demanded 100 per cent proof that blood and blood products were contaminated with AIDS before acting, recipients of those products could be denied compensation many years later on the basis of a subjective "balance of probabilities".

By August the assistant deputy ministers of health had cobbled together a package that they presented to the provincial chapter presidents of the CHS at a stormy meeting at Sutton Place Hotel in Toronto. The offer paled in comparison to Nova Scotia's. It included $30,000 a year for a maximum of four years, and a

$50,000 lump-sum payment to a spouse and $10,000 to each child upon the victim's death. The offer was about one-third of what the CHS had asked for, and included a waiver that would force recipients to forgo any legal action against the provinces. It was rejected.

A month later, when the health ministers met in Edmonton, the offer had been increased markedly. The $30,000 annual payment was extended for life, and a $20,000 "signing bonus" was added. The payment to spouses was increased to $20,000 annually for four years after the death of the victim, and children were to be given $4,000 each year for the same period. But the waiver was also extended to include not only the provinces and territories (and their hospitals and doctors) but the Canadian Red Cross Society and eighteen insurance companies.[4] This was particularly irksome to the victims, many of whom singled out the humanitarian agency for blame — especially given the fact that the health ministers refused to say how much the Red Cross would contribute to the $139-million package.

After six years of battling the provinces, it was a bittersweet achievement. "This will never be a victory for us, never, because we've lost so much in terms of friends and in terms of the quality of our lives, things that can never be replaced by any amount of money," said John Plater, chairman of the Hemophilia Ontario committee that had lobbied for compensation. But the fight was far from over.

For the next three months, the bureaucrats tried to set up the administrative end of the Multi-Provincial-Territorial Assistance Program (MPTAP). The hold-up was that each recipient of the federal EAP had to fill out a form agreeing to release his or her file to the Canadian Blood Agency, which was charged with administering the MPTAP. But the delay — given that the tragedy had had its roots in delay — made victims furious, and they zeroed in on the shortcomings of the program. There were three major flaws. First and foremost was the absence of a subsidy for prescription drugs, which cost victims with full-blown AIDS about $20,000 annually. As well, about fifty "secondarily infected" victims across the country, like Bill and Billie Jo Decarie, received no payment for their own disease, just as they had not in the federal "humanitarian assistance" years earlier. Furthermore, the victims considered it incongruous that the provinces and territories kept insisting the offer was "compassionate" while continuing to demand a waiver of future legal action.

The CBA worked quietly in the back rooms to try to resolve these issues, but the provincial health ministers were intransigent. They were also growing impatient. In late November 1993, the deputy ministers of health of the provinces and territories put a new offer on the table. Since their previous offer, fifteen more victims had died. The "final offer" to the survivors contained two surprises. First, the compensation offered was increased modestly: the signing bonus was upped to $22,000 and the payments to spouses and children were extended to five years. The total program was now $151 million,[5] with the new money coming not from the provinces but from thirteen pharmaceutical companies, including the four largest (and their subsidiaries) whose blood products were used extensively in Canada — Connaught Laboratories Inc., Miles Laboratories Inc. (Cutter Biological), Baxter Travenol Laboratories Inc. (Hyland Therapeutics) and Armour Pharmaceuticals Ltd.[6] In return for $2,000 per victim up front, they were included in the waiver: cheap legal protection for a multinational company.[7] (In the U.S., the same pharmaceutical companies had offered hemophiliacs $20,000 U.S. to sign a similar waiver.) The second, and most unpleasant, surprise in the final offer was that it included a strict deadline for acceptance: March 15, 1994. The deadline, as calculated a manoeuvre as the health ministers' initial pact of inaction, was designed specifically to force victims to decide if the program was adequate before there was a judgment issued in a civil suit and, more important, before Mr. Justice Horace Krever could make any recommendations. (When the Commission of Inquiry had been announced in September 1993, an interim report had been expected by May 1994, and the final recommendations by the end of the year. When the provinces made their offer, however, testimony had not yet begun.)

The "take-it-or-leave-it" deal with its tight deadline was far from compassionate, and the "sign now and we'll hear the evidence later" approach showed blatant disrespect for the judicial process. Clearly, the provinces wanted the issue resolved before more incriminating evidence came to light at the public inquiry. They were trying to avoid litigation and the kind of scrutiny that could destroy political careers and bring down governments.

Victims knew they had little choice but to sign. The alternative — legal action — was just not practical for most. Numerous attempts at class actions had failed, and the deadline ensured that efforts to have a class-action suit filed under revised Ontario law would be fruitless. Most hemophiliacs, some of whom had used thousands of blood products during the 1978–85 period, couldn't pin down exactly when they had been infected, giving them little recourse in court.* And lawsuits were expensive, and much too slow, for people who were in most

---

* This is similar to the problem of prosecuting war criminals in recent years: evidence is difficult to verify. It's worth noting that many tainted-blood victims referred to the Krever inquiry as "Our Nuremberg".

cases poor and dying. Besides, the MPTAP, though modest, was sure money, and there were no precedents for winning such cases before the courts.

The first judgment in a civil suit didn't come until March 14, 1994 — the day before the deadline — when the Ontario Court of Justice issued its ruling on Rochelle Pittman's case. The award — in excess of $500,000 — looked good at first blush, but the fact that most of the liability was assigned to the doctor and hospital involved in the case, and that the judge largely absolved the Red Cross of responsibility on key issues, prompted most holdouts to accept the MPTAP. Still, the fact remains that the victims of a decade of indifference were, in a sense, given 24 hours to decide on financial arrangements that would affect the rest of their lives.

Another aspect of the waiver that got little attention was that it required the recipient's lawyer to sign a certificate attesting that the client was under no duress or pressure when signing the waiver. The Law Society of Upper Canada called the stipulation "entirely inappropriate, as a term of every one of these settlements, the requirement that lawyers certify a state of affairs which they will know, in most cases to be untrue." If dying of AIDS is not duress, what is?

Those who had begun lawsuits and then accepted the MPTAP found themselves saddled with thousands of dollars in legal fees. For example, of the $22,000 signing bonus, some had to pay $5,500 to their lawyer. Counsel Kenneth Arenson, for example, said he would take the same or more, on the annual payments. The fees left a number of victims embittered, and cost Arenson clients he had represented for years. The settlement didn't include any provision for paying legal expenses, though the court action had certainly helped force the hand of the government. In an unrelated legal action before the Supreme Court later in 1994, Red Cross lawyers would reveal that 160 recipients had taken legal action against the humanitarian agency; 103 accepted the MPTAP; only 15 "discontinued for other reasons", a euphemism for settling out of court. An integral part of all those cases — including the seven hemophiliacs infected by heat-treated Armour concentrate, and a smaller group who were infected in 1985, when the Red Cross was virtually without insurance — was a strict non-disclosure clause, though at least one of the tainted-blood victims settled for close to $3 million — the amount government lawyers had predicted years earlier the lawsuits could cost.

*   *   *

As the deadline for the MPTAP approached, Randy Conners was rushed back to Victoria General Hospital with pneumonia. His condition deteriorated so severely that doctors gave Janet a choice: Randy could be put on a respirator, from which he would probably never be removed, or he could be given a morphine drip to make his impending death less painful. Janet kissed Randy, she thought, for one last time. He smiled weakly and she chose the respirator. A few weeks later, Randy flew to Toronto and testified at the Commission of Inquiry. His testimony was barely audible, as his throat had been torn up by the respirator tube. He had trouble talking. But he wanted to tell his story for the record and, above all, he wanted to underline the injustice of the compensation program that had been imposed on other hemophiliacs. He denounced it as "shameful and disgraceful" because it failed to cover drug costs. To prove the point, he produced his own drug bills, which had been paid by the Nova Scotia government. For 1993 the bill was $21,475 — and that was before he got really sick. Janet Conners, one of only two infected spouses who received compensation as victims themselves, said the treatment of the secondarily infected was contemptible. "The package doesn't provide a decent level of care; it condemns people to die in poverty and suffering."

After their testimony, Randy and Janet Conners returned home to Dartmouth, a CBC camera crew in tow, determined to leave the limelight and enjoy the little time they had left together. But something always came up: funerals, rallies, new causes. When Nova Scotia premier John Savage announced that a $150-million fractionation plant would be built in Bedford, Janet Conners attended the ceremony and stood in silent protest. The obsession with building a plant in Canada so that governments could take credit for job creation had got a lot more attention over the years than the safety of blood products, and now, in the midst of a public inquiry to decide how the system could be reorganized to avoid new tragedies, the main players were starting their antics all over again.

As a boy, Randy had been shackled to a bed and denied his dream of seeing the Beatles. As a man who had spent a lifetime shaking off the constraints of disease, he refused to be tied down by AIDS. On Victoria Day 1994, for example, Randy celebrated his thirty-eighth birthday by travelling to Montreal for a concert by the rock group Pink Floyd. Aside from trips down to the local fishing hole, it would be his last outing.

In the summer Randy fell ill with another bout of pneumonia. Friends thought he would bounce back again, as he had already done seven times. But it was not to be.

At the end, Randy's voice was gone but his hollowed cheeks and pleading eyes spoke volumes. Hours before his death the TV cameras were there, recording the death-dance of palsy, wheezing and tears. He wasn't bound by convention, nor was he, like so many, shamed into silence by AIDS.

The very public suffering of Randy and Janet Conners was difficult to watch, particularly because they had touched so many. But that was what they chose. A conspiracy of silence had been the root cause of much of his suffering, and of that of another 1,200 victims of tainted blood, and Randy was determined to go, not silently, but kicking and screaming at the injustice of it all.

11

UNDER THE MICROSCOPE
INQUIRIES, LAWSUITS AND JUSTICE

There is nothing covered, that shall not be revealed;
and hid, that shall not be known.

Matthew 10:26

Erma Chapman, Winnipeg

Because AIDS is such a physically devastating illness, its psychological impact on other family members is often overlooked, Erma says. Her husband, Jim Smyth, is a hemophiliac who learned shortly after they were married that he was infected with the AIDS virus.

"I am not the person with hemophilia or HIV, so I have not been the person who matters in all this. Whether it was lack of information from the hemophilia treating team who knew my husband and I were trying to start a family, or assistance packages which disregard the need for family respite or recovery, or a health care system which expects a spouse to act as a parent/nurse/24-hour care giver, or even family who focus on the needs of the infected individual, the message has been consistent: I am the one who will live, I am not the one who is ill, so I have nothing to complain about. . . . .

The impact of my husband's infection has been devastating to my life. What remains is a profound sense of loss. HIV-AIDS is isolating. While others mark their years with children's birthdays, career progress and plans for a future together, I mark my life with CD4 counts [a marker for the progression of AIDS] and funerals.

*There are no children. My career is on hold until things are 'over' and I am plan-
ning what I will do when my husband is gone. My life waits for his to be over.*

*It is no surprise to me at all that, with the exception of a couple who married
recently, I am the only spouse left in Manitoba of a person with hemophilia and
HIV. The other women, with whom I forged a bond 10 years ago, are widowed, or
separated and getting on with their lives. They have already faced the loss of their
loved one. I continue to anticipate, with dread, the loss of mine."*

(*June 15, 1994*)

GRACE THOMPSON'S HAND TREMBLED as she scrawled the heartfelt note that
accompanied the large, multisided cardboard valentine she had constructed. It
was her first Valentine's Day without Sam. Her son had died a few months earlier of AIDS, at age thirteen, and the card was a tribute to him. The giant
blood-red hearts were decorated with mementoes of the child — class photos,
syringes for infusing concentrate, and stuffed toys — and Thompson clutched
them tightly as she waited for Mr. Justice Horace Krever to arrive for the first
day of the Commission of Inquiry hearings. She had travelled from Regina to
Toronto to deliver the accompanying note.

"They took my son and all I got was this inquiry. Please make it count,"
read the mother's valentine to the judge. After years of silent suffering, the
most profound wish of the victims of Canada's tainted-blood tragedy was that
the public be told how and why a thousand people had received a gift of death
instead of the "Gift of Life"[1]: "I could never give Sam any answers as to what
happened. I've seen a lot of people die and I feel like that's been forgotten.
Maybe we can give them some answers," Thompson says.

It was somehow fitting that the long-awaited hearings should start on
February 14, 1994. There had, after all, been so much heart-break and longing
throughout the whole saga. Yet Judge Krever, the one-man panel of inquiry,
was far from sentimental. He was obviously uncomfortable with Thompson's
valentine offering, and opened the proceedings with a stern warning that "this
is not and will not be a witch-hunt. I will make a finding of fact. It's up to others to decide what action is warranted."

The hemophiliacs and transfusion patients who were the victims of tainted
blood would soon learn that Judge Krever, despite his tough exterior, had his
heart in the right place. He vowed that all victims who wanted to testify would
have the opportunity to do so, and the commission travelled across the country

to be more accessible and visible. The long-time Ontario Supreme Court justice was also determined to take all the time and money necessary to get to the bottom of the story. Keeping his promise to listen to those whose concerns had so long been ignored was time-consuming, but it marked an important turning-point in the evolution of the tragedy; for those who had been affected by tainted blood, testifying was both cathartic and empowering. Day after day for the next ten months, people with AIDS and their family members, from teenagers to seniors, from raging to resigned, from the dying to those bursting with life, would step down from the witness stand with their heads held high, possessed of a new dignity — a dignity that was far more precious to them than any amount of compensation.[2]

If many viewed their testimony as an emancipation, it was because they had remained hidden so long, and the public inquiry had been a long time coming. The irony was that, in a tragedy exacerbated by bureaucratic foot-dragging and a ponderous decision-making process, nothing took longer for the administrators of Canada's blood system to agree on than how their actions would be investigated.

The first call for a public inquiry had come in a *Medical Post* editorial almost nine years earlier. The editorial said the delay in testing blood for the AIDS virus had been unacceptably long and, aside from being a scandal in itself, pointed to major structural problems in the country's blood system. This was hardly news; the Canadian Hematology Society had identified significant flaws in the organization of the blood system as early as 1972. *The Medical Post*, while concentrating on the testing issue, provided an accurate summary of the contributing factors in the tragedy, chief among them the "lack of urgency" in the official response to AIDS. The provinces, the editorial noted, could barely agree on dates for meetings, let alone serious matters; the federal health department showed a glaring "lack of leadership" while the Red Cross was guilty of complacency, of not "putting up a stiffer fight" against dawdling bureaucrats. *The Medical Post* was largely ignored by those in positions of power. Only the Canadian Society of Clinical Chemists — scientists who shared the view that the introduction of AIDS testing had taken far too long — called for a "high level review" of the delay.[3] The Ontario chapter of the Canadian Hemophilia Society, the most militant branch of the national organization, took up the call for an inquiry. But the national office of the CHS didn't want to draw attention to its infected members, not with the growing persecution of people with AIDS. It's worth noting that the CHS, like the Red Cross, received virtually all its funding from federal and provincial ministries of health.

The media also failed to recognize the implications of the AIDS virus having entered the blood supply. At the time the AIDS test was being phased in, journalists took at face value the assurances of the Red Cross that the infection rate was negligible and that the deaths of hemophiliacs and transfusion patients that had occurred had been inevitable. Only the feisty *Medical Post* tackled the issue.

Activist Ontario hemophiliacs, for their part, went underground. After their visit to the eye-opening joint conference of the Canadian Hemophilia Society and the U.S. National Hemophilia Foundation in Houston in October 1985, they turned their energies to documenting the tragedy and producing the Archival Study, and shifted their tactics from calls for public scrutiny towards compensation for the afflicted.

In 1985 the Canadian Bar Association investigated the legal implications of AIDS. The Red Cross official who appeared before the panel was Dr. John Derrick. The lawyers were shocked to hear him say that Canadians needn't worry too much about their blood system because of the voluntary nature of blood donation. The only Canadian users of blood products who were infected were hemophiliacs whose concentrate had come from the United States, he claimed. By the time the CBA report was published in April 1986, testing for the AIDS virus had already been implemented, and the law group singled out blood donation as an area where testing should be mandatory. It also emphasized the need to do contact tracing of HIV-positive donors and of recipients of blood, and the need for more public education. The CBA view was that existing laws allowed adequate resolution of lawsuits. The problem, of course, with trying to resolve public health issues before the courts is that the law imposes liability only on the basis of existing standards of care. More important, judges don't recommend improvements to avoid repetition of problems.

One of the earliest and most discreet investigations of the implications of tainted blood had come in 1985, when insurance companies for the Red Cross and Connaught had set out to determine their liability in lawsuits. By that time there had been a number of suits launched in the U.S. against the pharmaceutical companies that manufactured concentrate. Under special protection granted by Congress, blood banks were exempt from product liability claims; to sue a blood bank successfully in the U.S., a litigant had to demonstrate negligence. The situation was similar for the Canadian Red Cross, because product liability claims are difficult to pursue in Canada. Insurance company investigators, however, didn't like what they found, so in June 1985, when Connaught decided to build the new fractionation plant to produce heat-treated concentrate, it was unable to get insurance. Connaught asked the Red Cross to provide indemnification, but the society had had its own insurance woes; in a single year premiums jumped from $158,000 tp $1.4-million, so the charitable agency cancelled its insurance. Had it been an airline, it would have been shut down by regulators; being the Red Cross, it continued operating — without insurance and without restrictions. In theory it was "self-insured", but the agency wasn't setting aside money for the purpose.

In June 1987, Bud Sharpe, a mild hemophiliac who had likely been infected with AIDS during surgery, sued the Red Cross Blood Transfusion Service, the first person to do so.* In the next few months the infection of seven hemophiliacs in Alberta and British Columbia who had been using heat-treated concentrate prompted more lawsuits. Because all seven had tested negative for the AIDS virus early in the year, and had used products from only one company (Armour), they had strong legal cases. The seven civil suits were resolved quickly in out-of-court settlements, with the money coming from the "self-insurance" plan of the Canadian Blood Committee — that is to say, the provincial treasuries. These incidents, more than eighteen months after hemophiliacs had been assured that their products were AIDS-free, also prompted the Ontario branch of the CHS to call once again for a public inquiry. William Mindell, chairman of the group's medical, scientific and public health issues committee, wrote that the Armour incident and the "actions taken and not taken by the blood authorities in Canada raise serious questions about the management and decision-making processes involved in the vital blood supply system." The committee called for a public review by a "recognized uninvolved and unbiased authority" but got no response from the federal minister of health.

In 1987 the Royal Society's panel to study the AIDS question established four subcommittees to review the crisis: medical, epidemiological, research and legal-ethical. The latter committee made the first independent recommendation of compensation when its report *AIDS: A Perspective for Canadians* was released in early April 1988, but it didn't raise the subject of a public inquiry.

In 1989, when federal regulations reclassified blood as a drug under the terms of the Food and Drug Act, the legal situation changed dramatically. Previously, though products like factor concentrate had been regulated, components like red cells and platelets had been, for all intents and purposes, unregulated. As a result of the change, the Bureau of Biologics had to determine if the Red Cross should be licensed. One would assume that a manufacturer whose products had left more than a thousand people infected with a deadly disease, even accidentally, would be subject to particular scrutiny by regulatory officials, yet the bureau never conducted its own investigation of the tainted-blood

---

* There had been some lawsuits over infection with hepatitis over the years, but they had been settled for "nuisance amounts", token payments of a few thousand dollars.

tragedy. The federal regulator didn't even inspect all seventeen blood centres before it granted the licence. Instead, the Red Cross standard operating procedures in blood centres, including self-inspection, were adopted as federal regulations. The bureau never questioned the past or current safety of blood, never investigated the efficiency of the trace-back and look-back system, didn't examine the state of donor records. It granted licence number 183, for the collection and distribution of all blood in Canada, in May 1989, without question.

After the Extraordinary Assistance Plan was announced in December 1989 (including a waiver preventing legal action against the federal government, but no provision for an investigation of the tragedy, either internal or external), most of the lawsuits fell by the wayside. Ottawa's timing was good. Within months, a jury in Arizona awarded the family of a 5-year-old boy infected by blood concentrate a whopping $28.7 million U.S. ($37.5 million Canadian). Shortly after, a court in Australia, where the legal system is almost identical to Canada's and the blood system is comparable, awarded a woman who contracted AIDS during surgery $880,000 ($885,400 Canadian).

To the government's delight, the assistance plan attracted very little media attention. But because the provinces and the Red Cross hadn't agreed to compensate anyone, the threat of the issue exploding before the courts was very real. As hemophiliacs and transfusion patients pushed the provinces to come through with financial aid, they also began to demand a formal review of the tragedy. In September 1990, for example, a Saskatchewan woman, a mother of two who had been infected with AIDS by her hemophiliac husband, told the province's health minister she would drop her lawsuit if he would call for a national public inquiry.*

In 1991 the provinces and territories created the Canadian Blood Agency to replace the hapless Canadian Blood Committee. There were a number of reasons for the change: as an incorporated body the CBA, unlike the CBC, would have limited legal liability; as the costs of the blood program soared, the funders wanted more direct control over the Red Cross. The new agency, while it vowed not to repeat the errors of its predecessor, didn't undertake any formal investigation of them. The provinces wanted to forget their past mistakes. The victims of tainted blood wouldn't let them.

* * *

By 1991 some victims — mostly hemophiliacs — were finally going public with their stories. Some of the stigma surrounding AIDS had dissipated, but

---

* According to a September 14, 1990, briefing note from Albert Liston, assistant deputy minister of Health and Welfare, to federal health minister Perrin Beatty.

the victims' anger had not, and they were getting sicker. The big change was the growing number of former transfusion patients who were finding out that they too had been infected with the AIDS virus.

In January 1991, Toronto businessman Jerald Freise was contacted by his insurance agent and told that a policy he had applied for was being refused because his wife, Marlene, was infected with a contagious disease. She had been infected with the AIDS virus in November 1982, when she received a blood transfusion to treat anemia. The couple's world fell apart. Their greatest fear was that their three-year-old, Whitney, would also be infected. While Freise and his daughter both tested negative, the stress was unbearable. In 1991 the couple attended their first meeting of the HIV-T Support and Information Service,* and were shocked to find so many families in a similar situation. Freise, who in private enterprise had been accustomed to having his questions answered promptly and seeing people who failed in their responsibilities unceremoniously fired, was astonished to learn that no one had ever been held accountable for the tainted blood, and that virtually the same blood system remained in place a decade after AIDS had come to Canada.

Freise not only sued the Red Cross, the province and the hospital, but he became a tireless activist, forming the HIV-T Group (Blood Transfused). Unlike the hemophiliacs, who had for the most part been tested early, transfusion AIDS victims focused their efforts on notification issues like trace-back and look-back. To Mr. Freise and his group members, it seemed unconscionable that there could be hundreds of people who had been infected with AIDS during blood transfusions who were still unaware that they had ever been at risk.

* * *

The events of fall 1992 — the scandal over France's blood system, the review of Dr. Stanley Bain, the death of Arthur Ashe — brought the whole tainted-blood issue into the limelight. After the Canadian Hemophilia Society's press conference in November, a spirited debate took place among a group of reporters who were divided on the news value of tainted blood. One side felt it was an old story, one that had been covered adequately when AIDS testing was introduced in 1985, and again when the EAP had been announced in 1989. Others argued that it always bore repeating that a thousand Canadians had been infected with AIDS by blood and blood products. Besides, no one had really investigated how the whole disaster had unfolded.

---

* A service offered to transfusion AIDS victims by the Canadian Hemophilia Society.

Two weeks later, *The Globe and Mail* published a two-part series on Canada's tainted-blood tragedy. The first story focused on contaminated factor concentrate, the slow introduction of heat-treated products and the resulting plight of hemophiliacs. It featured the story of Claude Blanchard, a hemophiliac from Allardville, New Brunswick, whose three older brothers, François, Roger and Gérald, had all died of AIDS within six months of each other. Claude and his wife, Raymonde, were also infected with the virus, and the stress of the dreadful disease had destroyed the entire Blanchard family, both financially and emotionally. The second story told of the unwillingness of blood system administrators to screen donors at the outset of the epidemic, and examined the troublesome delays in the introduction of testing.

The articles in *The Globe and Mail* and *La Presse*, which coincided with the return of Parliament, did what the four hundred deaths from tainted blood had not: they brought the issue firmly into the political arena. Opposition members of Parliament demanded a full public inquiry. New Democrat Chris Axworthy, who had lobbied in the back rooms on behalf of a number of infected hemophiliacs and transfusion patients in his Saskatchewan constituency, led the charge in the House of Commons. The government, he said, "must face its responsibility to explore the valid questions surrounding this medical catastrophe." In an open letter, Axworthy urged the Minister of Health to "respond to the cries of an outraged nation" and call an inquiry into the "misdirected and mismanaged healthcare policies. How could the warning signs have been ignored so long?" he asked. "Is it possible that a health scare of this magnitude will happen again?" Dr. Rey Pagtakhan, the Liberal critic for Health and Welfare, focused his attention on the issue of compensation and called for the Standing Committee on Health and Welfare to "get to the bottom of this issue."

Health minister Benoît Bouchard, obviously uncomfortable with the questions, said he wasn't yet convinced that an inquiry was necessary. He repeated what his briefing notes told him, that there was nothing new in the information (true for the bureaucrats, not for the public), and that Ottawa had fulfilled its obligations to the victims with its compensation package (partially true, but ignoring the fact that the provinces had not). Bouchard also left unanswered the most important question: could a similar tragedy happen in the future?

George Weber, secretary-general of the Red Cross, said the agency was "willing to assist in an open examination of how decisions concerning the blood program are made in Canada", but insisted that a public inquiry wasn't the appropriate forum for "complex legal and medical issues". Weber also lashed out at *The Globe and Mail*, saying its in-depth articles "risk misleading the public into believing there is a safety problem right now in Canada. There isn't. Our blood system is one of the safest in the world." Rather than taking issue with the content of the articles, the secretary-general, who had headed the agency in 1984 and had had the final say on some of its most controversial decisions — the refusal to spend Red Cross money on testing, the policy of non-notification of recipients, the refusal to contribute to compensation and the staunch opposition to a public inquiry — attacked journalists for not being Red Cross boosters. "Screaming headlines like 'Tainted blood scandal' concern us because we have six million Canadians on our donor lists and a lot of financial donors that are crucial to our operation." Weber's response encapsulated the approach of the humanitarian agency during his reign: the interests of the Red Cross were paramount, even when they conflicted with the public interest. Keeping the blood system running smoothly served Canadians well in the short term, but in the long term the lack of openness and the unwillingness to change would be costly.

Even more telling was the fact that Bouchard called Weber, the head of the Red Cross, to offer his co-operation should the agency voluntarily undertake a review of events in the 1980s. Over the years the federal regulator had often deferred to the Red Cross on crucial issues like heat treatment of concentrate, introduction of testing and trace-back and look-back programs. Somewhere along the way, the ministry and its minister had lost sight of who was ultimately responsible for the safety of the nation's blood. In 1992, as in 1982, the Minister of Health was still deferring to an agency that was accountable to no one.

Dr. Stan Wilbee, a maverick Conservative MP and chairman of the Commons Sub-Committee on Health Issues, didn't share his boss's hands-off approach. One week after the *Globe and Mail* series, on November 26, 1992, the subcommittee opened hearings to "study HIV infected blood and other related matters", the first public examination of the tragedy. The first witness was Jerald Freise, whose HIV-T Group had called for a public inquiry the day before in Toronto. "The people before you have been sideswiped by a system where the driver has yet to come forward. As we have asked questions about the system and who is in charge, the sounds of doors closing in front of us have been deafening. It appears to us like a hit and run," he told the MPs. Freise was accompanied by his wife, Marlene, Rochelle Pittman and Pierre Desmarais, a 30-year-old Montreal man with a minor platelet deficiency who had been infected during elective surgery in May 1984, and who was telling his story publicly for the first time. The subcommittee heard testimony every Thursday for ten weeks — a total of thirty witnesses — just scratching the surface of the tainted-blood issue.

On May 18, 1993, *The Globe and Mail* published details of a leaked copy of the subcommittee's final report, including nine recommendations on three major topics: a public inquiry, compensation and trace-back. The four MPs[4] on the all-party subcommittee recommended a full-scale judicial inquiry; they suggested that the terms of reference be drafted by the federal, provincial and territorial ministers of health but that, if there was no quick consensus, Ottawa should proceed alone. They recommended that compensation to victims be increased and that a process be established "as a matter of urgency" to locate former transfusion patients who might be infected. The day the report was leaked, Bouchard again rejected the need for a public inquiry, saying, "It could last two, three, four years and be very expensive. I'm not sure the state of the system today demands that very, very strong approach." But during the next week, as media attention focused on the fact that hundreds of Canadians might be infected and unaware of their status, the health minister changed his mind.

Within hours of the official release of the subcommittee report, Bouchard announced there would indeed be a judicial inquiry. "I listened, I heard, and I learned that, for better or for worse, public confidence in the blood system has been profoundly shaken. When that happens, we must act," the minister said. The years of obfuscating, foot-dragging and denial were finally catching up with the administrators of the blood system. Donations had begun to drop, and the system itself was threatened.

The Red Cross, more than any other group, recognized the cost of the sudden media interest. George Weber had jetted off to be Secretary-General of the International Committee of the Red Cross and had been replaced by Douglas Lindores, a former mandarin with the Canadian International Development Agency who had long been involved with the Salvation Army and had served as an officer in the RCAF. His job was damage control, and the position of the humanitarian agency changed markedly. He not only welcomed the public inquiry but said the Red Cross would use the forum to recommend sweeping changes in the administration of the blood system. "The current blood system requires major change. We have come to the conclusion that something more than goodwill is needed, and the system must be fixed," he said. The Canadian Hemophilia Society had also, in the previous few months, become an ardent proponent of an inquiry, but the group's president, David Page, had been around long enough to realize that the federal health minister, despite his announcement, would face some major hurdles. "Please, no more foot-dragging. Action is long overdue," he said, worrying aloud that federal-provincial bickering would kill the inquiry before it got off the ground.

The fears were well founded. History showed that making a decision was difficult enough in Canada's leaderless blood system, but implementing it was a whole other matter. Once again, the culprits were the provincial ministers of health. For the next months, the senior bureaucrats of the provinces' health ministries used all manner of stalling tactics. The sad truth was that the ministers had no interest in having their prior actions, and inaction, scrutinized, because they knew that an inquiry would inevitably lead to a call for provincial compensation.

For the Canadian Hemophilia Society the issue was a monetary one for those already infected, but a public health matter for the new generation of hemophiliacs, who could finally expect to live normal lives. But the CHS had learned the hard way that negotiation was pointless without public pressure. They had already gone back to the files, dug up the Archival Study and fleshed it out with documents obtained under the federal Access to Information Act. Those revelations had embarrassed the federal government and garnered media attention, contributing to the inquiry being called. The ongoing lawsuit by Rochelle Pittman also kept the issue in the news. But the story that captured media and public attention in the summer of 1993 was compensation. With victims of tainted blood dying at a rate of three a week, the drama was being played out all across the country. When Nova Scotia agreed to compensate Randy and Janet Conners, the story became even more compelling.

In fact, news coverage of the tragedy grew at an exponential rate; *The Globe and Mail*, for example, ran 21 tainted-blood stories in 1992 and 111 in 1993. The visibility of the Red Cross — its symbol is synonymous with blood collection and transfusion in Canada — began to work against it as it became the scapegoat for all the failings of the blood system. The agency that could once do no wrong could suddenly do no right. Meanwhile, the federal regulator (the Bureau of Biologics), the Canadian Blood Agency and the provincial ministers of health went virtually unscrutinized. So in August 1993 the Red Cross hired Government Policy Consultants (GPC), a lobbying firm with impeccable Tory credentials. The two-year contract was worth up to $1 million, unprecedented for the penny-pinching organization and an indication that it felt it was literally fighting for its survival. Lindores said hiring GPC was necessary to counter the bad press the Red Cross was getting, and to shift attention to the other players. "I wouldn't say we are feeling overwhelmed, but we are feeling challenged," he said. Yet, for the victims, many of whom were convinced that their death sentence was due to the Red Cross's unwillingness to spend a few extra dollars to ensure their safety, the $1-million contract was salt on their wounds.

After Health Minister Benoît Bouchard was shuffled out of the cabinet post, his successor, Mary Collins, soon learned that getting the twelve provincial and territorial ministers of health to agree to anything was a chore. The provinces wanted a two-tier investigation: a judicial inquiry to look at past events, and an administrative inquiry to recommend reforms to the system. They didn't want an outside party suggesting changes to the system because they feared a loss of power, and a number of ministers wanted the judicial inquiry announced but then postponed indefinitely, until all the cases before the courts had been resolved. Victims wanted a more sweeping investigation under the terms of the Inquiries Act, which would give the commissioner the power to subpoena reluctant witnesses and give lawyers the right to cross-examine. More militant groups, like one in Quebec led by lawyer Guy-Henri Godin, wanted criminal prosecutions of senior blood system administrators, as in France. But above all the victims wanted the exercise to begin quickly. Jerald Freise summarized the frustration in having the health ministers draft the terms of reference among themselves. "Right now it looks like the foxes are controlling the hen house, the same foxes who raided the hen house in the first place."

The one balancing force was Collins. While she publicly professed patience, behind closed doors she twisted arms and threatened that the federal government would unilaterally call an inquiry. On September 15 she lost patience with her dithering provincial colleagues. In an interview with *The Globe and Mail*, she served notice that, like it or not, there would be a judicial inquiry. "I understand this will make some people nervous but we have to understand the events of the past in order to ensure something like this does not happen again," she said. The foresight was refreshing, and the timing of the comments was perfect; the next morning, provincial and territorial health ministers were meeting in Edmonton. It had been a full eighteen weeks since Bouchard's announcement, but the new federal minister was telling the provinces that the waiting was over.

The Edmonton meeting was an eventful gathering. On the first day the provincial and territorial ministers of health announced a $139-million compensation package. And on the second day they reluctantly agreed to give their support "in principle" to a public inquiry. The inquiry was to review all aspects of the blood system in Canada, past and present, including the mandate, organization, management, operations, financing and regulation of the system. The ministers stressed, however, that there would be no findings of fault, and that individuals would not be singled out. The inquiry was supposed to be completed within a year, and a paltry $2.5 million was budgeted, with Ottawa agreeing to pick up half the tab. Quebec refused to consent to the hearings; publicly the Quebec government argued that healthcare was strictly a provincial jurisdiction, but behind closed doors health minister Marc-Yvan Côté said he would agree to an internal review but didn't want provincial actions on trial.

The provinces, to say the least, were not enthusiastic about the prospect of an inquiry, and they immediately tried to make an end run around it, appointing a task force of their own members to review the roles of the Red Cross, the Canadian Blood Agency and the Bureau of Biologics. They gave themselves a ninety-day deadline in the hope that they could make their own changes to the system, to pre-empt any recommendations coming out of the federally sponsored process. Again territorialism and petty politics took precedence over vision.

*   *   *

Three weeks after the public announcement of the inquiry, Mr. Justice Horace Krever of the Ontario Court of Appeal was named to head the commission.[5] As a lecturer in a number of legal and medical faculties, with a strong background in AIDS-related issues and a reputation for being thorough and unsparing in his judgments, he was ideal for the job. Judge Krever had been co-chairman of the Royal Society's panel on AIDS from 1987 to 1988, and a member of the Royal Commission on the Confidentiality of Health Records between 1977 and 1980.[6] He had served as chairman of a committee on the Human Tissue Gift Act (which regulates the donation and use of organs but specifically exempts blood) from 1971 to 1975. Before that, as a lawyer in private practice, he had served on a three-member Ontario committee that examined the educational programs and regulation of more than fifty healthcare professions, so he was experienced in disentangling complex bureaucracies and seeing through turf battles. The committee's executive assistant back then had been Mary Collins, who now chose Judge Krever to get to the bottom of the tainted-blood tragedy. She remembered the Montreal-born lawyer as someone who rigorously studied issues and was never distracted by emotional or tangential matters. While not a crusader, he had revealed himself over the years as a jurist who appreciated the social implications of the law and medicine while remaining careful and conservative.

Given his experience with public hearings, Judge Krever also knew the importance of good support staff, and he hired two lawyers who had distinguished themselves in that forum. Marlys Edwardh had served as counsel on two of the country's most politically charged public inquiries of recent years: the 1990 Royal Commission on Donald Marshall Jr., which found that the Micmac native had been wrongfully convicted of murder by a racist justice system, and the 1987 Commission of Inquiry into the Facts of Allegations of Conflict of Interest Concerning the Honourable Sinclair M. Stevens, which had found that the former industry minister had violated conflict-of-interest rules. Edwardh had a reputation as a formidable courtroom lawyer, one whose incisive questioning could pin down the most elusive witness. Céline Lacerte Lamontagne was her mirror image, a quiet jurist who had published numerous works in legal and scientific journals. In 1988 she had served as counsel to the Gagnon Commission on allegations of sexual abuse of children at a Montreal psychiatric hospital. A francophone, Lamontagne would ensure that the commission could function publicly in both official languages. Because many of the underlying issues in the inquiry involved controversies of science and health administration, Judge Krever also appointed a scientific advisor. Dr. George Connell, a former president of the University of Toronto, was a distinguished scientist, a biochemist with a specialization in immunology. While he would be out of the spotlight, he would play a key role supervising the research and overseeing a management committee that studied the present-day safety of the Canadian blood supply. The inquiry also hired two retired RCMP officers as investigators. Their job was to locate witnesses, do preliminary interviews and ferret out documents. In fact, the most difficult task would turn out to be getting the provinces to surrender all the relevant documentation.

Even before the hearings got under way, Judge Krever warned that the mandate to table a report by September 1994 was unrealistic. "I do not intend to do this sloppily. I do not intend to do what, in the jargon of the street, is called 'quick and dirty'," he said. "If the time that is set out . . . proves to be unreasonable, as I quite frankly think it may well prove to be, I do not intend to sacrifice the quality in order to meet the time limit." In November 1993 the Commission of Inquiry on the Blood System in Canada made its first public appearance, at Ottawa's Congress Centre, where the Consensus Conference on Heat-Treated Factor VIII had been held eight years earlier.

While the first two days were reserved for examining a single technical issue — to determine which groups would be entitled to have their legal fees subsidized — it turned out to be an explosive beginning that would set the tone for the many months of hearings to come. To make the point that the voices of consumers of blood products were essential to the inquiry, CHS president David Page revealed that more than 3 million units of Factor IX blood concentrate imported by Immuno Canada Ltd. from UB Plasma in Germany had recently been withdrawn because they were manufactured with plasma that hadn't been tested for AIDS antibodies. The news, he charged, had been suppressed by the Bureau of Biologics and the Red Cross, who still chose to keep such matters hush-hush. In fact, just two weeks before, the bureau and the Red Cross had said publicly that no products made from untested stock at UB Plasma — a company that had vampire operations in Eastern Bloc countries like Romania — had been imported into Canada. (German health officials had shut down UB Plasma and senior management faced criminal charges.) The news that the potentially dangerous products had indeed entered the country, and that the system reacted slowly to the threat, served to underline the importance and timeliness of the inquiry. It also frightened users. Daniel Baribeau, the father of a young hemophiliac, was beside himself. His son, born in late

1986, had been using Immuno products all his life, and he had been assured time and time again that there was no danger. As a parent and a consumer Baribeau demanded answers, but he was faced with a lot of official shoulder-shrugging. "It's 1993 and everyone is still passing the buck, you still can't get any straight answers," he said.

On the second day, Judge Krever made news himself, making an unusual public plea to the federal cabinet to increase his budget. He had granted financial aid to seven groups representing victims and donors to cover their legal costs, even though his budget for intervenor funding was only $500,000; the Canadian Hemophilia Society alone estimated that a hundred days of hearings would cost it $750,000. Judge Krever also granted standing, which conferred the right to cross-examine witnesses and obtain documentation, to ten other interested parties. Most of them, including Health Canada, the provinces, the Canadian Blood Agency and the Red Cross, would also have their legal costs paid by taxpayers; only two players would attend the hearings at their own expense, Connaught Laboratories Inc. and Miles Inc. — the principal suppliers of factor concentrate in the 1980s.

The real hearings didn't begin until Valentine's Day 1994. Just days before he turned sixty-five — an age when many people retire — Judge Krever began the inquiry into Canada's worst preventable public health tragedy. It was, as one media commentator put it, a job that required the wisdom of Solomon and the patience of Job.*

---

* By the summer of 1995, the commission budget had been increased to $11.025 million and intervenor funding increased to $2.5 million. In addition, the Red Cross asked the Canadian Blood Agency for $10.5 million to pay its legal, technical and public relations costs.

<u>12</u>

GLOBAL CONNECTIONS
TAINTED BLOOD AROUND THE WORLD

The only thing necessary for the triumph of evil is for good men to do nothing.
Edmund Burke

Carole Brunet, Edmonton

Carole says her husband, Marcel, died a horrible, undignified death from AIDS, and she has decided to tell his story at the public inquiry to restore some of his dignity. Marcel had a car accident in March 1982 and was transfused with 12 units of blood to treat a severe nose bleed. Marcel died on July 4, 1992, less than two weeks after he was first tested for the AIDS virus.

"My husband would kill me for being here today. His mother worked for the Red Cross for 30 years. And his father, in the 1950s, was chairman of the board and medical director for one of the hospitals in the city (Misericordia). . . . I don't know who else can speak for me. I don't know if anybody will be listening in the end. There is nobody but me left to speak up for Marcel. I just want to know the truth. . . .

He asked to be taken off the life support system. The doctors refused. They told me that he had been given so much morphine that his judgment could not be trusted. So he refused any kind of pain killer for 24 hours, until they would listen to him. He couldn't talk. He used an Etch-A-Sketch. I had to beg three more doctors, then some poor schmuck of a cardiologist finally pulled the plug. . . . "

(April 22, 1994)

A DRIVING SUMMER RAIN FELL on the protesters sprawled in bloody puddles on the Paris courthouse steps like corpses, as lawyers and journalists rushed by hurriedly. Inside the Thirteenth Chamber of the Paris Court of Appeals, the judge was about to deliver sentence on four senior administrators of France's blood system who had been found guilty on criminal charges for actions and inaction that had contributed to thousands of hemophiliacs and transfusion patients being infected with the AIDS virus. But the rain, like the tears and the sentences, could only partially wash away the angry words that members of ACT-UP had scrawled in blood at the foot of the statue of Justice: "Tainted Blood: In France, you can murder with impunity."

The message would have surprised the four men on trial on July 13, 1993. They had already been discredited and vilified and now they stood, one by one, to hear their sentences. Dr. Robert Netter, former director of the National Health Laboratory, received a one-year suspended sentence for "failure to assist a person in danger". Jacques Roux, former director-general of the Ministry of Health, received a three-year suspended sentence on the same charge. Dr. Jean-Pierre Allain, director of research at the National Blood Transfusion Centre, received a four-year penalty, with two years suspended, on a fraud charge, "deception over basic product quality". Dr. Michel Garretta, former director of the transfusion centre, received the maximum sentence for the same charge, four years in prison. While France remains the only jurisdiction where public health officials have been tried for, and convicted of, failing to respond adequately to the threat of AIDS-tainted blood, the verdicts that made headlines around the world were strangely unsatisfying, raising more questions than answers.

The victims, like the convicted bureaucrats, knew that the four were fall guys, and that many misdeeds, notably those of the political bosses who had ultimately approved the crimes, would go unpunished. In fact, the principal line of defence was that the four were scapegoats for a system that had failed, not only in France, but internationally. "Why four? Why not thirty? Or three hundred on trial?" asked lawyer François-Xavier Charvet. "These are the sacrificial lambs of tainted blood." Charvet compared his principal client, Dr. Garretta, to another famous physician, Jean-Baptiste Denis, who in 1668 had been charged with murder after a patient died of an experimental blood transfusion, and centuries later was hailed as a persecuted genius.

The other major question prompted by the convictions was, if the same mistakes had been made, with slight variations, around the world, why had only the French criminal justice system responded? An estimated fifty thousand hemophiliacs and transfusion patients in the developed world were infected with the AIDS virus through tainted blood and blood products between 1980 and 1985. The epidemic of blood-borne AIDS first hit the United States in the early 1980s.[1] Countries like France and Canada, which both imported large quantities of factor concentrate from the U.S. and had gay communities with a small core of sexually active international travellers, were hit by the next wave of the epidemic, about eighteen months later. The French and the Canadian blood systems were also quite similar: the National Blood Transfusion Centre collected volunteer blood (donated mostly in hospitals and mobile clinics) and distributed blood products for much of the country, while regional centres did the same work in outlying areas. The National Health Laboratory was responsible for monitoring safety, just as the Bureau of Biologics was in Canada, and the whole system was overseen by the national Ministry of Health. (In France, unlike Canada, the regulatory body didn't have to contend with the problem of federal-provincial power struggles.)

If initial investigations of the tainted blood were non-existent in Canada, in France they were merely plodding, but in both cases the politicians didn't act until the story exploded in the media. An internal inquiry by the French Ministry of Health had begun in early 1988, around the time the government first considered compensation, but it was conducted strictly in private and with no sense of urgency. But an article in the magazine *L'Événement du jeudi* on April 25, 1991, by journalist Anne-Marie Casteret, which included sensational excerpts from the minutes of a meeting on May 29, 1985, at the National Blood Transfusion Centre, set off a chain reaction that speeded up the process considerably.

The minutes revealed Garretta telling senior officials of the transfusion centre that distribution of non-heat-treated blood products to hemophiliacs would continue until stocks were used up or until they were explicitly forbidden by law. He knew at the time that 6 in 1,000 donations were infected with the AIDS virus and that, as a result, virtually 100 per cent of factor concentrate was contaminated, but he chose to withhold that information from the hemophilia association and the Ministry of Health. Between that meeting in May and October 1, 1985, when non-heat-treated concentrate was outlawed, at least 16 million units of Factor VIII and Factor IX were distributed. When, in Garretta's words, "unfortunate publicity" made some hemophiliacs aware that heat-treated concentrate was safer, the complainers were given the new product and the concentrate they returned was reissued to others. In the end, more than 1,200 of France's 2,500 hemophiliacs were infected with the AIDS virus.

The infection rate among hemophiliacs in Canada (44 per cent) is almost identical to the rate in France (45 per cent) and, not coincidentally, the transition from non-heat-treated to heat-treated concentrate was remarkably similar, although Canada continued to import half its factor concentrate from the U.S. after France had banned the practice because the products were considered too risky. The only "positive" was that Canada made the switch to heat-treated slightly more quickly, in July 1985 rather than in October. But in both countries the motivation for delay was the same — to use up stock to save money. The Canadian health system saved less than $2 million; the French blood system saved almost $4 million.

The second aspect of the tainted-blood scandal in France, the one that led to the convictions for "failing to assist a person in danger", was the slow introduction of testing of blood. The approval of the Abbott test kit by the U.S. Food and Drug Administration in March 1985 was the talk of blood program administrators around the world. Abbott, trying to cash in on its discovery, asked for the product to be licensed in France. At first, health ministry officials stalled. Then, at a meeting of the National Health Laboratory in early May, a decision was made to delay approval of the American test kit until scientists at France's Pasteur Institute had developed their own test kit. On May 9, 1985, a committee of cabinet ministers decided approval of the Abbott test should be "withheld for a while". The decision was a mixture of economic protectionism, promoting local products over imported ones, and scientific pettiness, revenge of sorts for the U.S. having claimed discovery of the AIDS virus. Pasteur didn't have its test kit ready until the end of June and the Abbott test wasn't approved until a month later. In the interim there was no testing in France, not even of high-risk groups like gay men and hemophiliacs. Universal testing of donations followed relatively quickly, with all blood being tested by August 1, 1985. But because the AIDS infection rate was growing exponentially at the time, it's estimated that hundreds of France's 3,500 transfusion AIDS victims were infected between March and August. During that same period, in Britain — a country with a similar population, but one which instituted testing almost immediately — there were 75 new transfusion AIDS cases. In Canada the introduction of testing took seven months — even longer than in France — and the delay is known to have resulted in the infection of at least 55 transfusion recipients.

While the similarities in the responses of the two countries are shocking, there were additional elements to the French blood scandal that don't appear to have a parallel in Canada. Dr. Allain, for example, had conducted research on hemophiliacs as early as 1983 in which he studied the effects of various heat-treated and non-heat-treated concentrates. Yet even before that he had decided that a hemophiliac boy he had adopted would receive only heat-treated concentrate because it was safer.* There was also a level of financial impropriety at the National Blood Transfusion Centre: Dr. Garretta was a major shareholder in Haemonetics, a major supplier of concentrate, and funnelled more than $1 million to phony biotechnology companies that he controlled. In Canada, no individual appears to have profited personally, but the Red Cross invested blood program surpluses and scooped up hundreds of thousands of dollars in interest.

The principal difference between the Canadian and French situations is the seriousness with which the concerns of the victims have been investigated. Even before Casteret's revelations, the inspector-general of Health Affairs, Michel Lucas, had launched an internal investigation. He eventually worked for more than three years, along with four other inspectors, to gather evidence. In Canada, by contrast, the only government investigation conducted prior to media reports in November 1992 was the study of the Extraordinary Assistance Plan conducted by the Program Audit and Review Directorate that was completed in October; and investigators didn't even interview anyone outside the Department of Health and Welfare, for fear of drawing attention to the issue.

In both cases, the impetus to investigate the causes of the tragedy came from the victims themselves. Research for the Archival Study began in late 1985, and by the summer of 1987 some victims had initiated lawsuits. Yet five years later, when the story made headlines, there were still no results except for the dozen or so cases that had been settled out of court, whose terms were kept secret. In the summer of 1991, shortly after the death from AIDS of his older brother Barry, Winnipeg businessman Ed Kubin approached the RCMP and asked them to investigate the possibility of criminal charges against administrators of the blood system. Police investigators listened politely but dismissed the idea. In France, however, criminal prosecutions can easily be initiated by individuals. By coincidence, shortly after Kubin approached the RCMP in Winnipeg, formal charges were sworn against the senior blood system administrators in France. Edmond-Luc Henry, an accountant, had taken his concerns to the Gendarmerie in Paris three years earlier, and since then Colonel Jean-Louis Recordon, a senior investigator, had been working on the case. The facts he uncovered served as the basis for prosecution.

Curiously, the charges sworn by Henry didn't attract that much attention initially. Henry tried to have Dr. Garretta and Dr. Allain, along with three cabinet ministers and a host of other bureaucrats and administrators of the blood system, charged with manslaughter and poisoning. The legal action was considered

---

* John Wilson, a hemophiliac from Osgoode, Ontario, says that Dr. Roger Perrault, whom he had known since his days as an intern, warned him in early 1983 to avoid using concentrate, but he did not heed the casual advice.

too radical by victims and journalists alike, and he was widely dismissed as an eccentric. It wasn't until a judge ruled that there was enough evidence to send the four administrators to trial on lesser charges that the press and the afflicted came on board, and even then they worried about the impact on the system.

"I don't care who or how much it hurts," Henry said at the outset of the trial. "I want the world to know the wrong we have suffered. And I want those who betrayed us to be judged for their acts."

In the end, it hurt a lot. Due to the negative publicity, blood donations plummeted, causing severe shortages and forcing the cancellation of elective surgery for thousands of people.

But the good largely outweighed the bad. The criminal trial, while resulting in fairly light sentences for a few scapegoats, was cathartic for the victims. The process also led to a compensation package unmatched in the world, and to dramatic reform of the blood system that was the root of the problem. Aline Boyer, a Paris lawyer who represented the interests of HIV-positive transfusion patients, likened the trial to life-saving surgery. "There is only one way to remove a tumour, radical surgery. Without it, the tumour would still be spreading, we would still have a diseased system. Now the healing can begin."

Francis Graeve, honorary president of the French Association of Hemophiliacs, who was initially a proponent of a public inquiry but opposed to putting administrators on trial for the failure of the healthcare system, also came to feel that criminal charges were the best route to justice. "The prospect of jail tends to cure bureaucratic amnesia. You may be able to rationalize the deaths of others, but the fear of your own career and life being ruined — it focuses the mind." What Graeve and many others really wanted was to see the politicians stand trial. Members of the National Assembly have immunity from prosecution, but the political wrangling caused by "l'affaire du sang contaminé" almost resulted in criminal trials for three of the most senior cabinet ministers at the time of the lethal decision to delay AIDS testing. Prime Minister Laurent Fabius, health minister Edmond Hervé and social affairs minister Georgina Dufoix and their political aides were hauled before the courts in late 1992 on charges of "failure to assist a person in danger", after they agreed to waive their immunity. The case was dismissed for lack of evidence because cabinet secrecy prevented access to documents and blocked their testimony. But angry victims tried again in late 1994, bringing the much more serious charge of "conspiring to poison" against Fabius and senior aides.

A public relations gesture by Dufoix, in which she donated the first unit of blood to be tested for AIDS and then declared the blood system to be the safest in the world thanks to a made-in-France blood test, became symbolic of the political cynicism at the heart of the tainted-blood scandal. Years later she declared, "I feel responsible, but not guilty." Disgust over the treatment of hemophiliacs and transfusion patients contributed to the defeat of the country's Socialist government, a message to politicians that they would, ultimately, be held accountable for their acts.

So far, in Canada, only the Red Cross has suffered from the fallout of tainted blood. Donations of blood and money have dropped, and its image has suffered irreparable harm. Politicians and their bureaucrats, on the other hand, have escaped such scrutiny and punishment at the hands of the electorate. When the Commons Sub-Committee on Health Issues held its public hearings in 1993, Benoît Bouchard refused to appear before his fellow MPs. Similarly, not a single provincial minister of health testified at the Commission of Inquiry on the Blood System in Canada, and bureaucrats were so reluctant to surrender public documents that Judge Krever threatened to take legal action to pry the papers out of their hands. The ministers who drafted the terms of reference for the investigation of their own actions (a blatant conflict of interest) ordered that Judge Krever only make findings of fact, and that he not be allowed to apportion any blame.

In France, the most dramatic result of the criminal-civil prosecution (the French legal system allows both to proceed simultaneously, so when the four were convicted they were also ordered to pay damages) was a substantial increase in compensation to victims. In 1989, insurers for the pharmaceutical companies had offered hemophiliacs the equivalent of $25,000 each if they waived their right to sue. The next year, a court awarded almost $600,000 to Émilienne Courtellemont, a woman infected by transfusion AIDS after a traffic accident. In response, the French government offered HIV-infected hemophiliacs and transfusion patients about $75,000, while infected spouses and children were offered $25,000; insurers matched that offer.

After the charges were laid, the government quickly agreed to the establishment of an independent compensation tribunal. Its awards, based on actual losses of income, averaged almost $500,000 per infected person. The European Court of Human Rights condemned the French government for the slow claims process, ruling that, because the victims of tainted blood had a fatal disease, they were entitled to swift compensation. The European court ordered additional payments of $30,000 to each of the claimants. In the civil part of the trial of Dr. Garretta, the National Blood Transfusion Centre was ordered to pay $3 million to seventy hemophiliacs who had brought suit. (The French statute of limitations on fraud is three years, so only those on record as infected when the internal investigation began in 1988, less than three years after non-heat-treated concentrate was phased out, were eligible.) And there were other actions that made the compensation more just. France has universal healthcare but, unlike most Canadian provinces, it pays for experimental AIDS drugs, removing a major financial burden from victims. In order to cut its liability and to avoid future claims, the French government undertook the most thorough search of transfusion records of any country in the world. In December 1992, health minister Bernard Kouchner ordered that every patient who had received a transfusion between 1981 and 1985 be contacted and urged to get an AIDS test. The process uncovered dozens of former patients who didn't know they were infected.

One of the most important rulings, in terms of precedent, came from an administrative tribunal that ruled that the state, and more particularly the Ministry of Health, had failed in its duty to transfusion patients by failing to protect the blood supply adequately. About four hundred transfusion AIDS complainants (mostly people who were infected after a test was available but before testing was implemented) were awarded, on average, about $450,000 each. The Ministry of Health "has committed grave errors in the exercise of its functions as the health police," the tribunal concluded. "The breadth of this health catastrophe demanded that the distribution of contaminated blood and blood products be halted without delay and in an authoritative manner." The judgment was appealed but the French equivalent of the Federal Court of Canada upheld the principle underlying the decision: that bureaucrats can't hide behind the argument that they are powerless to act without the approval of their political bosses. "Some errors are so grave that they become the responsibility of the state at all levels," the court wrote.

*　　*　　*

Aside from France, the only country where the tainted-blood tragedy led to criminal charges against blood system administrators was Switzerland. (In Germany five senior employees of the company UB Plasma were charged with causing personal injury for failing to test blood adequately, a case that rippled over into Canada when Immuno concentrate was withdrawn in late 1993.) Dr. Alfred Hassig, director of the Red Cross central laboratory in Geneva, was charged with inflicting grievous bodily harm for allowing the use of possibly infected blood. In April 1985 part of a shipment of plasma sent to the U.S. for fractionation tested positive for the AIDS virus, but the Swiss Red Cross ignored the warning and continued to use and distribute untested and non-heat-treated concentrate for another twelve months. Then, after testing became mandatory in May 1986 (later than in any other Western country), the Red Cross failed to recall products from clinics and hospitals. The justification for inaction in Switzerland, as in Canada, was that there was little risk of contamination in a volunteer donor system. The result was sixty-eight infected hemophiliacs and almost two hundred transfusion-AIDS victims. What made the charges against Dr. Hassig — they are still before the courts — particularly shocking was that the Red Cross was such a powerful symbol of what was right about Swiss society. "This was done by our beautiful Red Cross, a national monument beyond suspicion," said Jacques Barillon, a lawyer representing several tainted blood recipients. "Distrusting the Swiss Red Cross was like saying that Mother Teresa starved children to death." Switzerland is also the only country in the world where a recipient of tainted blood has successfully sued the donor.

While France responded to the tainted-blood scandal after dramatic legal actions, there were countries that took pre-emptive action to avoid the ravages of blood-borne AIDS. These good news stories are rarely told, but they show that many of the deaths and much of the suffering were preventable. One shining example of a jurisdiction that acted swiftly and decisively was Belgium. Public health officials had the same access to information in medical journals as their counterparts in Canada, but they opted for a "better safe than sorry" approach. Belgium, like Canada, announced screening measures to eliminate donors from high-risk groups in early 1983, but the Belgium administrators didn't back off when there were protests; instead, they redoubled their efforts by winning the co-operation of the gay and African communities, and by conducting a general education campaign to urge gay men, intravenous drug users and visitors to Central Africa not to donate. The strategy was planned and carried out by the Belgian AIDS Commission, not the Belgian Red Cross. More important, the Belgian Ministry of Health made a decision in early 1983 to switch all hemophiliacs from concentrate to cryoprecipitate. They didn't wait for 100 per cent scientific proof that concentrate was contaminated, and they didn't draft priority lists; they changed treatments and they told the hemophiliacs why. The result is that only 19 of 291 hemophiliacs in Belgium (6.5 per cent of the total) contracted the AIDS virus. Among those infected, five used foreign concentrate and two had other AIDS risk factors; not a single sexual partner or child was infected.

Belgians, like Canadians, are fiercely proud of their volunteer donor system, but their approach to self-sufficiency was to ensure that all blood transfused in their hospitals had been collected in their country. This resulted in a negligible number of transfusion AIDS cases, and allowed an easy switch to cryoprecipitate. When a test became available, cryoprecipitate donors were tested immediately, more than five months before testing became mandatory, in August 1985. That spring, when heat-treated concentrate became available, the Belgian Red Cross destroyed its six-month supply of non-heat-treated products. Hemophiliacs weren't returned to concentrate until May 1986, by which time the benefits of heat treatment had been proven beyond a doubt. Until that time, cryoprecipitate was heat-treated, and non-heat-treated concentrate that was used — mostly in surgery and for travel — was made with locally collected plasma from a small pool of "blue-chip donors" who had no known risk factors. The absence of imported U.S. and European concentrate was a considerable factor in Belgium's low infection rate; it was not outlawed, but not Belgian Red Cross practice. Around the world there is a direct correlation between the percentage of factor concentrate imported from the U.S. and the infection rate of hemophiliacs. Belgium, which imported no U.S. products, has an infection rate of 7 per cent; in Spain, which imported 100 per cent of its factor concentrate, a staggering 90 per cent of hemophiliacs were infected; Canada imported half its concentrate, and 44 per cent of hemophiliacs contracted the deadly disease.

The final irony is that, although Canadian administrators dragged their feet in an effort to save money, the Belgian actions saved the state millions of dollars. Aggressive screening reduced the donor pool by about 10 per cent and the switch to cryoprecipitate required an increase of almost 25 per cent in plasma collection. The public, kept abreast of the AIDS problem, responded to make up the shortfall. A decade later, the small investment in safety is repaying itself many times over; the tainted-blood victims negotiated a modest compensation plan but government officials were able to argue convincingly that they took every precaution. Further, their actions prevented the infection of hundreds of hemophiliacs with AIDS, a disease that costs some $200,000 per victim to treat.

Similarly, in Sweden victims of tainted blood have not received state compensation. But hemophiliacs who contracted the AIDS virus from concentrate there were the first in the world to get help, because the state, under the threat of prosecution, forced the insurance companies for the pharmaceutical manufacturers to compensate them. Sweden also instituted an early and strict screening program to weed out blood from high-risk donors. The state, known for its liberalism, also began explicit AIDS education programs that warned about the risk of blood-borne AIDS. Like all the Scandinavian countries, it practised self-sufficiency in collection of plasma rather than in the production of concentrate — that is, it shipped off local plasma to be manufactured into concentrate in other countries. The result was an infection rate of 16 per cent among hemophiliacs. While they weren't specifically compensated for the tainted blood they'd received, the state provides generous disability pensions for all people with AIDS.

The experience in Belgium and Sweden shows that self-sufficiency in plasma production — as opposed to self-sufficiency in manufacturing, the route

Canada pursued — was a key to minimizing the ravages of blood-borne AIDS. An analysis of blood collection world-wide reveals that only 20 per cent of plasma was collected by volunteer agencies like the Canadian Red Cross, while almost three-quarters was collected for U.S. pharmaceutical companies, and much of it was purchased and resold by blood brokers — members of a multi-billion-dollar industry that was largely unregulated. Stocks of plasma were also (and continue to be) purchased from Third World vampire shops, where donors receive a fraction of the price they are paid in the U.S. Canada, despite the monopoly afforded the Red Cross, did not escape such blood. Faced with shortages provoked by its industrial failures, Connaught Laboratories increased its purchases of plasma on the open market as the AIDS crisis grew. In a letter published in *The British Medical Journal* in March 1985, Newcastle hemophiliac clinic director Dr. Peter Jones said plasma purchased in Africa was funnelled into the U.S. via Montreal and Zurich, then used in the production of factor concentrate. Thomas Hecht — president of Continental Pharma Cryosan Inc. of Montreal, one of the largest plasma brokers in North America — dismissed the theory that concentrates were infected by African plasma. "To the best of my knowledge, no African plasma has ever come into the United States or Canada," he said at the time.

Because of regulation by the U.S. Food and Drug Administration, plasma imported to the U.S. came almost exclusively from North and Central America, from countries like El Salvador, Belize, Colombia and Mexico. There was no doubt, however, that some of the plasma collected in AIDS flashpoints like Central Africa — as well as Haiti — went to European manufacturers. Those products were sold in Asia and parts of Europe, and may have made their way to North America. Although France banned the import of U.S. concentrate because of the danger of AIDS, it secretly imported plasma from vampire shops in Brazil and elsewhere to meet its production goals. There is increasing evidence, thanks to new genetic testing techniques, that the early infection of concentrate was due to plasma collected in Central Africa and Haiti.

*   *   *

Often forgotten in this international tragedy is the fate of hemophiliacs and transfusion patients in the developing world. While tens of thousands of recipients of blood and blood products in the developed world contracted the AIDS virus in the early to mid-eighties, the problem of blood-borne AIDS was virtually resolved in Western countries by the end of 1985. When France made mandatory both heat treatment of concentrate and testing of blood in the fall of 1985, the respected pharmaceutical company L'Institut Mérieux simply began exporting non-heat-treated and untested products to other countries. Even though it was known that the blood concentrates were likely infected with AIDS, they were sold to at least eleven foreign countries, including Saudi Arabia, Argentina, Italy, Greece and Iraq. A single export of fifty vials of Factor VIII (which could be one treatment for a hemophiliac in the West) left six patients infected with AIDS in Tunisia. In Japan, where more than half of the country's 4,000 hemophiliacs are infected, Green Cross Corporation, a giant pharmaceutical company, imported plasma from U.S. blood brokers while other manufacturers imported untested and non-heat-treated concentrates from the U.S. after they were deemed unacceptable by Americans. To this day, sales of blood and blood products remain unregulated, and domestic regulations often don't apply to exports.

Declan Murphy, former executive director of the Montreal-based World Federation of Hemophilia, has pointed out that stocks of concentrate "destroyed" in the developed world actually found their way onto the black market. In India, for example, non-heat-treated, untested concentrate that was manufactured in the U.S. could be purchased on the streets years after they had been outlawed in the West. Another fact conveniently overlooked, Murphy noted, is that the numbers and suffering of victims in the developed world pale in comparison to the situation in the developing world. "You can't dismiss the tragedy of tainted blood, but it's a tragedy of the rich. Eighty per cent of hemophiliacs in the world still have no access to treatment. They live their lives in constant pain, and they die at adulthood." In India alone there are 80,000 hemophiliacs, and only a handful are rich enough to pay for treatment. (A year of treatment with factor concentrate for a moderate hemophiliac costs about $80,000 U.S.; if the person has inhibitors,* which require more specialized products and frequent hospitalization, the cost can exceed $500,000.) Even in relatively affluent countries like El Salvador there are no blood concentrates and the average age of death of hemophiliacs is twenty-five — as it was in Canada four decades ago. As Murphy observed: "Here, some of the decisions taken by government to protect the blood supply were questionable. But many governments elsewhere simply allow people to die of the underlying deficiency."

Transfusion patients are only slightly better off. Many developing countries — including China, the world's most populous nation, and Zaïre, with the

---

* Inhibitors are antibodies that develop to the foreign clotting factor. They not only render concentrate useless but can eat away at a hemophiliac's natural clotting factor, becoming life-threatening.

highest AIDS infection rate in the world — still don't screen blood for AIDS antibodies. In China almost 20 per cent of transfusion recipients contract hepatitis, an indication that a tainted-blood tragedy of unparalleled proportions could be on the horizon. Horror stories are only now beginning to emerge from Eastern Bloc countries. In Romania 2,376 orphans who were treated routinely with blood transfusions are known to have been infected with AIDS while in post-Communist Russia the blood trade is unregulated and unscrupulous. In Kenya, where family members are responsible for donating blood to relatives, entire families have been wiped out, while in Uganda paid blood collection has attracted some of the sickest and most desperate. The only mitigating factor is that, in some developing countries, many of the blood components used in hospitals are donated by the International Committee of the Red Cross, whose policy is to screen donations.

In the industrialized world, the tainted-blood scandal seems to have run its course — as far as AIDS is concerned. Hundreds of millions of dollars have been paid in state compensation, tens of millions more to settle civil lawsuits, and a handful of public health officials have gone to jail. But one can question whether the lessons have really been learned. The extent of blood-borne hepatitis-C infections is only now beginning to emerge; there were many more than AIDS, and they continued into the nineties. If some sinister new virus slips into the blood supply a few years hence, will administrators act decisively? Or will they once again wait and see? It is not clear that Western blood agencies have reformed themselves sufficiently to be ready for the next AIDS. And none of the knowledge about the need for early and decisive action to prevent blood-borne epidemics has been exported to the developing world, where the World Health Organization estimates that there may be as many as 1 million transfusion AIDS cases.

13

CALL TO ACTION
REBUILDING THE SYSTEM

Where there is no vision, the people perish.

Proverbs 29:18

Rita Marche, West Bay Centre, Newfoundland

One of the worst symptoms of AIDS, Rita says, is the stigma and the related isolation it causes. She learned her son Justin, a hemophiliac, was infected with the AIDS virus in the fall of 1985 when he was 12. Justin died in January 1992, but not before suffering dementia alongside a host of other diseases. Despite his multitude of problems, Justin was treated with the utmost respect by the care-givers at Western Memorial Hospital in Corner Brook, Rita says, allowing him to die with dignity.

"His friends never came to see him, never once in the hospital, never sent a card, nothing. . . .

I have nothing but praise for the medical staff, from the nursing supervisor down to every one of the personal care attendants who worked with my son. They treated him like he was their own son. They attended his funeral. He had no more friends, so they were the pallbearers. They made me feel like I had some control over my life again."

(August 19, 1994)

WHEN I FIRST INVESTIGATED the tainted-blood scandal for *The Globe and Mail*, my colleague Rod Mickleburgh and I were shocked by the breadth of the tragedy. Tainted blood was the worst public health disaster since the influenza epidemic that followed the First World War. The early stories touched on all the major contributing factors, and concluded that the root cause of the deaths of 1,200 Canadians was a painfully complex decision-making structure adminis-tered by foot-dragging bureaucrats. In brief, the system was sorrily lacking in leadership, a situation summed up eloquently by public health official William Mindell: "What we needed was a Winston Churchill. What we got was a lot of Neville Chamberlains." All the major players — the federal and provincial health ministries, the Red Cross, the Canadian Blood Committee, even the Canadian Hemophilia Society — acknowledged that the response to AIDS was indeed slow but argued that very little was known about AIDS at the time, so it was unfair to judge them in hindsight. No need to dwell on the past, they insisted, because things are different now. "Today, Canada has one of the safest blood systems in the world," was the refrain.

The argument that "we didn't know how bad AIDS would be" is, on the surface, compelling. But digging into the records, immersing yourself in the debates and scientific knowledge of the time, as the thorough documentary work done by the researchers for the Commission of Inquiry on the Blood System in Canada allows, quickly reveals that the ignorance defence doesn't hold much water. By mid-1982, public health officials in the United States and Canada had important clues that AIDS was transmitted by blood in a similar, if not identical, manner to hepatitis B. By the end of that year they knew that users of blood products were in danger of infection.

Because the contamination of the Canadian blood system lagged behind that in the U.S. by some eighteen months, for various reasons, the problem was almost entirely preventable in this country. Even if we accept that severe hemophiliacs, because of their early and heavy reliance on blood concentrate manufactured with U.S. source plasma, were doomed from the outset, it remains that eight or nine hundred AIDS-related deaths could have been avoided had public health officials demonstrated a little foresight and leadership. What they practised instead was a pattern of behaviour best described as "malicious inertia".[1]

Time and time again, strategies were proposed by various consumer and medical groups to minimize risks and save lives: stringent screening of donors, switching hemophiliacs from concentrate back to cryoprecipitate, collecting blood from women only and reducing the number of transfusions during surgery, to name only a few. Yet the powers-that-be argued that scientific proof of AIDS being transmitted by blood was lacking; and when incontrovertible proof was offered up, the argument quickly switched to resignation: hemophiliacs are already infected, so there's no need to rush in safer products. The chosen course was "business as usual", and consumers were kept in the dark about risks; stocks of concentrate that, without a shadow of a doubt, were contaminated were used up rather than destroyed. If that were not enough, when the time came to lend a helping hand to those who were infected, many politicians and bureaucrats redoubled their obstinacy, refusing to compensate victims and balking at calls for public health campaigns to locate the infected. This not only exacerbated the suffering of those infected with AIDS by blood, but led to the deadly disease being passed on to lovers, spouses and children — a whole new level of needless death.

Sadly, the chief reason that this ongoing abdication of responsibility was tolerated, or at least unchallenged, by bureaucrats, public health officials and politicians alike, was homophobia. Health officials reacted swiftly to adulterated Tylenol, tainted tuna, Legionnaire's disease, even ersatz Cabbage Patch dolls, but when it came to tainted blood and blood products they demanded more proof that they should spend money — more proof that AIDS was a threat to "normal" people. At a time when Canada was adapting to a new Charter of Rights and Freedoms, respect and rights were being denied those threatened by or infected with AIDS because it was viewed as a "gay disease". That people were relegated to second-class status because of the social origins of their disease is perhaps our greatest and most lasting shame. Diseases discriminate, but a public health system worthy of its name should not.

As a journalist I am expected to be objective, to tell both sides of a story — or however many sides there are — without passing judgment. That was easy at the beginning. But the more I learned, the more I became convinced, based on the evidence available at the time, that there was an ideological commitment to a wrong view — to the scientifically untenable argument that AIDS was a one-in-a-million risk, a negligible concern — that served the vested political and economic interests of the main players. I'm not suggesting that any one person was a criminal or that any institution was monstrously negligent, but the leaderless blood system allowed them all to wear blinkers, to conspire to neglect. By clinging to the false premise that AIDS wasn't really a problem, everyone could easily defend a business-as-usual approach: the regulator, the federal Bureau of Biologics, avoided a nasty confrontation with the Red Cross and the provinces; the Red Cross, the collector and distributor of blood, didn't have to change its way of doing business or approach penny-pinching governments for more money; the provinces, through their agency, the Canadian Blood Committee, could pursue their foolish goal of building fractionation plants as a job-creation tool. Only the consumers of blood and blood products were left out of the equation; this systematic contempt for the public was ultimately the reason we now have thousands of victims of tainted blood.

The knowledge that what occurred over the years wasn't merely a tragedy but, in large part, a scandal, has compelled me to go beyond the normal bounds of journalism, to advocacy. Too few lessons have been learned, and the result is that the tragedy of tainted blood could be repeated. The catchphrase of the 1980s, "AIDS is a one-in-a-million risk," has given way to an equally dismissive cliché for the 1990s: "We have one of the safest blood systems in the world."

Safe, yes, but ill prepared for the next threat, and unworthy of our faith. The blood system, as it exists, is outdated, unresponsive, patronizing and profoundly undemocratic.

*　　*　　*

The structure of Canada's blood system, as a group of angry hemophiliacs noted years ago in the Archival Study, is best compared to a "hydra, none of whose heads are connected to the others", and a Herculean effort will be required to tame the beast. The system can only be reformed through the consensus of thirteen ministers of health, and after an initial *mea culpa*, the danger is that the politicians will fall back on their deplorable habit of implementing half-measures. That is precisely the indication that came out of the Ministers' Review, the "quickie exercise" in 1994 that was designed to circumvent and undermine the public inquiry process. In that review, the ministers decided the blood system should remain more or less the same, and that all that was needed was a contract between the Red Cross and the Canadian Blood Agency. In April 1995, the Red Cross and the CBA accordingly signed a "Master Agreement" that clarified the financial arrangements between the provinces and the humanitarian agency — instead of block funding, the CBA will now pay for blood products on a per unit basis. The all-important leadership question remains up in the air. The Red Cross continues as "preferred supplier", effectively the sole agency for collecting and testing blood, the manufacture of blood products and their distribution to healthcare institutions. Both parties claim that safety will be improved by the arrangement, but the proof that the leadership vacuum continues can be found in Red Cross plans to build a fractionation plant, in open defiance of the CBA and the ministers of health, and consumers of blood products, all of whom have spoken out against the plans.

William Dobson, executive director of the Canadian Blood Agency, neatly summed up the process that resulted in the Master Agreement: "The arrangement is the best we can make given the frame we have to paint in. We were not given authority to remove the Red Cross or set up something different than existed originally." It is precisely this lack of imagination, this stubborn refusal to correct the flaws of the system itself, that exacerbated the tainted-blood tragedy of the 1980s.

The reality is that the Red Cross wants to work directly for the provinces and see the CBA eliminated from the picture. The CBA, for its part, imagines a landscape in which the Red Cross is clearly subservient to it, just one of a number of suppliers. Either option would be a slight improvement on the current system, but neither is the answer. The choices at hand are difficult ones, and they require singlemindedness and backbone — something the country's health ministers have shown a sorry lack of over the years. The response to hepatitis C — notably the refusal to introduce surrogate testing and failure to warn transfusion recipients of the risks both before and after testing began in May 1990 — was no better than the one to AIDS. Ultimately, more people will die of blood-borne hepatitis C than AIDS, and there is every indication that the next viral threat will be handled no better. There is no excuse to wait for hundreds or thousands more deaths before taking action. It's time to wipe the slate clean and design a new blood system, from the bottom up.

The Red Cross, naturally, is at the heart of the issue. Its charitable works have been remarkable in times of war and times of peace, and its Blood Transfusion Service is among its proudest achievements — a service that has provided a Gift of Life to millions of Canadians. But in the half century since the Red Cross began collecting and distributing blood, the nature of the relationship between the state and the humanitarian agency, between donors and recipients, has never been seriously re-examined.

Dr. Patrick Moore, who opened the first BTS centre in Vancouver in 1947, believes the Red Cross has strayed far from its original mandate. Blood plasma was desperately needed during the Second World War, and in the pre-medicare days, when major surgery could easily cost a year's salary. Back then, Red Cross volunteers worked alongside nuns in ministering to the sick. With the advent of medicare, charitable and religious organizations were eased out of the system, along with fee-for-service doctors. Though no one ever suggested that their work wasn't valuable and appreciated, times had changed, and the healthcare system evolved. Only the Red Cross remained as a bizarre anomaly, collecting blood as a charitable act (though increasingly subsidized by government) in a professional, state-controlled public health network. "You wouldn't think of giving medicare to the Kinsmen or Rotary clubs to operate," observes Dr. Raymond Guévin, medical director of the Montreal BTS centre from 1962 to 1984. And if you were building a blood system from scratch, you wouldn't put the Red Cross in charge of it.

Blood collection, fractionation and distribution is no longer a charitable activity; it's big business, at the cutting edge of science. The Red Cross, to its credit, recognizes this, and has been working in recent years to reinvent itself into a modern manufacturer. The New York Blood Center, an independent, not-for-profit blood bank with its own blood fractionation facilities, regulated by U.S. federal health authorities, is serving as the model for this reform.

The problem with the change in approach is twofold. First and foremost is the fact that, unlike the Canadian Red Cross, the New York Blood Center doesn't have a monopoly; not-for-profit blood banks in the U.S., which collect whole blood from volunteer donors but pay for plasma and sell its by-products to underwrite their charitable activities, operate within a system entirely different from Canada's state-controlled medicare system. Secondly, it's already odd enough to have the provinces paying a charity hundreds of millions of dollars annually to administer a cornerstone of the country's healthcare system; doing the same with a *de facto* private enterprise trading in blood is all the more dubious.

The underlying question, which the provinces and the Red Cross have too long avoided, is: do Canadians want a private or a public blood system? This, of course, is part and parcel of a much larger debate on state financing of the healthcare system. But regardless of one's view of the larger question, there should be general agreement that some services are so fundamental that they shouldn't be commercialized. Allowing private enterprise to operate a medical clinic is one thing; allowing it to trade in the blood of Canadians is quite another, just one step away from the trade in body parts.

Further, even if privatizing the blood system in whole or in part is the chosen option, it shouldn't be done through the back door, without public debate or assent, as is currently happening with the silent approbation of the provincial health ministers. This is an affront to Canadians. Equally unacceptable is the current system of contracting out blood services to a charitable organization neither accountable nor open to scrutiny the way an organization receiving more than $225 million a year in government money should be.

The time has come for the Red Cross to get out of the blood business, not as punishment for its failures in the recent tragedy — overall, it performed no better and no worse than public health authorities — but because it's time to create a blood system that better reflects the needs, concerns and philosophy of Canadians.

"To reach the people most in need of them, the Red Cross must have the courage to take its health services to the remotest frontier areas," Dr. Stuart Stanbury, the founder of the Red Cross blood service, wrote in the agency's 1961 annual report, the last one before his death. "Each program must be built according to the highest professional and technical specifications, but the Society must not hesitate to surrender its most successful model when the appropriate time comes. It must always have a vision of the future, so that with each succeeding development in the official health services, the Red Cross could pioneer areas yet unexplored." The very founder of the blood program, because he was such a staunch supporter of medicare, suggested that the charitable agency should not rest on its laurels but, when the state was ready, surrender control and take up other challenges. After three decades of universal medicare, the full integration of the blood system into the network of public health services is long overdue.

"Humanitarian and charitable organizations are often reticent to speak out, preferring their deeds to shout and their words to whisper," Douglas Lindores, secretary-general of the Red Cross, said in an address to the Canadian Club in early 1995. The actions of the agency, and its increasingly vocal demands that it maintain control of the country's blood system, should trouble its supporters. The same Lindores has threatened to withdraw from the blood system. The agency is forging ahead with its plans to build a fractionation plant. It has vigorously fought back against the accusations of hemophiliacs and transfusion patients who contracted AIDS from tainted blood, and it was a party to the strong-arm tactics that led to many victims accepting a compensation package that was clearly insufficient. The Red Cross even signed a $1-million public relations contract to improve its image. These are deeds far removed from the vision of Henri Dunant, the Swiss philanthropist who began it all; they betray a corporate attitude not befitting an agency whose guiding principles are supposed to be humanity, impartiality, neutrality, independence, voluntary service, unity and universality. That the Canadian Red Cross spends almost four times as much operating a national blood transfusion service as the $68 million a year it spends on international relief is a graphic indication that it has lost touch with its roots.

In 1996 the Red Cross will mark its hundredth year in Canada. This is a perfect time for a change of direction, a rebirth. It should walk away from the blood program with its head held high, albeit with a tinge of sadness for all the suffering the tainted-blood tragedy has caused. The Red Cross flag should be proudly displayed in this country, and around the world, but at the site of disaster and relief efforts — and if the agency agrees, it could remain as a symbol at volunteer blood donor clinics. Of late, that honourable emblem has seen far too much action in courtrooms and corporate boardrooms; those should not be the battlefields of a humanitarian agency.

* * *

The Red Cross has been synonymous with blood transfusion in Canada since the first volunteer donor clinics in 1940. If it is removed from the equation, the crucial question is: what will replace it? No one is suggesting that Canada's blood program, which has evolved over fifty years, should be discarded. The blood collection and distribution structure is sound, and the scientists are competent; what is required is a new administration. The Canadian Blood Committee had an abominable record as the administrator of the blood system; its replacement by the Canadian Blood Agency in 1991 was an improvement, but not enough of one. What started out as a hydra has become a two-headed monster, with the CBA and Red Cross both jockeying for control and the health ministers refusing to make a choice. "The animosity is destructive to sound governance of the Canadian blood supply system," according to an independent audit commissioned by the Commission of Inquiry on the Blood System in Canada. The auditors, a group of respected scientists and healthcare administrators, needed four months to figure out the confused lines of authority. By the end of it, Mr. Justice Horace Krever was asking, "Can we really call it a system?" The answer is clearly no. As the audit team noted, the bickering between the two main players has not only left Canada lagging years behind its U.S. and European counterparts, but has imperilled the safety of consumers. Meanwhile, public disillusionment is beginning to tarnish the image of the Red Cross and eat away at one of the most precious elements of the system, the generosity of donors.

A generation after AIDS, a dangerous new virus has infected the country's blood system: mistrust. As with HIV, the symptoms are rather slight and easy to overlook at the beginning: the man who, after years of participating, can't be bothered to join the office blood drive; the woman who, recovering from a difficult birth, refuses a transfusion that could speed up her recovery. A poll conducted by Compas Inc. for the Red Cross in the spring of 1995 found that a full 33 per cent of Canadians would refuse a transfusion because of fears about tainted blood. The 1994 annual report of the Red Cross Blood Transfusion Service showed that donations were down 16 per cent since the scandal became news. Canada's blood system, built on the twin pillars of generosity and trust, is now teetering. Most Canadians are no less willing to give than in the past, but they have lost faith, and for good reason.

What is required is a single agency — a streamlined amalgam of the Red Cross and the Canadian Blood Agency — that leaves no doubt who is in charge of the blood system. It could be called Transfusion Canada.* The medical side would come from incorporating, in their entirety, the Blood Transfusion Service, the seventeen BTS centres, the National Reference Laboratory and the Blood Donor Recruitment service of the Red Cross; the business side and the liaison with government would come from the CBA. In other words, Transfusion Canada would be run by the same people who are currently responsible for the daily operations of the blood system, but with their roles clarified. This is not to suggest, however, that the administration would simply be turned over to federal and provincial bureaucrats, who time and time again failed to act on the threat of AIDS.

When Dr. Stuart Stanbury inaugurated the blood program in 1947, he said the Red Cross was committed to getting safe, free blood from the donor to the recipient. Today that is no longer enough. Donor blood must be manufactured into products, and it must be possible to carry out public health functions like tracing donors and tracking recipients almost instantly. Safety and gratuity must be guaranteed from vein to vein and back again.

The big difference is that the new blood system *would be* a system, with clear lines of authority, and legal responsibility deriving from that authority. With a single agency there would be no room for buck-passing. And to avoid the foot-dragging that was so deadly at the outset of the AIDS epidemic, Transfusion Canada would be overseen by a community-based board of directors that would serve the essential functions of monitoring and public input that are now lacking. (Hospitals in many provinces already have this type of board of directors.) At present, the budget for Canada's blood program is equivalent to that of Vancouver General Hospital, and the CBA includes one delegate from each province, usually a senior official of the ministry of health who has no expertise in blood. When you consider that a single mid-level bureaucrat oversees the administration of hospital spending for all of Metropolitan Toronto — more than $2.5 billion — the excessive bureaucratization of the CBA is more than clear.

The board of Transfusion Canada, like that of a hospital, needs only a couple of provincial ministry of health representatives (the provinces could, among

---

* The name, which has been proposed independently by a number of individuals and organizations, seems to have its roots at the Red Cross itself. In the mid-1960s, when a wave of centennial patriotism swept across Canada, the Red Cross BTS uniform included a shoulder patch that bore the bilingual name Transfusion Canada.

themselves, choose the delegates with the most appropriate expertise). The majority of members should be appointees with practical medical expertise — a hematologist, epidemiologist and Medical Officer of Health with field experience — and representatives of users, including hospitals and patients. Given the fallout of the tainted-blood scandal, strong consumer representation is paramount if Transfusion Canada is going to be credible with the public in the all-important transition period; therefore, the board should include representatives of hemophiliacs, transfusion patients and blood donors. The Commission of Inquiry could provide the transition team; Dr. George Connell, its scientific advisor, is precisely the type of chairman Transfusion Canada needs — a remarkable scientist who also has administrative experience.

In France, where the tainted-blood scandal had the most dramatic political repercussions, there was a systematic reform of the blood system to ensure a swift response to blood-borne diseases and accountability for decisions that are made or not made. The National Transfusion Centre (which, like the Canadian Red Cross, had operated independently of government but with state funds) was dismantled and replaced by the Agence française du sang (AFS) — similar to the proposed Transfusion Canada. The AFS, whose executive director reports directly to the Minister of Health, is responsible for everything from collection through to distribution and follow-up testing. If something goes wrong, there is no doubt who is responsible; if a crisis arises, there should be no doubt who can and will act. The French agency, which depends solely on volunteer donations, employs thirty doctors who oversee the country's 163 blood collection centres, and the hospitals and clinics that collect and distribute blood. The decentralization of the collection function, with much of the responsibility falling to blood donor committees across the country, would work well in Canada. But the most substantial change in France, and one that Transfusion Canada would do well to adopt, is that the AFS has fifteen in-house inspectors and epidemiologists who constantly monitor the blood supply; they are prepared not only to react to the next viral threat, but to prevent new infectious agents from entering the blood system. Another laudable initiative of the French has been to introduce an element of competition in purchasing policies while maintaining an overall state monopoly: while the AFS is responsible for all product purchases, hospital transfusion committees and hemophilia clinics can demand products from a government-approved list, a mechanism designed to force the agency to keep up with product developments. "Safe, safe, and safer," was how health minister Bernard Kouchner described the revamped system when it was announced in the summer of 1993. "Given our history, the French people would tolerate nothing less."

The hiring of inspectors specific to the blood system would resolve many of the failings of the Bureau of Biologics, an agency that failed utterly in its public health responsibilities in the 1980s. But the new blood agency can't be entirely self-regulating; the federal health department must provide checks and balances to ensure vigilance. Standards for blood safety in Canada needn't be identical to those of the U.S. Food and Drug Administration — except in the case of plasmapheresis operations, because otherwise plasma can't be exported for fractionation — but they should be few, clear and conscientiously enforced, with centre shutdown as the penalty for serious failure. To do the job, the Bureau of Biologics, and there appears to be no other agency capable of providing the supervision required, needs a clear mandate — blood was only deemed to be a drug in 1989, and regulations are still incomplete — and it needs personnel. A change of attitude is also required, and that can only come from a major shake-up of the department — one that establishes consumer advocacy as a priority. To be effective as public health police, the government department must also have the backing of its minister. The inaction of the Bureau of Biologics in responding to blood-borne AIDS reflected all too accurately the will of its political bosses who, for far too long, simply didn't care about AIDS, a disease whose characteristics — a long incubation period and entry points in marginal communities — lent itself to short-term indifference.

The medical directors, nurses and laboratory technicians who work in the seventeen centres of the Blood Transfusion Service are, for all intents and purposes, employees of the state, not the Red Cross, and they have been for a long time. They are also dedicated professionals who should be allowed to continue their fine work. Most of them would welcome the change as well; Red Cross medical directors have themselves called for the transfusion service to be separate from the rest of the charitable organization. It makes no sense, they realize better than anyone, to report to a board of directors that treats blood transfusion and water safety as two branches of the same corporation, and whose rigid, military-like structure doesn't allow for free scientific debate. With an agency dedicated solely to blood, and answerable to the public, there is little doubt the type of initiatives that medical directors proposed in the early days of the AIDS epidemic would be acted upon, not ignored.

While the entire transfusion and donor recruitment services of the Red Cross would be transferred as a whole, Transfusion Canada would have to review the current allocation of resources. Many Red Cross decisions were made for purely political reasons. For example, some blood donor clinics were conducted to "fly the flag" in communities and give people the chance to donate blood, even if the clinics weren't cost-efficient. Similarly, it's difficult to justify the existence of permanent blood centres in both Regina and Saskatoon, and both in London and Hamilton. In other words, a strictly government-run blood system need not cost more, and it could be less bureaucratic than the existing confusing mix of agencies and committees. Charities like the Red Cross maintain an aura of efficiency which is not necessarily justified; one need only think back to the Red Cross in Montreal, where the administrators of transfusion and recruitment services were working at cross-purposes, or consider the fact that the AIDS issue was bandied about by 20 internal Red Cross committees.

The most pressing issue, however, is establishing a clear policy on self-sufficiency. One of the principal causes of Canada's tainted blood tragedy was the obsession with the fractionation of blood into blood products on Canadian soil. Hundreds of lives were lost, hundreds of thousands of litres of volunteer plasma were wasted and tens of millions of dollars were squandered because the country's ministers of health viewed blood as a job-creation tool, not a public health issue. Transfusion Canada's mandate should be clear: the priority must be self-sufficiency in supply of plasma; self-sufficiency in production capacity, if it is cost-efficient, can follow. Without adequate stocks of plasma, which Canada hasn't had since the boom in fractionation products in the 1960s, building a plant is a doomed exercise, financially and medically.

The fractionation plant being proposed for construction in Bedford, Nova Scotia, in conjunction with Bayer Inc., formerly Miles, should be shelved. The project is a desperate bid by the Red Cross to control all elements of the blood system, to make itself indispensable. Yet there is no justification for pumping public money — the original cost was $150 million, but that estimate has since doubled — into a manufacturing facility that will be operated by one of the world's largest pharmaceutical companies.[2] Bayer is taking no financial risk; it is providing technical know-how; if the project goes sour, the Red Cross will take the hit, and the provinces will be called on to bail out the agency. If there were a profit to be made from fractionating blood in Canada, private enterprise would have done it long ago. The only way the Bedford plant can work, given its proposed production capacity of 800,000 litres annually, is if it is awarded a monopoly on the use of Canadian plasma and also purchases plasma from the U.S. But that would leave the Canadian blood system with its hands tied, as they were with Connaught. Yet the CBA, despite its opposition to the plant, has granted the Red Cross "preferred supplier" status, an indication the blood agency has not retained the lessons of the previous débâcle. The time to invest in fractionation was in the mid-1970s, when commercial-scale production of factor concentrate began. Already, Factor VIII and Factor IX are being cloned, which largely eliminates concerns about plasma shortages. Even purer concentrate is being made synthetically,[3] a guarantee that it is free of viral contamination. The CBA, after hesitation about costs, has made the products available to Canadian hemophiliacs, and because of their purity they are especially invaluable to people with suppressed immune systems, such as those infected with the AIDS virus. A centrally-controlled blood system with a strong consumer bent would promote the judicious use of concentrate and reduce usage to a minimum when new threats to the blood system arise. For hemophiliacs the next step will be genetic surgery to insert the missing clotting factor, either in the womb or at birth. Researchers are also making progress in the bid to create artificial blood. But, as the past has taught us, these miracles could have a downside; there is a need to be vigilant for early problems.

Canada collects enough whole blood to meet all its needs for red cells, but it is short of plasma, the part of blood used to manufacture blood products. By ensuring an adequate supply of the raw material, plasma, screening and safety measures are easily instituted and production capacity can be found to produce products to specification, regardless of technological breakthroughs. When appropriate levels of blood collection have been determined by Transfusion Canada, self-sufficiency goals can be set, and an appropriate investment made in a plasmapheresis program. Over the years, the provincial health ministers refused to invest in plasmapheresis, although it would have cost a fraction of the money wasted on building failed plants.[4] If the new agency makes serious efforts to achieve self-sufficiency in plasma requirements, it could make our blood system safer and our supplies more secure, and save money as well. Increased production would also make Canada more attractive to a fractionation company; subsidies would not be required to woo them here.

If critics of the Red Cross have hesitated to say that the charity no longer has a place in the blood system, it is due primarily to the fear of what would happen to the voluntary blood donor system. There is, without a doubt, a certain mythology attached to the Red Cross symbol. But does it necessarily follow that the 1 million donors in Canada would give to the Red Cross but not to Transfusion Canada? Not at all.

"Whether the blood transfusion van carries a heart, as in the United Kingdom, or a cross, as in Canada, at the end of the day the blood donors, staff and volunteer helpers will continue to support the patient in the hospital bed, irrespective of the blood collection agency that happens to be involved," says Dr. Richard Huntsman, former medical director of the St. John's BTS. Canadians give blood to their fellow citizens in need; the Red Cross is but a vehicle. If the public is convinced that Transfusion Canada is more accountable to them and that the result will be blood and blood products that are safer, they will give generously. Better still, if their faith is restored in the system after the tainted-blood fiasco, the disillusioned donors will likely come back, and the fears of potential recipients will dissipate.

There is no need, as was proposed by the Canadian Hemophilia Society in early 1995, to pay donors for plasma while continuing to depend on donated whole blood. Creating a two-tier system, a semi-commercialization, would mark the beginning of the end of the system Canadians have embraced for half a century. Selling blood is dangerously similar to selling vital organs; it is unseemly. Free blood must be an unflinching commitment of Transfusion Canada, and giving blood an act of generosity towards fellow citizens and a gesture of faith in the healthcare system.

*   *   *

Aside from repairing the flawed blood system, federal and provincial governments have some unfinished business with the victims of tainted blood. The federal Extraordinary Assistance Plan —$120,000 in "humanitarian assistance" in the form of four annual payments of $30,000 — was for the most part well intentioned, but over time it has proven to be clearly inadequate. The plan covered four years because it was assumed that all the victims would be dead within that time; applications were not accepted from people infected after 1989 because it was assumed the problem had been fully resolved. We now know that, on average, people infected with HIV live fourteen years, many of them suffering a slow, steady decline in health that makes working impossible. Further, we know that there were dozens of infections after 1989, with HIV, hepatitis C[5] and possibly newer blood-borne contaminants like Chagas' disease. The EAP should be revisited, as recommended in 1993 by the Commons Sub-Committee on Health Issues, and quickly.

The Multi-Provincial-Territorial Assistance Plan is a whole other matter. The behaviour of the provincial ministers of health on the compensation issue has been a disgrace from beginning to end. The same ministers who readily agreed to generous compensation for Connaught Laboratories because it was unable to manufacture heat-treated concentrate also conspired to deny compensation to victims of tainted blood. The provinces exploited the stigma of AIDS to save their provincial treasuries a few dollars until 1994, when a civil suit was about to be resolved and a public inquiry was going to explain the underlying reasons for the tragedy; then they grudgingly cobbled together an assistance package encumbered by a waiver so that victims couldn't sue the Red Cross, major pharmaceutical companies or insurers. And the "humanitarian" package came with a signing deadline only weeks away — the ultimate in cynicism from a group whose inability to make decisions quickly had been one of the contributing factors to the tragedy.

The package itself was also designed to pinch pennies, not serve justice. Victims who were directly infected by blood and blood products were entitled to $30,000 a year for "life" (in reality, few of the victims will live to the turn of the century), but infected spouses and children were offered nothing. The MPTAP doesn't pay for AIDS drugs or homecare, stripping many victims of their right to die with dignity. The majority of the victims were primary breadwinners struck down in their prime, but there is no provision for retraining spouses or educating children. The program also doesn't pay for legal fees incurred, and thus punishes those whose lawsuits brought the issue to public attention.

The MPTAP was a settlement imposed under duress, an injustice that should be corrected. What is required is an independent adjudicator, preferably a judge experienced in civil matters, empowered to impose a settlement based on need. In the short term, due to the urgency of the matter, the adjudication process should be limited strictly to the victims of tainted blood. But it should also serve as a model for a permanent body dealing with all sorts of medical catastrophes. In 1990 Robert Prichard presented the country's deputy ministers of health with a report he was commissioned to prepare on liability and compensation issues in the healthcare field. As he pointed out, insurance costs alone exceed $200 million a year for Canadian healthcare institutions. He recommended that the right to sue remain because it contributes to reducing avoidable injuries, but that a no-fault system be developed to provide an alternative to victims. As it stands, only one in ten patients who suffer negligent injury are compensated, a chilling reminder that the victims of tainted blood are not alone in their suffering.

Public health officials still haven't made serious efforts to notify the 3.5 million Canadians who received blood transfusions between 1978 and 1990, to warn them that they were at risk of contracting AIDS and hepatitis C. The Sick Kids program showed that a significant number of former transfusion patients are infected with HIV but still don't know it. The Laboratory Centre for Disease Control published a study in August 1994 estimating that between 942 and 1,441 Canadians were infected with the AIDS virus by transfusion, many more than the 419 officially reported. Many presumably died of their original medical condition without their AIDS infection being diagnosed — but others must still be out there, at risk of spreading the disease. Yet only a handful of the country's 1,200 hospitals have systematically tracked down patients. The Canadian Hospital Association didn't issue guidelines on tracing former recipients until June 1994, and then it still ignored recipients of blood tainted by hepatitis C. The number of people who contracted hepatitis C from transfusions is no doubt many times greater than those who got AIDS and, while it isn't 100 per cent fatal, the disease can be debilitating and can be sexually transmitted, yet there has been no formal tracing or notification program.

There has been little examination of the role of professional associations in the tainted-blood tragedy. The Canadian Medical Association, for example, issued guidelines about "universal precautions" for physicians dealing with patients who could potentially have AIDS very early in the epidemic, but never pushed physicians to inform patients about the risks of blood, or the need for testing of former transfusion patients. Even today, people who test positive for AIDS are not systematically asked if they gave blood; this despite the fact that a 1994 Alberta study showed that patients who tested positive were happy to co-operate, and were remarkably accurate in their recollection of donation dates, making tracking very simple. Similarly, the Canadian Hospital Association, whose members transfused all the tainted blood, never spoke out, even when some hospitals, angry at the slow introduction of AIDS testing, took the unprecedented move of setting up their own blood-testing laboratories. Medical historian Dr. Mirko Grmek documented another important aspect of the slow reaction to AIDS: the manner in which medical journals systematically rejected or delayed articles about AIDS. Normally, papers that pertain to epidemics and matters of public health urgency are fast-tracked. The lack of documentation, in turn, convinced doctors and public health officials that there was no urgency; and far too many doctors dealing with the new disease were too proud to refer their patients to specialists, and too patronizing and ethically wanting to tell patients of their diagnosis. Hospitals and doctors, the primary providers of health services, must be on the front lines of the public health battle. They must make serious efforts to atone for their failings in the tainted blood tragedy, and play an active role in the proper functioning of Transfusion Canada to ensure a co-ordinated plan of prevention and a swift response to blood-borne infection agents, both in keeping patients informed, and relaying the concerns of users back to the system's administrators.

Even with the final report of the Commission of Inquiry on the Blood System in Canada in 1996 after proceedings that lasted almost two years, the victims of tainted blood will still have one important unanswered question. Many feel that there were criminal actions that contributed to their suffering, yet those charges have never been seriously investigated. The mandate of Mr. Justice Horace Krever specifically stated that he would not make findings of criminal wrongdoing.

Unlike France, it's difficult in Canada for a private individual to bring criminal charges against anyone. AIDS-related trials are still very uncommon in our courts. In 1989 James Charles Thornton was convicted of committing a common nuisance after knowingly donating blood infected with HIV at a November 1987 Ottawa clinic. In upholding the conviction and fifteen-month sentence in June 1993, the Supreme Court of Canada ruled that the Criminal Code imposes a "duty of care" on citizens which Mr. Thornton "breached by not disclosing his blood contained HIV antibodies. This common nuisance obviously endangered the life, safety and health of the public." In Newfoundland, Raymond Mercer was sentenced to eleven years in prison for failing to tell women that he was infected with the AIDS virus before he had unprotected sexual intercourse with them. (It is unclear how many women he infected, but Conception Bay has one of the highest infection rates in the country.) The question in the tainted blood scandal is whether the failure of public health officials to tell hemophiliacs and transfusion patients of the risks constitutes a similar violation of the "duty of care" — or worse. After a heated public debate about the legal and ethical difficulties involved in legislating sexual behaviour, Charles Ssenyonga was brought to trial in London, Ontario, in April 1993. Although he is believed to have infected at least twenty women, Ssenyonga was charged with one count each of criminal negligence causing bodily harm and aggravated sexual assault. He died before a verdict was delivered.

So much has been said, so many accusations have been levelled that the question of criminal charges should not be left unexplored. Once the commission has completed its work, the federal justice minister should appoint a senior Crown attorney to hear submissions from each of the parties with standing at the inquiry, and to examine the evidence independently to determine if charges are warranted. The senior RCMP investigators who gathered evidence for the inquiry could play an important role in assisting the Crown. The process proposed is unusual but necessary.

Another necessity is an apology to the victims — one read in Parliament and in every provincial legislature. Provincial and federal ministers of health should be ashamed of their actions, and the inaction of their bureaucrats in this sorry saga, and the least they can do is say they are sorry. The argument that an apology will unduly influence court proceedings is feeble at best; each of the remaining lawsuits can and will be judged on its merits. The hundreds of other victims need to hear a simple admission that things should have been done differently. Refusing to apologize and refusing to investigate the possibility of criminal charges would leave a dark cloud over the blood system. It would leave doubt in the minds of the public, doubt that would hamper the rebuilding of trust in the volunteer donor system — doubt that justice had been done.

* * *

Claude Labelle, forty-nine, had heart bypass surgery on November 5, 1991, at Montreal's Sacré-Coeur Hospital. He had heard the horror stories about tainted blood, had even lost a brother-in-law to transfusion AIDS a few years earlier. So, like a growing number of Canadians, Labelle didn't want blood. The operation, fairly routine, went well, but the recovery, always unpredictable, didn't. Three days after surgery, he was still in hospital, anemic, lethargic and exhausted. The doctor said a blood transfusion would get him back on his feet. Labelle refused. Later, a nurse tried to convince him that the treatment was necessary and safe. "It is really impossible to get AIDS from blood," she told him. "All the blood is tested." He gave in and was transfused with two units of red cells.

The Red Cross had, at that point, been testing all blood donations for HIV for more than six years. But what the nurse failed to tell Labelle was that the system wasn't foolproof. "Blood is inherently an unsafe therapeutic agent in that each unit of blood comes from someone who has been subject to a variety of environmental exposures and who may not remember occurrences of high-risk behaviour," says Dr. Peter Gill, a former scientist at the Laboratory Centre for Disease Control who now heads the National Reference Laboratory at the Red Cross. In other words, donors, while altruistic, do not always realize that they may have been exposed to infectious agents. In 1993, 1 in every 50,000 donors at Red Cross blood clinics tested positive for HIV. It is likely that others were not detected. It can be six weeks to eight months before the body of an infected person starts creating antibodies to HIV — and during that time, tainted blood can slip through undetected.

With concentrate, this risk is countered with heat treatment and solvent detergent methods of viral inactivation but, to date, heating most blood components to kill viruses has not been possible, nor practical. Platelets, for example, must be used within four days of donation or they lose their effectiveness. Heat treatment of red cells, which have a shelf life of about 35 days, destroys their oxygen-carrying function, so it is not feasible. The practical difficulty with treating most blood components is that the processes require large quantities of raw material to be cost-efficient. Experience has shown that the key to having a safe blood supply is having virus- and bacteria-free plasma. Clotting concentrate is pooled from the plasma of up to 20,000 donors, which greatly increases risks if an infectious agent survives, as occurred when dry-heat treatment was introduced in the early eighties. In the spring of 1995, the New York Blood Center applied for a licence from the U.S. Food and Drug Administration to be allowed to pool and virally inactivate its plasma destined for transfusion. While this would be a remarkable safety breakthrough, virtually eliminating the

226\ THE GIFT OF DEATH

risk of infections from all manufactured blood products and frozen plasma (together they account for more than three-quarters of all blood use), it set off a furious debate among scientists because the corollary is that, in the case of a failure or of a new infectious agent, the risk to patients would be many times greater. The compromise will likely be to limit pool size to find an acceptable risk-benefit ratio; the challenge for Transfusion Canada would be to decide if the process and pool size judged safe in the U.S. would be accepted in Canada, and whether the technology would be installed in all the country's blood transfusion centres, or just some.

Since mandatory testing of blood was introduced in November 1985, there have been at least thirteen confirmed cases of transfusion AIDS in Canada, and thousands more cases of infection with hepatitis C, including about thirty serious cases a year since screening began in 1990.* Today the Red Cross says the risk of a unit of HIV-infected blood slipping through is 1 in 225,000, while the risk for blood carrying hepatitis C is 1 in 40,000. The figures are theoretical ones, based on units screened with both questionnaires and AIDS antibodies tests. The HIV estimate comes from the Centers for Disease Control in Atlanta, based on mathematical projections. When you consider that patients receive, on average, five units of blood, the average risk increases to 1 in 45,000. One study in the U.S., however, gives even more reason to pause. Research published in the *Annals of Internal Medicine* in October 1992 found that when doctors tested 11,532 surgery patients from 1985 to 1991, both before and shortly after surgery, two patients had contracted HIV from blood. In total, 120,312 units had been transfused, putting the risk per person at 1 in 60,000 (given the average of 10 units received by those in the study). While that's far better than the 1 in 2,000 risk prior to testing in Canada, there is still reason to be cautious.

The blood Claude Labelle received in November 1991, against his better judgment, was infected with the AIDS virus. Within months, he developed meningitis, a result of his failing immune system. Labelle was diagnosed promptly and as a result his wife, Lina Laflamme, wasn't infected. The suspect unit of blood was also traced quickly, but the Red Cross never found the donor. By November 1993 Labelle was dead. Because he had been infected after 1989, the cut-off date for the EAP, he wasn't eligible for compensation.

---

* Auditors commissioned by the Krever inquiry estimated twenty-six to thirty-seven cases a year due to the window period.

*　　*　　*

The single best safety measure against blood-borne infections is reducing the amount of blood transfused. It's a cheap, efficient and healthy alternative. For a long time, blood transfusions were administered in a rather cavalier fashion — particularly in Canada, where blood is free. A study conducted at Kingston's Hôtel-Dieu Hospital found that almost half of all transfusions were unnecessary. The good news is that surgeons are changing their ways, largely because they fear litigation. At Toronto Hospital, where Kenneth Pittman received his fatal transfusion, the average use of red cells during heart surgery fell from 4.3 units in 1989 to 1.7 units in 1992. Still, there is much room for improvement. Dr. Kenneth Shumak, a hematologist and vice-dean of medicine at the University of Toronto, says too many surgeons still regard transfusion as routine. "I know of certain surgeons who, every time they do a hip replacement, give a routine order for six units of blood. No one ever considers whether that's right for that patient. I don't believe there should be anything like a routine transfusion order." The key, then, is changing the attitude of surgeons, and educating patients.

The Royal Society of Canada wrote in its 1988 report *AIDS: A Perspective for Canadians*, "The risk of becoming HIV infected by blood transfusion can be removed entirely for medically suitable patients who use their own blood banked in advance of elective surgery." Red cells keep for up to forty-two days and frozen plasma lasts for up to ten years, yet far too few hospitals permit autologous donations (blood stored in advance for the donor's own use), and the Red Cross has actively discouraged the practice. The major argument against autologous transfusion is that widespread use of this procedure could reduce the number of volunteer donors and thus the regular supply of blood. The obvious answer is that fewer donations are required in a system that keeps transfusions to a minimum.

Bloodless surgery is also, in many cases, a realistic alternative. Heart surgery is routinely done without transfusions; the process simply takes longer because it involves a lot of cauterizing to prevent bleeding. Doctors can also "recycle" blood ("intraoperative autologous transfusion")* so that blood that would otherwise end up on the floor is pumped right back into the body; they can employ hemodilution, boosting the blood volume with, for example, saline solutions, to conserve the patient's blood; and some hospitals have even taken to collecting a patient's blood lost during surgery and transfusing it during the recovery phase (post-operative salvage).

---

* Blood recycling was pioneered by Dr. Raymond Heimbecker of the University of Western Ontario.

The key to introducing these measures is a democratization of the medical process, a recognition that a patient's wish to minimize risk must be respected at all times. Patients should discuss their wishes with the surgeon before going under the knife. Mr. Justice Horace Krever has recommended that no one, except severe trauma patients, should receive a transfusion before signing a consent form. The exercise, he stressed, should not just be routine; it should involve a serious discussion of the risks and benefits of transfusion.

Anecdotally, we know that simple changes in treatment have saved lives — or could have. Lilliane Couture, a Burnaby woman with Crohn's disease, received blood transfusions annually until the early 1980s. Then she heard about AIDS in the media and asked to be treated with injections of iron instead. Her physician, a specialist, tried to talk her out of it. She insisted. Today Mrs. Couture doesn't have AIDS. Dr. Annette Poon, director of the blood bank at the Hospital for Sick Children in Toronto, decided to "wash" the red cells that were transfused regularly into patients with thalassemia and sickle cell anemia. (Washing consists of putting the unit of blood in a centrifuge to try to remove excess proteins that could cause reactions.) In the process she seems to have washed away the AIDS virus; despite receiving one or more transfusions per month during the years tainted blood went undetected in the Canadian blood system, not a single thalassemia or sickle cell patient was infected at Sick Kids. Bob Verreau, a Calgary hemophiliac, is living proof of the benefits of cutting back when blood quality is in doubt. An avid reader who browsed through medical journals regularly, he was alerted early to the possibility of contaminated factor concentrate and reacted by cutting his usage. In 1981 Verreau used 148,000 units of Factor VIII, but he reduced his intake each year to 1985, when he used a mere 16,000 units — virtually unheard of for a severe hemophiliac. The "party line" at the time was that you had to treat aggressively or risk being crippled, but Verreau rejected the scare-mongering and opted for the "better safe than sorry" approach. While he suffered tremendously at times — he had a shoulder hemorrhage so severe that his upper arm popped out of joint, but he still refused to inject concentrate — the Calgary man is one of the "15 per centers", the few severe hemophiliacs in Canada who escaped AIDS.

One can only imagine how many hundreds of transfusion patients and hemophiliacs could have avoided infection with HIV or hepatitis C over the years had improved screening been combined with more rational use of blood and blood products. Let us hope that, next time, action will come earlier, and that the only imagination required will be in the calculation of infections avoided.

* * *

Since the tainted-blood scandal began making headlines years ago, there have been ominous threats that the next viral epidemic will be worse than AIDS. But what will be the next serious blood-borne infectious agent? And how can we prepare for it?

There are more than twenty-five infectious agents known to be blood-borne, including various sorts of viruses, parasites, rickettsia, spirochetes and bacteria that can survive in blood outside the body anywhere from days to weeks. Currently, the Red Cross tests all blood donations for six agents:

- Testing for the spirochete *Treponema pallidum*, the cause of syphilis, has been routine since the early days of the blood program; today its incidence in blood is negligible and it is believed that cold storage kills the spirochete, making the test rather superfluous.
- Screening for HBV, the hepatitis B virus, which can cause serious liver damage in about 10 per cent of cases, began in 1970; this test also eliminates HDV, the hepatitis D virus, which can't replicate without HBV.
- Universal testing for HIV, the virus believed to cause AIDS, began in November 1985; factor concentrate is also heat-treated to kill HIV and HBV; yet it's estimated that at least two blood recipients a year still contract AIDS.
- Testing for HCV, the hepatitis C virus, began in 1990. The scope of infections is only beginning to emerge because the consequences, cirrhosis and liver cancer, develop from fifteen to thirty years after infection. It's estimated that twenty-five to forty transfusion patients still contract chronic hepatitis C each year.
- The test for HTLV-I (human T-cell lymphotropic virus type I), a disease that can cause leukemia and lymphoma twenty to forty years down the road, was quietly introduced in 1990.
- In 1992, testing began for HTLV-II, another retrovirus related to HIV, which causes chronic degenerative neurological disease after a long latency period. The incidence rate for HTLV-I and II (a single test is now conducted) is 3.8 per 100,000. It's still unclear how long a person can be infected before the disease shows up in testing.

The Red Cross doesn't routinely test for cytomegalovirus, but blood products destined for patients with suppressed immune systems are tested because the virus can pose a serious risk for them; some other members of the herpes family, Epstein-Barr virus (EBV) and human herpes virus type 6 (HHV-6) have a blood-borne phase, but tests are not conducted.

Moreover, the Red Cross tries to screen out many diseases with its questionnaire. Donors who have had mononucleosis are deferred temporarily, which eliminates most cases of EBV. Donors who have a history of tick bites are deferred for six months to avoid the spirochete *Borrelia burgdorferi*, the cause of Lyme disease; the organism can survive in blood for up to sixty days. To avoid the transmission of the parasitic infection malaria, donors who have travelled to endemic areas are deferred.

In 1995 the Red Cross began asking donors about Chagas' disease, and deferring those who had travelled to areas where the parasite, *Trypanosoma cruzi* (spread by bedbugs), is endemic. Chagas' disease, which attacks the heart muscle and kills more than 50,000 people a year in South America, is known to have killed one Canadian transfusion recipient in 1986, and is often cited as one of the big threats of the end of the century. While there are diagnostic tests, no blood screening test is yet available.

Another parasitic disease that should be setting off alarm bells is visceral leishmaniasis, caused initially by sandfly bites, but blood-borne. The threat of this disease has greatly increased since thousands of soldiers served in the Gulf War region, an area where it's endemic. The U.S. military, which operates its own blood collection and transfusion service, defers soldiers who served in the Gulf for three years, but there is no similar screening for leishmaniasis in Canada, despite the high proportion of Canadian Forces personnel who are donors.

In its February 1995 interim report, the Commission of Inquiry on the Blood System in Canada listed several other blood-borne pathogens that could pose a threat in the years to come.

- Human parvovirus B19 is a world-wide disease whose symptoms are only beginning to come to light; it is now suspected of causing leukemia. Transfusion-related cases have been documented, and it poses a particularly severe risk to hemophiliacs using concentrate; it can lead to erythema infectiosum, or severe joint pain. Parvovirus B19 also demonstrates the challenges a little-known disease can pose to public health efforts: when the virus is infectious and present in the blood, the carrier has no symptoms, making verbal screening virtually impossible; and screening for antibodies isn't useful because the presence of antibodies doesn't indicate that the donor is still infectious.

- Yersiniosis, a bacterial disease characterized by fever and diarrhea, can be transmitted months after symptoms disappear. The bacteria, *Yersinia enterocolitica*, multiplies efficiently in refrigerated red blood cells, and the concentrations can lead to post-transfusion sepsis, a type of blood poisoning that is almost always fatal. Worse yet, yersiniosis thrives in temperate climates like Canada's, and during cold season.
- Human T-cell lymphotropic virus type V, a newly discovered retrovirus that attacks the immune system, has been reported in Italy; like other viruses, it is most likely transmitted both sexually and by blood. The danger with retroviruses, from a public health point of view, is that they tend to attack specific populations at the outset, much in the manner AIDS did, raising civil rights concerns and the risk of complacency.
- HAV, hepatitis A virus, is a widespread illness that is rarely fatal. The infection of factor concentrate in several European countries in late 1992 demonstrated that Canada still didn't have a plan ready to deal with new viral outbreaks. When hemophiliacs asked what was being done to keep the concentrate from entering the country, neither the Red Cross nor the Bureau of Biologics had an answer.
- Lassa fever, caused by a virus carried by rodents in West Africa, has a high mortality rate and an incubation period of up to three weeks, a bad combination because blood is used quickly. Lassa's risk to the blood supply should also draw attention to a similar danger closer to home. There have been several outbreaks of hantavirus, linked to mice, in Canada.
- Bancroftian filariasis, a parasitic disease carried by mosquitoes in most tropical countries, can lead to elephantiasis, characterized by gross swelling, particularly in the legs and testicles. Sufferers can be infectious for five years or more after recovery.
- Creutzfeldt-Jakob disease, a fatal neurological disorder, is transmitted by tissue transplants and might also be blood-borne. The organism is unknown, but the disease's incubation period is thought to be as long as thirty years. In July 1995, news that two blood donors had been diagnosed with this prompted the Red Cross to conduct the most extensive withdrawal of blood products in Canadian history.

This is but a partial list. There are other threats like the flesh-eating filovirus Ebola that was the subject of the best-selling book *The Hot Zone* and the Hollywood movie *Outbreak*, or the many other "emerging viruses" that strike with lightning speed. In many ways they are easy to deal with, because they garner immediate media and political attention. The most dangerous disease is one that mimics AIDS: one with a long incubation period that fools the public into believing it's relatively harmless, with modes of transmission that include activities of daily life.

None of this is intended to create a panic, or to scare people who really need transfusions away from accepting blood. Blood truly is the Gift of Life to accident and burn victims, and many major surgery patients; we can't lose sight of that. But we must remember that — like almost everything else in the medical field — it can also bring harm.

"What we've learned over the past ten to twelve years is that communicable diseases will always be with us, and they will probably become increasingly challenging," says Dr. Sharon Macdonald, a professor of public health at the University of Manitoba. "There are new and emerging pathogens and it behooves a department of public health to have the skills to develop strategies against infectious diseases." Yet all across Canada, early intervention programs — the sentinel system that allows scientists to spot deadly new diseases — are being gutted, falling victim to budget cuts. One of the important lessons of the tainted blood tragedy is that surveillance, monitoring and epidemiological research are good investments. When a single donation of contaminated blood can infect fifty to a hundred people, there is no room for complacency.

A dedication to disease prevention requires, more than anything else, political will. As Jerald Freise, whose wife was infected with the AIDS virus by blood transfusion, says, "All the technology in the world is worthless unless you have the courage to get up and act." The time for patching and bandaging has long passed. Radical surgery is required, and urgently, from the creation of Transfusion Canada through to public education.

The next blood-borne virus could arrive at any time and, difficult as it is to imagine, it may well be even more insidious and more lethal than AIDS. We can never again lose sight of the fact that every deadly drop of blood affects a child, a family, a community — the toll is not just anonymous statistics. We owe it to them all, donors and recipients alike, to see that the tragedy of tainted blood is never repeated.

EPILOGUE

IN APRIL 1993 MRS. Z., a suburban mother of three, was listening to the news on the car radio on the way to work when a story caught her ear. Dr. Susan King of the Toronto Hospital for Sick Children was urging that children who had undergone heart surgery between 1978 and 1985 be tested for AIDS, because there was a slight risk that they might have been exposed to contaminated blood. The tainted-blood scandal had been in the news a lot of late, but AIDS just didn't seem like a worry to a happily married couple living on the outskirts of Toronto. Yet this kind of warning was getting dangerously close to home. "We thought that if it was possible that children in our society had HIV, then we should get our son tested," Mrs. Z. says.

Jason* had been born at Toronto's Mount Sinai Hospital in January 1985, nine weeks premature. Like all preemies, he looked and sounded fragile, weighing only three pounds nine ounces at birth, and his underdeveloped lungs needed the help of a respirator. The first six weeks of his life were spent in a hospital incubator, with his parents constantly at the boy's side, praying. The baby was a real fighter, the nurses said, so they nicknamed him the Little Warrior.

Despite a diagnosis of pulmonary valve stenosis, a heart murmur, Jason grew into a rough-and-tumble kid, the kind who broke an arm during summer vacations. Sometimes his lymph nodes swelled to the size of golf balls, but the doctors said not to worry. The boy took antibiotics to ward off any virus that could attack his weak heart, and the swelling went down. Since October 1992, however, Jason

---

* Jason Z. is a pseudonym designed to protect the boy's identity. No other aspect of his story has been altered.

had been quite ill with a nagging cough. The boy had visited countless specialists, but the best they could come up with was that he had respiratory problems; one said asthma, another said acute sinusitis and post-nasal drip. Jason was treated with antibiotics, bronchial dilators and steroids, but his condition grew worse and worse. He coughed every thirty seconds, twenty-four hours a day, for five months, to the point of retching and vomiting. The child could barely sleep and eat, and the rest of the family wasn't faring much better.

"Our son was only eight years old and he was coughing himself to death," Mr. Z. recalls. "The cough was killing not only our son, but ripping us apart. We felt each retching cough as if it were our own. It was sheer torture because we felt so powerless." Just weeks earlier, Jason had to be hospitalized for his "acute asthma". But he wasn't responding well, so doctors tested for tuberculosis, cystic fibrosis, lung cancer and virtually every other respiratory disease they could think of. Still he coughed.

Jason hadn't had heart surgery as a baby but, as the announcer had said, some parents weren't even aware that their children had received transfusions. "If in doubt, get a test" was the message Mrs. Z. retained from Dr. King's interview. Besides, they were at wit's end. They might as well have the boy tested for AIDS; if nothing else, they could scratch the disease off the list.

Just days after the radio broadcast, the couple asked the family doctor to test Jason for AIDS. The physician balked; there was no record of blood transfusion in the child's ever-growing medical file. They looked at the coughing boy, and they insisted.

On May 7 — Mother's Day, 1993 — the doctor phoned with the test results. Jason had AIDS. The nagging cough wasn't asthma, it was deadly PCP. "Our lives ended that day," Mr. Z. says. "All I could think was that someone murdered our son, our shining star, our reason to live." He was convinced that a homosexual pedophile had assaulted the boy. There was no other way he could have got AIDS.

The couple had been told that they were infertile, that they would never have children. The pregnancy in 1984 was an unexpected godsend, the difficult pregnancy and premature birth shrugged off as the foibles of a miracle baby who couldn't wait to get on with life. But three weeks after he was born, unknown to his parents, Jason was injected with sixteen cubic centimetres of red cells. Pediatricians call the popular treatment a "top-up", a little shot designed to put colour in the cheeks. The single tablespoon of blood was infected with the AIDS virus.

The parents had never consented to the blood transfusion, and no institution — not Mount Sinai, not the Red Cross, not Ontario public health authorities —

had ever made an effort to track the recipients of the contaminated donation. In a similar case at the Hospital for Sick Children, where doctors were giving "top-ups" to children recovering from surgery, a single unit of blood left four children infected with AIDS. There was already widespread knowledge that the blood system was infected, but no public health official had urged limiting transfusions to emergency surgery, and medical and hospital associations didn't think to advise doctors to reduce blood use to a minimum. The Red Cross had long ago backed off efforts to screen high-risk donors; the tablespoon of blood injected into the child came from an openly gay man, a "diamond donor" (seventy-five-plus donations) who was never turned away.

When the boy went to Sick Kids on May 8, the day after his test results came back, he had already missed out on a lifetime of treatment. The first thing doctors did at the AIDS clinic was a saline bronchoscopy, an examination of lung tissue and fluid. They were able to stop the cough immediately, because a proper diagnosis makes treatment possible.

By the time Jason went for tests at the infectious diseases clinic some months later, just after his eighth birthday, his CD4 count was 10. The count is a quick reflector of the body's immunity; the normal range is 500 to 1,500. The child had virtually no immune system left. Any childhood disease could easily kill him. Jason started the regime people with AIDS know all too well, a daily diet of AZT, antibiotics and antifungals, and monthly treatments with immunoglobulins (a blood product that boosts the immune system) and aerosolized pentamidine.

The parents — who, like many Canadians, thought of AIDS as strictly a homosexual disease — were forced to confront their prejudices. They quickly realized that AIDS had not only medical but social consequences. "We decided to cocoon against discrimination." They told family members the tragic truth, but in the community they hid behind the fiction of cancer. Social workers and counsellors urged them to keep the news from Jason's school, and from the boy himself. Kids can be too cruel, adults too reactionary.

The parents became frustrated with the professional help because it focused on getting them to deal with the fact that Jason had a fatal disease. Mr. and Mrs. Z. couldn't accept that until some basic questions had been answered. How and why had Jason ended up getting a transfusion of tainted blood? Those who ran the blood system had no satisfactory answers. Like so many families across the country, the couple suddenly found their lives spiralling out of control, and desperately wanted someone to talk to, to help them find answers. They turned to the HIV-T Group and soon became militant lobbyists for justice. Mr. Z. would drive around the highways of suburban Toronto, talking to Jerry Freise on his cell phone and bawling his eyes out. "People must have thought I was a maniac or something because I was breaking down all the time, but it was my only outlet." In the summer of 1993, when hemophiliacs and transfusion-AIDS patients were lobbying hard for provincial compensation, Mr. Z. told his story publicly for the first time, to *The Globe and Mail*. Every detail poured out, in a mixture of bitterness and sadness. "Why, why, why?" he kept asking.

Jason's story serves to underline the inadequacies of the "humanitarian assistance" offered by governments. Mr. and Mrs. Z. decided to accept the federal EAP, $30,000 annually for four years, largely because the boy's infection had put them on the verge of bankruptcy. Mr. Z. had been driven to despair by the AIDS diagnosis and, as he was self-employed, his business foundered. But they rejected the Multi-Provincial-Territorial Assistance Package for a number of reasons, chief among them that it doesn't satisfy the financial needs of parents with an HIV-infected child. There are no provisions for drugs and homecare costs while the boy is alive, no recognition of the losses in income or work experience and the possible need to relocate, not even money for funeral expenses. Because the MPTAP couldn't be collected until EAP payments were complete, Jason wouldn't have seen that money until 1997, and he is unlikely to live that long. But the ultimate insult, Mr. Z. felt, was the prerequisite waiver of legal action against the Red Cross, the hospital and the province. "I really question why it is called assistance when a seventeen-page waiver is required," he testified at the Commission of Inquiry on the Blood System in Canada. The family is one of a few dozen across the country who have pursued legal action, but it is unlikely their lawsuit will be heard in the boy's lifetime.

The couple's testimony at the public inquiry, on March 11, 1994, was among the most poignant. It was late Friday afternoon; many lawyers had skipped out early, and most of the journalists were gone. Jason didn't attend the hearings; he was in school. Instead, Mr. and Mrs. Z. put a photo of the boy on the table before them. He looked much younger than his ten years, more frail and frightened than words can describe. The camera, as was the arrangement when witnesses appeared confidentially, focused on Mr. Justice Horace Krever. That day he looked more like the father of four he is than a learned judge as he watched Mr. Z., in a quivering voice, read a statement. The summary of the family's sorry tale, punctuated by tears, ended with an angry denunciation.

"In closing I would like to say that the system which continues to deny to accept responsibility is criminal. It reeks of complicity. We must now live with this legacy of deceit. Our pain is excruciating and endless. It is a system that can rob us of our trust. It can steal away our very faith, usurp us of our will to live. It cheats us of our humanity; it plunders our morals and rapes our ethics, defrauds and bilks us of our very existence. It snatches away our hopes and shatters our dreams. It leaves us to wallow in despair, hopelessness and pain.

"The system even attempts to circumvent our legal rights. It has murdered our son, and may get away with it. But there is something that this corrupt system can never — and, I repeat, never — take away from us, and that is the unconditional, undying, unfathomable love and devotion to our son and the other people who have been racked by this tragedy."

The family has remained anonymous for the sake of Jason, who has yet to be told he has AIDS. The doctors say such a revelation should be "age appropriate", delivered when the child is about twelve and can understand the consequences of a fatal disease. "It would kill me to tell him," Mr. Z. says. "We want him to have a normal kid's life." The Children's Wish Foundation has helped, sending Jason and his dad salmon fishing in British Columbia.

But because he received a gift of death, there is little hope Jason will make it to that birthday in 1997 — the year the peacetime blood program will mark its fiftieth anniversary. Jason and most of the other 1,200 victims of AIDS-tainted blood won't live to see its evolution.

The legacy of the tragedy should be a safer, more responsive blood system — one that will restore the faith of Canadians, and ensure safe transfusions of blood and blood products for many, many years to come. That would truly be a Gift of Life.

GLOSSARY

ACT-UP: AIDS Committee To Unleash Power, an international AIDS group known for its acts of civil disobedience.

AHG: freeze-dried anti-hemophilic globulin, the precursor to factor concentrate.

AIDS: Acquired Immune Deficiency Syndrome, a disease characterized by opportunistic infections such as Kaposi's sarcoma and PCP in an HIV-positive person. A person with a CD4 count of less than 200, or who has suffered from PCP, is said to have AIDS. Researchers estimate that contaminated blood will transmit HIV about 90 per cent of the time; approximately one-third of children contract the virus in the womb if the mother is HIV-positive; the risk for injection drug users is about 1 in 100; the risk of contracting AIDS during intercourse range from 1 in 100 for anal intercourse to 1 in 1,000 for vaginal intercourse, though the receptive partner is at greater risk and the risk of transmitting the virus are greatest when CD4 counts are low.

AIDS-related complex: a term, no longer in use, used to describe the early symptoms of AIDS infection such as swollen lymph glands, night sweats and persistent fever. It is now referred to as seroconversion illness.

ARC: AIDS-related complex.

AZT: azidothymidine (now called zidovudine), a drug used to treat people with HIV-AIDS, it is believed to slow the replication of the virus.

Anemia: a condition characterized by below-normal hemoglobin levels and destruction of red cells; the most common cause is lack of iron, but the condition can be hereditary. See sickle cell anemia, thalassemia.

Antibody: an immune or protective protein, either existing naturally or prompted by an antigen. The existence of an antibody often indicates the existence of an antigen, i.e., blood is tested for the presence of HIV antibodies to determine if the virus is present.

Antigen: a substance capable of inducing a specific immune reaction, i.e. toxins, foreign proteins and bacteria. The presence of an antigen will evoke the existence of an antibody.

Anti-HBc test: anti-hepatitis-B core test, one of the tests that can identify a person infected with hepatitis B. It was suggested as a surrogate test to identify persons at high risk of AIDS before the HIV antibody test was developed.

Apheresis: the process of bleeding a donor but retaining only a specific component of blood and returning the rest of the blood back into the body; i.e., plasmapheresis, plateletpheresis, cellpheresis.

Archival Study: a document prepared by members of the Canadian Hemophilia Society to back their demands of compensation, it is considered the first detailed examination of the tainted-blood tragedy.

Asymptomatic: showing no symptoms; used to describe the condition of a person infected with HIV but showing no signs of illness.

Autologous transfusion: transfusion with blood or blood components originating from the recipient; also called self-donation.

BDR: Blood Donor Recruitment, the branch of the Red Cross responsible for organizing clinics and recruiting volunteer blood and plasma donors.

BTS: Blood Transfusion Service, the branch of the Red Cross responsible for collection, testing and distributing blood and blood products. It has operated since 1939.

Blood: whole blood, which is now rarely used in transfusions, consists of red cells (45 per cent) and plasma (55 per cent), and tiny portions of white cells and clotting factors.

Blood components: the natural components of whole blood: red cells, plasma, platelets, leukocytes.

Blood donation: a donation of whole blood is 450 millilitres, a donation of plasma 225 millilitres. Blood can be donated every 70 days, plasma weekly.

Blood products: the generic term for products manufactured using parts of plasma after fractionation, including cryoprecipitate, factor concentrate, sera and vaccines.

Bureau of Biologics: a division of the Health Protection Branch of Health Canada, it is responsible for the testing and approval of blood products, the inspection of blood collection and plasmapheresis centres.

CBA: Canadian Blood Agency, an incorporated non-profit agency with representatives from each province and territory; created in 1991, it oversees the blood program on behalf of health ministries.

CBC: Canadian Blood Committee, an unincorporated body with representatives from the federal and provincial governments; created in 1981 and disbanded in 1991, it served as an advisory group to the ministers of health on blood-related issues.

CD4 cell: a receptor on the surface of T4 cells, it plays a key role in the body's immune system. AIDS infection begins when a protein on the surface of the HIV binds to the CD4 cell and then merges with T4 lymphocytes, a process likened to getting a foot in the door to force one's way into a house. Damage to the immune system is monitored by counting CD4 cells; a normal count ranges from 500 to 1,500, but when the count falls below 200, a person is susceptible to opportunistic infections and considered to have AIDS; see T4 cells.

CDC: U.S. Centers for Disease Control in Atlanta, Georgia (now known as the U.S. Centers for Disease Control and Prevention); an agency of the U.S. Public Health Service.

CHS: Canadian Hemophilia Society (founded in 1953).

CUE: confidential unit exclusion, a screening program pioneered by the New York Blood Bank, that allowed high-risk donors to designate their blood "for research purposes only" if peer pressure forced them to donate.

Canadian Blood Agency: see CBA.

Canadian Blood Committee: see CBC.

Canadian Hemophilia Society: see CHS.

Canadian Red Cross Society: see Red Cross.

Centers for Disease Control: see CDC.

Christmas disease: hemophilia B, characterized by a deficiency of clotting factor IX. Named after Canadian Stephen Christmas.

Cryoprecipitate (cryo): Factor VIII derived from frozen plasma by thawing it and skimming the factor-rich crystals off the top; a bag of cryo contains 80 to 100 international units of Factor VIII.

DDAVP (desmopressin): a drug that boosts the amount of Factor VIII in blood; an alternative treatment for hemophiliacs, particularly those with inhibitors.

Dry-heat treatment: a method of killing by heating factor concentrate in its powdered form; dry-heat stopped being used in 1987 when it was discovered that it was not 100 per cent effective at killing the HIV. It was replaced by wet-heat treatment.

EAP: the Extraordinary Assistance Plan, a "humanitarian assistance" plan announced by the federal government in 1989 that paid victims of tainted blood $120,000 over four years.

ELISA: enzyme-linked immunosorbent assay, the initial screening test for detecting the HIV antibody; if a blood donation tests positive for HIV antibodies, it is then re-tested using the Western Blot method.

Endemic: present in a community at all times; usually refers to a disease of low morbidity that is constantly present, like influenza.

Epidemic: a disease that attacks many people in a region at the same time and is widely diffused and rapidly spreading; usually refers to a disease of high morbidity and that is only present occasionally.

Epidemiology: the medical science concerned with specific causes of localized outbreaks of infection, and with the relationships of the various factors determining the frequency and distribution of diseases.

Factor concentrate: concentrated form of blood factors, most commonly Factor VIII and Factor IX; small vials of white powder to be reconstituted with distilled water. Vials contain between 200 and 1,200 international units; a moderate hemophiliac requires about 40,000 international units annually.

FDA: Food and Drug Administration, a U.S. regulatory agency.

Factor VIII: a blood clotting factor, or a concentration of that factor; see factor concentrate and hemophilia A.

Factor IX: blood clotting factor similar to Factor VIII; see factor concentrate and hemophilia B.

Federal Centre for AIDS: a branch of the Canadian Department of Health and Welfare that was responsible for AIDS research and prevention programs, it has been disbanded.

Fibrinogen: a protein essential to coagulation, it is found in plasma.

Fractionation: the process of breaking down blood into components using a centrifuge.

HIV: human immunodeficiency virus, the agent believed to be responsible for AIDS.

HIV Information Project: a research project by the Toronto Hospital for Sick Children that sought to contact cardiac patients from 1978 to 1985 and have them tested for AIDS.

HIV-T Group (Blood Transfused): a Toronto-based support group for former transfusion patients with AIDS.

HTLV: human T-cell leukemia virus, type I is a retrovirus that can cause adult T-lymphocyte leukemia between 10 and 30 years after infection. HTLV-II causes chronic degenerative neurological disease 10 to 20 years after infection. The virus called HIV was originally known as HTLV-III.

Heat treatment: process of heating plasma or factor concentrate to kill bacteria and viruses in a manner similar to the pasteurization of milk; see dry-heat treatment and wet-heat treatment.

Hemoglobin: a compound found in the red cells that carries oxygen to cells throughout the body and carries away carbon dioxide; also a measure of the blood's ability to carry out its key function of transporting oxygen, referred to commonly as the "iron level".

Hemophilia: a hereditary deficiency, or total absence, of a specific blood clotting factor. (There are 13 clotting factors, but Factor VIII and Factor IX are the most common deficiencies.) Characterized by spontaneous or trauma-related subcutaneous (below the skin) or intramuscular hemorrhages. One in 5,000 males is a hemophiliac, but the clotting deficiency may be mild, moderate or severe.

Hemophilia A: a deficiency of clotting Factor VIII.

Hemophilia B: a deficiency of clotting Factor IX, also known as Christmas disease.

Hemorrhage: severe bleeding, internally or externally.

Hepatitis A: an infectious liver disease spread by a bacteria, it is not blood borne, but associated with unclean water supply; it is the least severe form of hepatitis.

Hepatitis B (HBc): an infectious liver disease spread by a virus, the symptoms can vary from mild discomfort to cirrhosis. It can be transmitted by blood or by sexual contact, but a vaccine has been available since 1981.

Hepatitis C (HCV): an infectious liver disease spread by a virus, the symptoms can vary from mild discomfort to cirrhosis or liver cancer. Transmitted by blood. The virus was not discovered until 1989; until then the condition was known as non-A-non-B hepatitis. There is no vaccine, nor cure.

Human t-cell leukemia virus: see HTLV.

Kaposi's sarcoma: a cancer that was rare prior to the appearance of AIDS; it causes multiple bluish-red patches which are the most visible manifestations of AIDS infection.

LAV: lymphadenopathy-associated virus, the name initially given the AIDS virus by French researchers.

Laboratory Centre for Disease Control: a division of the Health Protection Branch of Health Canada, it is responsible for disease surveillance, and serves as an early warning system for new outbreaks. It publishes *Canada Diseases Weekly Report*.

Look-back: the procedure when a blood donor is identified as HIV-positive; his or her past donation record is checked and recipients are contacted to be tested.

MPTAP: Multi-Provincial-Territorial Assistance Program; announced by the provinces in 1993, it paid some victims of tainted blood $30,000 a year for life.

MSAC: Medical and Scientific Advisory Committee of the Canadian Hemophilia Society.

Mild deficiency: in hemophilia, factor activity ranging from 6 to 50 per cent of normal; hemorrhages are caused by major trauma or surgery, and this level of hemophilia is often not discovered until adulthood. Treatment with concentrate is rare, usually after a serious accident.

Moderate deficiency: in hemophilia, factor activity ranging from 1 to 5 per cent of normal; hemorrhages are caused by moderate trauma. Treatment with concentrate is occasional, rarely more than weekly.

Multi-Provincial-Territorial Assistance Program: see MPTAP.

NACAIDS: National Advisory Committee on AIDS, an advisory body to the federal Minister of Health and Welfare (formerly called the National Task Force on AIDS).

Opportunistic infection: an infection that does not normally occur in healthy people, but may be found in persons whose immune systems are not functioning at full capacity; PCP is an example.

PCP: *pneumocystis carinii* pneumonia, a previously rare form of pneumonia that is common among people with AIDS.

Plasma: the yellowish liquid that constitutes about 55 per cent of blood; it is used primarily to treat shock. Plasma is also fractionated into various proteins that form the basis of more than two dozen specialized blood products. Prior to factor concentrate, fresh frozen plasma was the treatment of choice for Factor IX hemophiliacs.

Plasmapheresis: a process in which only a donor's plasma is kept; the other blood components are injected back into the donor. The advantage is that plasma can be donated weekly, and it is in much greater demand than whole blood.

Platelets: an element of blood that aids clotting, commonly referred to as the "sticky part of blood"; used to treat leukemia.

Pneumocystis carinii pneumonia: see PCP.

Prophylaxis: preventive treatment.

Rh factor: the rhesus factor; a person's blood is either Rh-positive or Rh-negative and blood must be matched by Rh type to permit a safe transfusion. Rh-positive babies born to Rh-negative mothers subsequent to their first pregnancy require immediate transfusion, unless the problem has been treated before birth.

Red cells: the red liquid that constitutes about 45 per cent of blood. Red cells carry oxygen so they are often administered during surgery.

Retrovirus: a virus that needs a special enzyme (the reverse transcriptase) to reproduce; HIV is a retrovirus and while it is easy to find its chemical footprint (the enzyme), it is difficult to find the retrovirus itself, which explains why researchers have been unable to develop a vaccine and why drugs used to treat AIDS, like AZT, interfere with the enzyme's reproduction.

Self-donation: see autologous transfusion.

Sera: see serum.

Seroconversion illness: when HIV first begins attacking the immune system and cells are seroconverting from HIV-negative to HIV-positive, many people suffer a first bout of flu-like illness characterized by fever, chills and night sweats. See ARC.

Serum (plural *sera*): a derivative of blood that, like plasma, contains no red cells or platelets; serum (often called antiserum) usually contains specific antibodies and is used to make vaccines.

Severe deficiency: in hemophilia, factor activity level less than one per cent of normal; spontaneous bleeds occur in muscles and joints, and even minor trauma can provoke severe hemorrhage. Severe hemophiliacs use prophylaxis to prevent bleeds, and infuse concentrate as often as daily.

Sickle cell anemia: a hereditary blood disorder, occurring mostly in blacks, in which abnormal hemoglobin causes red cells to become sickle-shaped, hampering their iron-carrying function, leading to anemia; treatment consists primarily of regular transfusions of red cells, on average monthly.

Surrogate test: a substitute test; for example, before there was a test for antibodies to HIV, HBV antibodies were used as a surrogate because virtually everyone with AIDS had a previous bout of hepatitis B.

T4 cells: a set of white blood cells (lymphocytes) that play a crucial role in the body's defence against disease by orchestrating other parts of the immune system. HIV enters T4 cells, multiplies and destroys the T4 cells; see CD4 cells.

Thalassemia: a hereditary form of anemia, usually in people of Mediterranean origin, that leads to iron accumulation and retarded growth; treatment consists of regular transfusions of red cells.

Trace-back: the procedure when an HIV-positive person is identified as a recipient of a blood transfusion; the blood unit numbers are identified and donors traced so they can be tested.

Universal precautions: the routine use of barrier devices (gloves, gowns, masks) to prevent the transmission of infectious disease.

Von Willebrand's disease: a hereditary deficiency of the Von Willebrand factor, a protein in the blood associated with platelet stickiness and with Factor VIII clotting activitity. Treatment is virtually identical to that for hemophilia A.

Western Blot: a confirmatory test for AIDS antibodies.

Wet-heat treatment: a method of killing viruses by heating plasma before it is freeze-dried and manufactured into factor concentrate; there have been no documented cases of HIV from wet-heat-treated concentrate. See dry-heat treatment.

Window period: the time between infection with the HIV and the body's production of antibodies; during this period, up to six months, the virus can go undetected by the ELISA test.

CHRONOLOGY

DATE	EVENT
Jan. 29, 1940	First blood donor clinic opens at Grace Hospital in Toronto.
June 4, 1940	First transfusion of Canadian blood serum into soldier, at Dunkirk.
Nov. 10, 1942	Red Cross allows women to donate blood for the first time.
1943	Hundreds, perhaps thousands of units of dried plasma contaminated by bacteria.
Aug. 15, 1945	Wartime blood clinics shut down, just after VJ Day.
Feb. 1947	First peacetime Blood Transfusion Service Centre opened in Vancouver.
1953	Canadian Hemophilia Society founded by Frank Schnabel.
1954	Blood fractionation plant built at Connaught Laboratories in Toronto.
1955	First adult hemophilia treatment centre is established at St. Mary's Hospital in Montreal.
1959	Freeze-dried anti-hemophilic globulin (AHG) is made available, in limited supply, for "treatment of intractable cases of haemophilia".
April 1960	First Canadian treated with factor concentrate from Connaught Laboratories.
Jan. 1965	First treatment centre for hemophiliac children established at the Ontario Hospital for Sick Children in Toronto.
1965	Cryoprecipitate replaces transfusion of whole blood for treatment of hemophiliacs.
1967	Medical journals begin reporting cases of hepatitis in users of blood concentrate.
1968	Factor VIII concentrate licensed for treatment of hemophilia-A patients.
1968	Frank Schnabel founds World Federation of Hemophilia.
1969	Factor IX concentrate licensed for treatment of hemophilia B patients.
1970	Red Cross begins testing blood for hepatitis B antibodies.
1972	Connaught Laboratories sold to Canada Development Corporation, a Crown corporation.
Feb. 26, 1973	Health ministers establish Federal-Provincial Programme and Budget Review Committee and increase financial support to Red Cross to strengthen voluntary blood donor system.
1974	Red Cross introduces quality control program to ensure safety and efficiency of use of blood products, in particular Factor VIII and platelets.
1975	Red Cross introduces first questionnaire for blood donors.

1976	Consultant recommends Red Cross build and operate a fractionation plant. Red Cross makes a formal request to federal government.
1977	Manual establishing the criteria for blood donor selection is distributed to blood donor service centres.
1978	First cases of AIDS are reported in U.S.
1979	First AIDS case diagnosed in Canada.
1980	Behringwerke produces Factor VIII heat-treated for hepatitis B.
Sept. 30, 1981	Health ministers establish Canadian Blood Authority, later the Canadian Blood Committee.
Jan. 1982	First confirmed AIDS death in Canada, a homosexual man in Windsor.
	A Miami hemophiliac dies of AIDS, indicating the disease is blood-borne.
July 16, 1982	*Mortality and Morbidity Weekly Report* reports three cases of PCP in U.S. hemophiliacs and warns that "cases suggest possible transmission of an agent through blood".
July 27, 1982	The name AIDS coined at a meeting of U.S. government scientists, blood bankers, gay groups, hemophiliacs. High-risk groups reject donor deferral measures.
Aug. 6, 1982	Bureau of Biologics warns Red Cross of the "theoretical risk that an unknown transmissible agent present in [blood products] may be responsible for AIDS" and asks the agency to step up surveillance. At the time, there are eight AIDS cases.
Oct. 1982	U.S. National Hemophilia Foundation recommends screening out high-risk donors, homosexual men specifically.
Dec. 2, 1982	First meeting of the Ad Hoc AIDS Group.
Dec. 10, 1982	*Mortality and Morbidity Weekly Report* reports San Francisco baby developed AIDS after a transfusion of platelets.
Dec. 11, 1982	*Canada Diseases Weekly Report* publishes preliminary report showing 70 per cent of hemophiliacs have reduced cellular immunity, an early sign of AIDS.
Jan. 4, 1983	U.S. Centers for Disease Control holds meeting to demand response to blood-borne AIDS.
Jan. 13, 1983	American Red Cross, American Association of Blood Banks and Council of Community Blood Centers issue an alert about possible, but still unproven, transmission of AIDS by blood transfusion. They reject screening out homosexual men.
	The New England Journal of Medicine suggests hemophiliacs be switched from concentrate to cryoprecipitate.
Jan. 14, 1983	U.S. National Hemophilia Foundation issues recommendations on prevention of AIDS in hemophiliacs, including screening and surrogate testing.

Jan. 17, 1983	Medical director of Ottawa blood transfusion service expresses concern that blood products for hemophiliacs are not safe.
Feb. 10, 1983	Red Cross medical directors unanimously endorse joint statement of U.S. blood bankers of Jan. 13, including symptom specific questions. They later reverse that decision.
Feb. 17, 1983	Medical and Scientific Advisory Committee of Canadian Hemophilia Society proposes reducing use of concentrate by switching hemophiliacs to cryoprecipitate and DDAVP, better screening to eliminate high-risk blood donors and increasing collection of plasma in Canada to avoid U.S. imports.
March 10, 1983	Red Cross makes first public plea to high-risk donors not to give blood.
March 22, 1983	A Montreal baby dies of AIDS contracted during transfusion in October 1982.
March 24, 1983	FDA issues guidelines for screening blood donors. Only some blood banks implement these measures.
March 31, 1983	A B.C. mill worker becomes the first Canadian hemophiliac known to have died of AIDS.
May 5, 1983	National Advisory Committee on AIDS (NACAIDS) holds its first meeting.
May 20, 1983	Dr. Luc Montagnier of France's Pasteur Institute announces discovery of LAV, lymphadenopathy-associated virus, as cause of AIDS.
May 23, 1983	France bans import of U.S. blood products. (By year's end, eight other European countries follow suit.)
July 1, 1983	Stanford University Blood Bank starts screening for AIDS, using surrogate testing. The measure adds 10 per cent to the cost of a unit of blood.
July 1983	Miami woman dies of AIDS, the first wife of a hemophiliac known to have died.
July 23, 1983	Red Cross issues second press release urging high-risk donors to not give blood.
Aug. 1983	"There is no evidence that blood is any less safe now than prior to the appearance of AIDS," Red Cross says in a brief prepared for public health officials.
Aug. 1, 1983	Chairman of transfusion committee of the FDA and American Association of Blood Banks blames public concern about transfusion AIDS on "overreacting press".
Sept. 8, 1983	*The New England Journal of Medicine* says while the cause of AIDS is unknown, high-risk groups have been identified and blood donations by their members should not be accepted.
Oct. 31, 1983	Cutter withdraws 13 lots of Factor VIII and one of Factor IX after a donor dies of AIDS.
Nov. 22-25, 1983	World's top AIDS experts gather at WHO headquarters in Geneva

for first meeting on the international implications of AIDS, a disease reported in 33 countries on five continents.

Nov. 23, 1983   Baxter-Hyland receives licence to sell heat-treated Factor VIII in Canada; heat treatment kills hepatititis B.

Jan. 1984   *The New England Journal of Medicine* publishes a study of seven transfusion patients who died of AIDS.

Feb. 1984   Four babies in Australia receive blood from a gay man infected with AIDS. (By year's end all four babies are dead.) Queensland legislature passes law imposing stiff fine and two-year prison sentence on any member of a high-risk group who donates blood.

AIDS now the leading killer of hemophiliacs in the U.S., with 16 dead to date.

March 1984   Health and Welfare Canada distributes 200,000 AIDS pamphlets saying the risk of contracting AIDS from blood is 2 in 1 million.

April 1984   Red Cross issues pamphlet "An Important Message to Our Blood Donors", the first information on AIDS. It makes no mention of AIDS symptoms.

April 23, 1984   Discovery of human T-cell lymphotropic virus type III (HTLV-III) as cause of AIDS is announced by Dr. Robert Gallo at U.S. National Institutes of Health.

May 1984   Red Cross issues pamphlet for blood donors that includes general health questions and description of AIDS symptoms.

June 1984   Tests by U.S. Centers for Disease Control find 72 per cent of hemophiliacs with no signs of AIDS are infected with LAV, and 90 per cent of those who infuse more than once a month.

July 1984   Preliminary research reveals that 55 per cent of hemophiliacs test positive for HTLV-III.

July 7, 1984   *The Lancet* reports 64 per cent of hemophiliacs treated with concentrate at a Danish hospital test positive.

July 13, 1984   *Mortality and Morbidity Weekly Report* reveals 72 per cent of asymptomatic hemophilia patients using Factor VIII concentrate test positive.

Sept. 1984   U.S. blood banks begin large-scale clinical trials using ELISA test.

U.S. Centers for Disease Control reports 80 cases of transfusion AIDS and 52 hemophiliacs with AIDS, a quadrupling of confirmed cases in eight months.

National Hemophilia Foundation reports Factor VIII use down 20 to 30 per cent; hemophiliacs would rather risk uncontrolled bleed than AIDS.

Sept. 10, 1984   Canadian Hemophilia Society meets major suppliers of Factor VIII to state concerns about lack of heat-treated product and general shortage of Factor VIII.

Sept. 29, 1984   *The Lancet* publishes a study by Cutter Laboratories confirming efficacy of heat treatment in inactivating HIV-like virus.

Oct. 5, 1984	Red Cross submits position paper on blood testing to NACAIDS, saying need for testing unproven and citing "very serious psycho-social implications to instituting such testing prematurely".
	B.C. coroner's jury criticizes public health officials for failing to prevent the infection of hemophiliacs with AIDS virus.
Oct. 11, 1984	Canadian Hemophilia Society demands immediate cancellation of Connaught contract. Red Cross continues to doubt efficacy of heat treatment.
Oct. 13, 1984	U.S. National Hemophilia Foundation recommends immediate switch to heat-treated products.
Oct. 26, 1984	Senior Red Cross official writes in Hemophilia Ontario newsletter that "evidence that coagulation factor therapy carries a significant direct risk of AIDS" is less than conclusive.
Oct. 30, 1984	Red Cross has two-month inventory of Factor VIII and enough "plasma already in the pipeline" to produce 8 million units more; switching to heat-treated products would mean financial loss.
Nov. 13, 1984	Cutter Laboratories granted a licence to heat-treat Factor VIII concentrate.
Nov. 16, 1984	Bureau of Biologics issues directive to all manufacturers of Factor VIII and IX requiring that they provide heat-treated products as soon as feasible.
	New Zealand's Minister of Health announces all blood donations will be tested and stocks of untreated factor concentrate withdrawn.
Nov. 22, 1984	*Nature* reports Factor VIII gene has been cloned, meaning clotting factor can be produced without human plasma.
Nov. 26, 1984	Red Cross informs Connaught that, as of Dec. 1, plasma will be redirected to Cutter for heat treatment. Red Cross asks that Connaught continue supplying untreated products until March 31, 1985, to use up plasma already provided.
Dec. 1984	Health authorities in England report at least 55 Britons treated with blood contaminated with AIDS virus. Testing in West Germany reveals two-thirds of hemophiliacs are infected.
Dec. 10, 1984	American Association of Blood Banks, American Red Cross and Council of Community Blood Centers issue joint statement about need for tracing and notifying recipients of potentially tainted blood.
	Consensus conference on heat-treated Factor VIII endorses introduction of new products "as soon as it is feasible before May 1985".
Dec. 12, 1984	Red Cross announces plans to order 40 million units of heat-treated concentrate, a one-year supply.
Dec. 21, 1984	Travenol Laboratories offers Red Cross royalty-free license to manufacture heat-treated factor concentrate in Canada.
Feb. 1985	The Red Cross begins clinical trials with blood-testing kits.
Feb. 14, 1985	U.S. National Hemophilia Foundation recommends all blood be tested for AIDS.

Feb. 18, 1985	Bureau of Biologics receives first two lots of Cutter heat-treated Factor VIII for review.
March 2, 1985	FDA licenses first HIV-antibody test kit. By the end of March, 99 per cent of whole blood is screened, but source plasma used for Factor VIII is not fully screened until November.
March 7, 1985	NACAIDS task force recommends Red Cross prepare plan for implementation of HIV screening by March 30.
March 15, 1985	First supply of heat-treated Factor VIII (from Cutter) is released by Bureau of Biologics.
March 20, 1985	Director of blood products services tells regional Red Cross centres that 40 million heat-treated units ordered but says distribution will take place from May to July.
April 1985	After one month of testing, American Red Cross reveals that, nationally, 1 in 500 donors tested positive for AIDS.
April 1, 1985	First HIV-antibody test kit approved for sale in Canada. A second kit is approved on April 18.
April 12, 1985	Armour becomes second manufacturer licensed to sell heat-treated Factor VIII.
April 20, 1985	Canadian Hemophilia Society approves priority list for distribution of heat-treated coagulation products.
April 25, 1985	Canadian Hemophilia Society medical and scientific advisory committee requests immediate institution of HIV testing.
April 29, 1985	Red Cross advises its regional medical directors each centre "will be supplied with a limited amount of heat-treated factor concentrates" and that the "majority of hemophilia patients should continue to receive non-heat-treated coagulation factor products until July 1st".
April 30, 1985	First heat-treated coagulation products distributed.
May 1, 1985	Red Cross presents blood-screening plans to the Canadian Blood Committee, suggesting screening begin Aug. 1, pending budget approval by provinces.
May 8, 1985	Red Cross admits, for the first time, that two transfusion recipients contracted AIDS. Both men died earlier in 1985.
May 15, 1985	NACAIDS accepts Red Cross plan to start testing blood 10 to 12 weeks after funding received. (Canadian Blood Committee approves in principle on June 4.)
May 30, 1985	Red Cross tells regional medical directors that "routine centres requirements for Factor VIII concentrate can only be met with untreated products . . . because there is currently an insufficient supply of heat-treated products to fill all routine requests".
	Letter to Red Cross from Abbott Laboratories reveals that testing of 3,000 otherwise healthy donors found 1 in 270 (or .37 per cent) reactive to the ELISA test.
June 3, 1985	The Red Cross has 15 million units of heat-treated Factor VIII in inventory.

June 14, 1985	Red Cross granted $20 million by Ottawa and provinces for construction of a new national headquarters.
July 1, 1985	Heat-treated Factor VIII fully replaces the old product.
July 4, 1985	Provincial health officials agree that Red Cross screening plan should be implemented by Oct. 14, if Canadian Blood Committee approves budget by July 12; they also agree each province will designate one or more labs for HIV testing.
July 17, 1985	Canadian Blood Committee members approve screening program, with exception of Ontario and Manitoba. Ontario provides funding Aug. 1.
Nov. 4, 1985	All Canadian blood donations now screened for AIDS.
Jan. 1986	Connaught granted a licence to sell heat-treated Factor VIII.
April 1986	Insurance companies for manufacturers of blood concentrate in Sweden provide compensation to hemophiliacs in out-of-court settlement.
May 31, 1986	Letter in *The Lancet* warns of "caution in the reliance on dry heat inactivation" of factor concentrate.
June 19, 1986	Canadian Blood Committee advised by Red Cross that the problem with look-back program is unavailability of blood bank records beyond a couple of years, but that 450 recipients annually might be involved in look-back procedures.
June 30, 1986	Armour voluntarily withdraws 206 lots of heat-treated Factor VIII made from unscreened plasma after infections reported.
Feb. 27, 1987	Cutter withdraws 34 lots of Factor VIII and Factor IX concentrate made with unscreened plasma.
March 19, 1987	ABC television program "20/20" airs report on AIDS in blood supply, with emphasis on hemophiliacs infected with AIDS.
May 3, 1987	Bureau of Biologics recommends no further purchases of dry-heated products.
July 1987	Red Cross begins limited look-back program.
Sept. 1987	Infection of seven hemophiliacs in B.C. and Alberta who used heat-treated concentrate exclusively is revealed.
Nov. 1987	Hemophiliacs infected with HIV in Britain receive financial compensation.
Dec. 15, 1987	Bureau of Biologics recommends dry-heat-treated coagulation products be replaced with wet-heat-treated products.
April 1988	Self-help group for HIV-infected by transfusion is formed in Calgary.
Sept. 1988	Canadian Hemophilia Society requests Catastrophe Relief on behalf of HIV-infected hemophiliacs.
Sept. 1989	Blood classified as drug and placed on Schedule D of Food and Drugs Act, giving the Bureau of Biologics regulatory control over blood as well as blood products.

Ministers of health establish Canadian Blood Agency to replace Canadian Blood Committee. Federal government not directly involved in the new agency.

Dec. 14, 1989   Health and Welfare announces a federal program for "compassionate" financial assistance for HIV-infected hemophiliacs and blood transfusion recipients, $120,000 over four years.

May 1990   Red Cross begins testing blood for the hepatitis C virus.

Nov. 26, 1992   Commons Sub-Committee on Health Issues begins public hearings on the tainted-blood tragedy.

April 1, 1993   Most tainted-blood victims receive their final cheques under federal compensation plan.

May 25, 1993   Commons Sub-Committee on Health Issues recommends judicial inquiry on tainted blood, and measures to track down Canadians who may have been infected.

June 15, 1993   Toronto Hospital for Sick Children announces preliminary results of trace-back program. A total of 17 of 1,700 cardiac patients tested positive.

Aug. 11, 1993   Nova Scotia health minister announces compensation plan for tainted-blood victims.

Sept. 15, 1993   Other provinces offer compensation package of $30,000 annually to victims of tainted blood. The Multi-Provincial-Territorial Assistance Program has March 15 deadline.

Sept. 16, 1993   Federal health minister Mary Collins announces public inquiry to examine the events underlying tainted-blood tragedy and recommend revamping of blood system.

Oct. 1993   Red Cross announces it will build fractionation plant in conjunction with Bayer Inc.

Nov. 22, 1993   Commission of Inquiry on the Blood System in Canada convenes for the first time, but the hearing is only to determine which groups will be given standing.

Dec. 1993   Pharmaceutical companies and the Red Cross are included in the MPTAP compensation plan; victims must waive legal proceedings against them to get money.

Feb. 14, 1994   Commission of Inquiry on the Blood System in Canada opens its public hearings.

Mar. 14, 1994   Ontario Court of Justice awards Rochelle Pittman $515,000.

Mar. 15, 1994   Deadline for accepting Multi-Provincial-Territorial Assistance Program.

June 1994   Canadian Hospital Association urges Canadians who received blood transfusions between 1978 and 1985 to be tested for AIDS.

Summer 1994   Number of Red Cross regional blood centres fail FDA inspections.

Feb. 24, 1995   Commission of Inquiry on the Blood System in Canada issues interim report, urging greater efforts to track down 3.5 million Canadians who received blood between 1978 and 1985.

252 \ THE GIFT OF DEATH

April 10, 1995	Red Cross and Canadian Blood Agency sign a master agreement.
April 19, 1995	Canadian Hemophilia Society calls for plasma donors to be paid, as part of revamping of blood system.
May 1995	Estimated cost of Red Cross-Bayer fractionation plant jumps to $300 million.
June 7, 1995	Bureau of Biologics announces it will conduct annual inspection of Red Cross BTS centres.
July 1995	News that two blood donors suffering from Creutzfeldt-Jakob disease prompts largest recall ever of blood products.
Dec. 31, 1995	Deadline for final report of Commission of Inquiry on the Blood System in Canada.

ENDNOTES

1: GIFT OF LIFE: KISS OF DEATH

1. Donald Francis, expert on AIDS epidemiology and etiology, formerly of the Centers for Disease Control in Atlanta, testified during the civil lawsuit that Kenneth Pittman's odds of being transfused with tainted blood in December 1984 may have been as high as 1 in 4. His calculation was based on the fact that Pittman received 46 units of blood and using the results of a clinical trial with the Abbott test kit that found 17 of 3,000 samples collected in the Toronto area tested positive for HIV. The Red Cross argues that the clinical trial results do not accurately reflect the level of contamination of the blood supply because the samples were not collected randomly and infected units may well have been screened out.

2. CD4 lymphocytes are the centre of the body's immune response. The CD4 is often likened to the conductor of the orchestra and "if the conductor is taken out, the orchestra falls apart," explains Dr. Alex Klein.

3. In an unusual move, the court visited Toronto Hospital in April 1992 to record Mr. L.'s testimony, fearing he might die before the case went to trial. The Red Cross provided him with legal counsel. Mr. L. died in January 1993, almost three years after Kenneth Pittman.

2: BLOOD TIES

1. On Dec. 6, 1917, the French munitions ship *Mont Blanc* caught fire in the Halifax Harbour and exploded with the force of 2,800 tons of TNT. More than 1,700 people were killed and another 4,000 wounded.

2. The flag hoisted at the Battle of Batoche is now on display at Canadian Red Cross Society headquarters in Ottawa.

3. In Canada, as in Great Britain, the Red Cross and St. John Ambulance were closely linked, the former giving medical aid in wartime and the latter in peacetime.

4. In 1917, a Wisconsin state official who complained that the American Red Cross was being run by wealthy New York businessmen — it was — was convicted under the Espionage Act and served six months in Leavenworth Penitentiary.

5. The Canadian Red Cross, unlike its U.S. counterpart, did not discriminate based on skin colour; in southern U.S. states, miscegenation laws prevented not only inter-marriage but the mixing of blood of different races.

6. The most notable early use of plasmapheresis was at the University of Winnipeg, where Dr. Bruce Chown took women with Rh antibodies and created a vaccine. The drug produced by the Rh Institute, WinRho, became world-renowned for virtually eliminating dangerous reactions at birth, a problem that arises when Rh-positive babies are born of Rh-negative mothers who have previously given birth. If the incompatibility is discovered only after birth, multiple transfusions are administered to change the baby's Rh factor.

3: BOYS WHO BLEED

1. A woman can have hemophilia if she has the hemophilia gene on both her X chromosomes. This can happen only if her father is a hemophiliac and her mother a carrier, or if she develops a mutation on her X chromosome.

2. Factor VIII deficiency is referred to as hemophilia A, or classic hemophilia. Factor IX, the next most common blood disorder, is known as hemophilia B, or Christmas disease. (Clotting Factor IX was discovered in 1952 in tests on the blood of Stephen Christmas of Toronto.)

4: DEATH TOUCHES DOWN

1. The first official acknowledgement of AIDS in the medical community came in the July 4, 1981, edition of *Mortality and Morbidity Weekly Report*, but doctors with a substantial gay clientele had been aware of a new disease for at least two years prior to that article.

2. The hypothesis that AIDS originated in Africa, probably as a mutant strain of a disease affecting primates, was formulated by the French AIDS Task Force and presented at a seminar in Boston in February 1983 by Dr. Jacques Leibowitch.

3. At a May 1983 meeting of the Haitian Physicians' Association in Paris, research was presented that revealed that 30 per cent of Haitian men said they had had anal sex with foreign tourists. The admission came only when they were questioned by Haitian doctors; when questioned by foreign researchers, they denied any such sexual contacts.

4. In July 1982, the Centers for Disease Control defined a case of AIDS as a "disease, at least moderately predictive of a defect in cell-mediated immunity, occurring in a person with no known cause for diminished resistance to that disease. Such diseases include Kaposi's sarcoma, pneumocystis carinii pneumonia and other serious opportunistic infections. The full spectrum of AIDS may range from absence of symptoms (despite laboratory evidence of immune deficiency), to non-specific symptoms, to specific diseases that are insufficiently predictive of cellular immunodeficiency to be included in incidence monitoring. Risk factors identified so far include male homosexuality, intravenous drug abuse, Haitian origin, and perhaps hemophilia A."

5. The antibody test for AIDS was a simple laboratory process: plastic beads were coated with the AIDS virus and, when a drop of blood was added to the small well where the beads rested, antibodies to the virus latched onto the virus; the beads were then washed with various dyes and chemicals and those that turned purple indicated a positive test.

5: LETHAL INDIFFERENCE

1. Red Cross headquarters were located on the periphery of the gay "ghetto" and only one block away from the country's first and largest AIDS-prevention group, the AIDS committee of Toronto.

2. In April 1983, the Toronto-based group Gays in Health Care, also produced a pamphlet but Dr. Derrick said it could not be distributed at blood clinics because it was too explicit.

3. Randy Shilts, *And the Band Played On*, p. 406.

4. The term "homophobia-phobia" was coined by John Plater, president of Hemophilia Ontario.

6: BLOOD MONEY

1. Hemophilia was one of the first human disorders for which the gene responsible for the disorder was identified and cloned, setting the stage for the development of factor concentrate that did not require human blood derivatives. Recombinant products are produced by genetically engineering the Factor VIII enzyme to ensure they are disease-free. Monoclonal products are derived from plasma but treated with detergent to kill all viruses before the Factor VIII is cloned.

2. The first heat-treated Factor VIII concentrate was developed by Behringwerke AG, a German company, in 1980. The Baxter Company (also known in Canada as Hyland) received a Canadian licence to sell Factor VIII concentrate heat-treated to kill the hepatitis B virus on November 23, 1983. Factor VIII heat-treated specifically to kill the AIDS virus was not licensed in Canada until November 13, 1984.

3. On a number of occasions, federal health officials didn't even bother urging withdrawal of concentrate manufactured with AIDS and hepatitis-tainted plasma.

4. Connaught purchased plasma from a Montreal blood broker that purchased it from the Arkansas Department of Corrections and from a blood bank in San Francisco, among others. Cutter had equally dubious sources including plasmapheresis centres along the Mexican border and in Oakland.

5. Had it invested the losses it incurred in penalty clauses in plasmapheresis, the Canadian blood program could have increased Canadian-source production by 10 per cent, providing 1.5 million units of safer concentrate annually.

6. To this day, a tiny minority of hemophiliacs refuse to treat their bleeds with cryoprecipitate or concentrate. William Hall, a beekeeper from Nipawin, Saskatchewan, and a Jehovah's Witness — his faith forbids blood transfusions — uses a combination of ice packs, magnets, herbal remedies and prayer, and he is in his late seventies.

7: CONSENSUS FOR INACTION

1. "There is no reason . . . to not have had pasteurized products on the market by 1980, had reasonable and prudent research and development been used," Thomas Drees, former head of Alpha Therapeutics Inc., a U.S. manufacturer, said in an affidavit filed in a 1988 lawsuit by a patient known only as Jane Doe.

2. While Dr. Michael O'Shaughnessy tested the samples using antibodies tests supplied by the CDC, the samples had come from the research being conducted by Dr. Christos Tsoukas since early 1982. The 55 per cent of hemophiliacs whose blood tested positive were not informed of the results, nor were those who tested negative.

3. Connaught Laboratories Inc., long affiliated with the University of Toronto, was in 1984, a wholly owned unit of CDC Life Sciences, a subsidiary of the Canada Development Corporation, which was in turn 47 per cent owned by the federal government.

4. The offer of a five-year, royalty-free licence to manufacture and sell heat-treated concentrate in Canada was made in a December 21, 1984, letter from Dale Smith, vice-president of Travenol, to Roger Perrault of the Red Cross.

5. While most attention has focussed on Factor VIII, it should be noted that 10,000 vials of heat-treated Facto IX sat in a Cutter warehouse from November 28, 1984 until they were delivered to the Red Cross on May 31, 1985. During that period, two children at Sick Kids in Toronto contracted AIDS from non-heat-treated Factor IX.

6. Total inventory of concentrates withdrawn after the switch to heat-treated products was 1,815,685 AHF units, according to analysis by Craig Anhorn, Red Cross manager of Blood Products Services, September 27, 1985.

7. An audit by Deloitte & Touche management consultants recommended that the laboratory repay $14,256,469 for failing to meet its production goals and another $500,000 for exceeding operating expenses in its final year of operation, but the Canadian Blood Committee never collected the money.

8. At least 206 lots of heat-treated Armour concentrate and 34 lots of Cutter concentrate were recalled, according to documents released under the Access to Information Act.

8: ONE IN A MILLION

1. The average adult male has 5.5 litres of blood flowing through his body, while the average woman has only 3.5 litres in her body. A donation of whole blood is 450 millilitres, for both men and women.

2. In June 1984, six weeks after the the discovery of the AIDS virus was announced, the U.S. Department of Health and Human Services selected five companies to develop an AIDS test, and provided them with samples of the virus. They were Abbott Laboratories; Electro-Nucleonics Inc.; Litton Bionetics Inc.; Travenol/Genentech Diagnostics; and Biotech Research Laboratories Inc. in conjunction with E.I. du Pont de Nemours and Co.

3. In the U.S., kit manufacturing insisted on "unlinked" testing to avoid legal liability. The Canadian Red Cross adopted this practice, meaning that blood that tested positive in clinical trials was used, and donors were not notified.

4. Conservatives Keith Norton, Philip Andrewes and Alan Pope, and Liberal Murray Elston, all served, in turn, as Ontario Minister of Health during the first six months of 1985.

5. In fact, during the blood-borne AIDS crisis from 1981-1985, the blood program underspent its budget by $11 million. The Red Cross itself was also flush with cash. In 1985, the year heat treatment of concentrate and AIDS testing were delayed, the agency's investment portfolio increased to $19.5 million from $16 million.

6. Studies in the U.S. have shown that donors are more forthright about their medical and sexual history when donating anonymously than with directed donations, largely because the knowledge of the rejection of their blood within the family could result in the revelation of potentially embarrassing personal details.

10: MONEY CAN'T BUY ME LIFE

1. Randy Conners's grandfather, the Reverend Hollis Kimball, was a Wesleyan minister who preached throughout New Brunswick, Nova Scotia and Maine, and often travelled by snowshoe to minister to his followers. He was one of the longest-lived hemophiliacs in Canada, and perhaps the world. Reverend Kimball died in 1985 at the age of eighty-three.

2. Although the Archival Study prepared for the Canadian Hemophilia Society has no authors' credit, those who contributed included Robert Gibson (deceased), Stephen Christmas (deceased), Robert O'Neill (a CHS director who now works with The AIDS Project in Vancouver), Ann Harrington (a nurse at St. Michael's Hospital in Toronto), William Mindell (a former City of Toronto public health official) and Santo Caira (a former employee of Hemophilia Ontario). It was put together, in the form of a legal brief by law student Mark Hauer, who worked as a summer student at the CHS.

3. The order-in-council creating the Extraordinary Assistance Plan was P.C. 1990-4/872, an order respecting ex gratia payments to persons infected with the human immunodeficiency virus (HIV) through blood or blood products in Canada.

4. The eighteen insurance companies included in the MPTAP waiver are: Canadian Medical Protective Association, Commercial Union Assurance Company of Canada, The General Accident Insurance Company of Canada, The Guarantee Company of North America, Halifax Insurance Company, Manitoba Public Insurance Corporation, Royal Insurance Company of Canada, Quebec Assurance Company, Western Assurance Company,

Saskatchewan Government Insurance, The Dominion of Canada Group, The Casualty Company of Canada, The Canadian Indemnity Company, The Canadian General Insurance Company, Traders General Insurance Company, Scottish & York Insurance Company, Victoria Insurance Company, Toronto General Insurance Company.

5. The $151-million contribution to the Multi-Provincial-Territorial Assistance Program includes a minimum of $109 million from the provinces, up to $42 million from fractionators and insurance companies and $3 million from the Red Cross. The Canadian Blood Agency, which is not covered by federal or provincial Access To Information laws, refuses to reveal these details publicly, but sources who participated in the negotiations say the fractionators will kick in about $12 million.

6. The thirteen pharmaceutical companies included in the MPTAP waiver are: Miles Canada Inc., Miles Inc., Bayer AG, Armour Pharmaceutical Co., U.S.V. Canada Inc., Rorer Group Inc., Rhone-Poulenc Rorer Inc., Baxter Healthcare Corp., Baxter Corp., Baxter International Inc., Baxter World Trade Corp., Connaught Laboratories Ltd., Connaught Biologics Ltd. and their related corporations.

7. The contribution of the pharmaceuticals, paid proportionally to the amount of their product used by Canadian hemophiliacs from 1978 to 1985, was a combination of cash and factor concentrate.

11: UNDER THE MICROSCOPE

1. Paradoxically, it appears that Sam Thompson contracted the AIDS virus from cryoprecipitate — a treatment much safer than concentrate — that he was afforded because he was a "virgin hemophiliac". The donor was the wife of a hemophiliac, whose blood was never refused despite her being at high risk of contracting AIDS. The woman's donations of plasma for cryoprecipitate are believed to have infected four Saskatchewan hemophiliacs.

2. The first phase of the Commission of Inquiry ran from February 14 to December 7, 1994. A total of 312 people testified, including 166 victims (and their family members) and 146 "experts".

3. The Canadian Society of Clinical Chemists was interested in the tainted-blood issue largely because one of its executive members was Frank Terpstra, a hemophiliac.

4. The members of the Commons Sub-Committee on Health Issues were: Dr. Stan Wilbee (PC, Delta), Jean-Luc Joncas (PC, Matapédia-Matane), Dr. Rey Pagtakhan (L, Winnipeg North) and Chris Axworthy (NDP, Saskatoon).

5. The Commission of Inquiry on the Blood System in Canada was formally constituted by order of cabinet P.C. 1993-1879 on October 4, 1993.

6. The Royal Commission on Confidentiality of Health Records was called after the RCMP was implicated in using confidential medical records for disruptive purposes. Judge Krever went to court to compel RCMP informants to testify, and extended the inquiry to look at the conduct of doctors who used confidential files in an abusive fashion. He produced a 1,626-page report in 1980, but the provinces ignored virtually all the recommendations.

12: GLOBAL CONNECTIONS

1. Blood-borne AIDS hit first and hardest in the U.S.; some concentrate was contaminated as early as 1977 and some transfusion patients were at risk by 1980. More than 10,000 U.S. hemophiliacs and 15,000 transfusion patients were infected even though the country was among the first to introduce heat-treated products and testing of blood.

13: CALL TO ACTION

1. The term "malicious inertia" to describe the reaction of public health officials to blood-borne AIDS was coined by Dr. Edgar Engleman, former medical director of the Stanford University Hospital, where the most transfusions in the world are performed each year.

2. Bayer Inc. is a subsidiary of Bayer AG, the multinational pharmaceutical company best known for making Aspirin headache tablets.

3. Recombinant factor concentrate is manufactured by inserting the human Factor VIII gene into the kidney cells of, for example, a hamster, then "growing" the clotting factor in the lab.

4. Dr. Roger Perrault calculated that, between 1980 and 1995, an additional $699 million was spent due to the lack of self-sufficiency in plasma, including more than $50 million building inefficient plants.

5. The hepatitis C infection rate among Canadian blood donors is 66 per 100,000, compared to 30 per 100,000 for hepatitis B and 2 per 100,000 for HIV.

SOURCES

PREFACE

Hamara, Gregory, "In Critical Condition: The Media Treatment of Canada's Blood Issue", an address to the annual law luncheon of the Public Legal Education Society of Nova Scotia, April 12, 1995.

Huntsman, Richard, address to the Annual Scientific Meeting of the British Blood Transfusion Society, Southampton, Sept. 16, 1994.

Picard, André, "Could the media have done a better job covering the tainted blood tragedy?", address to the Canadian Association of Journalists, Ottawa, April 8, 1994.

——, "Federal payments ending for hemophiliacs with AIDS: Victims of tainted blood scandal feel abandoned", *The Globe and Mail*, April 1, 1993, p. A1.

1: GIFT OF LIFE: KISS OF DEATH

Blackwood, Kelly, testimony at the Commission of Inquiry on the Blood System in Canada, Vol. 15, Toronto, March 11, 1994.

Downey, Donn, "AIDS a minefield, woman tells hearing: Decision deferred on penalty for doctor who didn't tell patient of infection", *The Globe and Mail*, Jan. 28, 1993, p. A6.

——, "AIDS safeguards failed, court told: Man died after receiving transfusion of tainted blood", *The Globe and Mail*, March 9, 1993, p. A14.

——, "Red Cross slow to guard blood, court told: Lawyer says Canadian branch not aggressive enough in screening donors", *The Globe and Mail*, March 10, 1993, p. A8.

——, "Risk of HIV infection 'horrendous,' court told: MD says test should have been offered", *The Globe and Mail*, April 20, 1993, p. A12.

——, "Tainted blood risk was 1-in-4, court told", *The Globe and Mail*, May 21, 1993, p. A18.

L., Mr., testimony in the case Pittman *vs* Bain *et al.*, April 30, 1992.

Lang, Madam Justice Susan, judgment in civil suit Pittman *vs* Bain *et al.*, Toronto, March 14, 1994, pp. 312.

Mickleburgh, Rod, "AIDS infection 'abject horror': MPs hear testimony from Canadians who received tainted transfusions", *The Globe and Mail*, Nov. 27, 1992, p. A10.

——, "Doctor guilty of misconduct: Patient not told he may have received AIDS-infected blood in operation", *The Globe and Mail*, Nov. 26, 1992, p. A1.

——, "Official said AIDS warning not obligatory, MD testifies: Doctor says he believed patient 'too fragile' to be told of condition", *The Globe and Mail*, Oct. 10, 1992, p. A10.

——, "Risk of virus transfer focus of AIDS hearing: No-sex statement called insufficient", *The Globe and Mail*, Oct. 23, 1992, p. A11.

Picard, André, "HIV-infected widow wants assisted death: Change law, woman at blood inquiry urges", *The Globe and Mail*, March 12, 1994, p. A4.

Pittman, Rochelle, testimony at the Commission of Inquiry on the Blood System in Canada, Vol. 15, Toronto, March 11, 1994.

——, testimony at the Commons Sub-Committee on Health Issues, Nov. 26, 1992.

2: BLOOD TIES

Bator, Paul Adolphus, and Andrew James Rhodes, *Within Reach of Everyone: A History of the University of Toronto School of Hygiene and Connaught Laboratories*, Vol. I, 1925 to 1955, Canadian Public Health Association, Ottawa, 1990.

Gibbon, John Murray, and Mary Mathewson, "The Canadian Red Cross Society", in *Three Centuries of Canadian Nursing*, Macmillan, Toronto, 1947, pp. 341-351.

"The Gift of Life, available to those who need it", pamphlet, Canadian Red Cross Society, 1985.

Gordon, P.H., "The Blood Transfusion Service", in *Fifty Years in the Canadian Red Cross*, self-published, 1967. (Courtesy: Canadian War Museum.)

Guiou, Norman M., "WWII On The Home Front", in *Transfusion: A Canadian Surgeon's Story in War and Peace*, self-published, undated, pp. 105-120. (Courtesy: Canadian War Museum.)

Hutchinson, John, "The history of the Red Cross is anything but dull", *Canadian Medical Association Journal*, Vol. 141, Aug. 15, 1989, pp. 336-39.

"The ICRC's origins", pamphlet, International Committee of the Red Cross, ICRC Publication and Documentation Service, Geneva.

Perrault, Roger, *The Canadian Red Cross Blood Programme from 1974 to 1990, A Report to the Canadian Hematology Society*, Canadian Red Cross Society, Dec. 1990.

"Red Cross Society", *The Canadian Encyclopedia*, Hurtig Publishers, Edmonton, 1988, p. 1835.

Ryerson, George Sterling, "The Canadian Red Cross Society", in *Looking Backward*, Toronto, Ryerson Press, 1924, pp. 112-124.

Stanbury, Stuart, "Origin, Development and Future of the Canadian Red Cross Transfusion Service" (brief presented to the Royal Commission on Health Services, May 22, 1961), Canadian Red Cross Society, 1961.

Valpy, Michael, "Public health at issue in Connaught merger", *The Globe and Mail*, Sept. 27, 1989, p. A8.

Whitby, Sir Lionel, "The Army Blood Transfusion Service", in *The Army Medical Services, Administration*, Vol. II, ed. F.A.E. Crew, Her Majesty's Stationery Office, London, 1955, pp. 372-420.

3: BOYS WHO BLEED

Burns, Sheila, "A History of Blood Transfusion", *American Medical Writers' Association Journal*, Vol. 8, No. 4, 1993, pp. 132-135.

Gottlieb, A. Matthew, "History of the First Blood Transfusion", in *Transfusion Medicine Reviews*, Vol. V, No. 3 (July) 1991, pp. 228-35.

Isaac, Barry M., "The Canadian Hemophilia Society: The Historical Challenge", *Hemophilia Today*, Vol. 29, No. 1, Nov. 1993, pp. 47-65.

——, "A Consumer's View: The History and Future of Blood Transfusion in Canada", *Hemophilia Today*, Vol. 29, No. 1, Nov. 1993, pp. 66-72.

——, testimony at the Commission of Inquiry on the Blood System in Canada, Vol. 35, Edmonton, April 22, 1994.

Kubin, Edward, testimony at the Commission of Inquiry on the Blood System in Canada, Vol. 50, Winnipeg, June 15, 1994.

Littell, Robert, "Bearer is a Hemophiliac: Frank and Mazie Schnabel's demonstration of high courage against a sinister disease", *Reader's Digest*, April 1959. (Reprinted in *Hemophilia Today*, Vol. 29 No. 1.)

Maluf, N.S.R., "History of Blood Transfusion", *Journal of History of Medicine*, Vol. 9, 59:107, 1954.

Miller, Connie, "Inheritance of Hemophilia", pamphlet, National Hemophilia Foundation, 1992.

Oberman, Harold A., "The History of Blood Transfusion", in *The Clinical Practice of Blood Transfusion*, pp. 9-28.

Page, David, testimony at the Commission of Inquiry on the Blood System in Canada, Vol. 5, Toronto, Feb. 18, 1994.

Schmidt, P.J., "Transfusion in America in the eighteenth and nineteenth centuries", *The New England Journal of Medicine*, 279:1319, 1968.

Shumak, Kenneth, testimony at the Commission of Inquiry on the Blood System in Canada, Vol. 1, Toronto, Feb. 14, 1994.

Webster, C., "The Origins of Blood Transfusion", *Journal of History of Medicine*, 15:387, 1971.

4: DEATH TOUCHES DOWN

Anderson, R.M., and H.J. Barrie, "Fatal pneumocystis pneumonia in an adult: Report of a case", *American Journal of Clinical Pathology*, Vol. 34, No. 4, Oct. 1960, pp. 365-370.

Centers for Disease Control, "Possible transfusion-associated acquired immune deficiency syndrome (AIDS)—California", *Mortality and Morbidity Weekly Report*, 1982; 31:652-54.

Compas, Jean-Claude, "Pourquoi Haïti?", *Le Monde*, July 7, 1984.

Curran, James, *et al.*, "Acquired Immune Deficiency Syndrome (AIDS) associated with transfusions", *The New England Journal of Medicine*, Jan. 12, 1984, 310: 69-75.

Garfield, Simon, "How They Spread the Bad News", *The Independent on Sunday*, Nov. 13, 1994, pp. 16-20.

——, "The End of Innocence: Britain in the time of AIDS", *The Independent on Sunday*, Nov. 6, 1994, pp. 4-8.

Grmek, Mirko D., *History of AIDS: Emergence and Origin of a Modern Pandemic*, Princeton University Press, Princeton N.J., 1990.

Jett, J., M.D. Kuritsky, J.A. Katzmann, *et al.*, "Acquired Immunodeficiency Syndrome associated with blood-product transfusions", *Annals of Internal Medicine* 99 (1983): pp. 621-624.

Johnstone, Tim, testimony at the Commission of Inquiry on the Blood System in Canada, Vol. 24, Vancouver, March 29, 1994.

Montagnier, Luc, *et al.*, "Isolation of T-lymphotropic retrovirus from a patient at risk for AIDS", *Science*, May 20, 1983, pp. 868-70.

Murray, Terry, "Blood banks' hidden bomb: AIDS", *The Medical Post*, Dec. 28, 1982, p. 1.

Shilts, Randy, *And the Band Played On: Politics, People and the AIDS Epidemic*, Penguin, New York, 1988, pp. 640.

Tsoukas, Christos, *et al.*, "Immunological dysfunction in patients with classic hemophilia receiving lyophilized Factor VIII concentrate and cryoprecipitate", *Canadian Medical Association Journal*, Vol. 129, Oct. 1, 1983, pp. 713-17.

5: LETHAL INDIFFERENCE

Alcindor, Antony, testimony at the Commission of Inquiry on the Blood System in Canada, Vol. 78, Montreal, Sept. 26, 1994.

Guévin, Raymond, testimony at the Commission of Inquiry on the Blood System in Canada, Vol. 73-4, Montreal, Sept. 19-20, 1994.

Hollobon, Joan, "Red Cross, AIDS group discuss blood donations", *The Globe and Mail*, July 21, 1983, p. P5.

Huntsman, Richard, testimony at the Commission of Inquiry on the Blood System in Canada, Vol. 67, St. John's, Aug. 17, 1994.

MacKenzie, Hilary, "Hemophiliacs, patients getting blood transfusions at risk: The struggle against AIDS", *The Globe and Mail*, June 11, 1984, p. M6.

Noble, James, testimony at the Commission of Inquiry on the Blood System in Canada, Vol. 55, Saint John, July 13, 1994.

Wigod, Rebecca, "B.C. moves 'reduced risk' of HIV-tainted blood", *The Vancouver Sun*, March 30, 1994, p. A3.

——, "Suspect blood dumped, probe told: Suspected addicts, gays 'screened'", *The Vancouver Sun*, April 7, 1994, p. A3.

Willoughby, Brian, testimony at the Commission of Inquiry on the Blood System in Canada, Vol. 30, Vancouver, April 8, 1994.

6: BLOOD MONEY

"Blood derivatives sold while in shortage", *The Globe and Mail*, Feb. 4, 1976, p. 1.

"Connaught's hunt for profit", *The Globe and Mail*, Feb. 28, 1976, p. 4.

"Contamination problems, danger of infection reported at Connaught: Federal regulations violated", *The Globe and Mail*, Feb. 27, 1975, p. 4.

Curran, Peggy and Michael Doyle, "Brokers deny African plasma spread AIDS", *The Gazette*, March 27, 1985, p. A3.

Golt, Lolly, "Blood and Money", *Weekend Magazine*, May 6, 1978, pp. 4-5.

Keddy, Barbara, "Red Cross won't give in on plasma deal", *The Globe and Mail*, Sept. 16, 1980, p. P4.

Laver, Ross, "Ministers shut door on Red Cross ambition to set up blood plant", *The Globe and Mail*, Oct. 1, 1980.

Levy, Jay A., Gautam Mitra and Milton Mozen, "Recovery and inactivation of infectious retroviruses from Factor VIII concentrates", *The Lancet*, Sept. 29, 1984, pp. 722-23.

Landry, Anne-Marie, testimony at the Commission of Inquiry on the Blood System in Canada, Vol. 55, Saint John, July 13, 1994.

Landry, Normand, Testimony at the Commission of Inquiry on the Blood System in Canada, Vol. 55, Saint John, July 13, 1994.

"Money needed to revive firm, critic tells Connlab powers", *The Globe and Mail*, Feb. 27, 1976, p. 4.

Picard, André, "An accident waiting to happen? Family fights to ensure pain not in vain", *The Globe and Mail*, Sept. 6, 1993, p. A1.

——, "Red Cross continued purchasing: Letter to lab dated after Ottawa ordered switch to heat-treated blood", *The Globe and Mail*, July 22, 1993, p. A4.

7: CONSENSUS FOR INACTION

"Blood Transfusion, Haemophilia, and AIDS", editorial, *The Lancet*, Dec. 22-29, 1984, pp.1433-35.

Department of Health and Human Services, "Update: Acquired Immune Deficiency Syndrome (AIDS) in persons with hemophilia", *Mortality and Morbidity Weekly Report*, Oct. 26, 1984, p. 589.

Evenson, Brad, "The forgotten ones: Focus on AIDS victims of blood transfusions ignores other sufferers", *The Citizen*, Sept. 17, 1993, p. A2.

——, "Hepatitis C, not AIDS, may be the worst legacy of tainted blood", *The Citizen*, March 26, 1994, p. A1.

Gaul, Gilbert M., "America: OPEC of global plasma industry", *The Philadelphia Inquirer*, Sept. 28, 1989, p. A1.

Hornbrook, Michael, "No Shortage of Heat-Treated Blood Products", World at Six, CBC Radio transcript, Feb. 11, 1994.

Perrault, Roger, "The Canadian Red Cross Blood Programme from 1974 to 1990, A Report to the Canadian Hematology Society", Canadian Red Cross Society, December 1990.

——, testimony at the Commission of Inquiry on the Blood System in Canada, Toronto, Vol. 123-144, May 8-June 13, 1995.

Picard, André , "Ottawa knew blood tainted: AIDS specialist warned of contamination a year before action taken", *The Globe and Mail*, July 20, 1993, p. A1.

"Sanguine: Blood transfusions", *The Economist*, Jan. 21, 1995, p. 89.

8: ONE IN A MILLION

Alberts, Sheldon, "Transfusion killed husband", *The Calgary Herald*, April 23, 1994, p. A1.

Bowen, Beverley, "Red Cross confirms its blood had AIDS", *The Globe and Mail*, May 10, 1985, p. M1.

Brennan, Brian, "Tainted Blood Cut Short Blackie Couple's Dream", *The Calgary Herald*, May 3, 1994, p. B2.

Curran, James, *et al.*, "Acquired immunodeficiency syndrome (AIDS) associated with transfusions", *The New England Journal of Medicine*, Jan. 12, 1984, pp. 69-74.

Davey, Martin, "Demographic and Donor Profile, Anti-HIV Screening, for the Period November 1, 1985 to November 30, 1986", The Canadian Red Cross Society, Jan. 6, 1987.

——, testimony at the Commission of Inquiry on the Blood System in Canada, Toronto, Vol. 123-144, May 8-June 13, 1995.

Department of Health and Human Services, "Five pharmaceutical firms identified to develop AIDS test", *Plasma Quarterly*, June 20, 1984.

Lett, Daniel, "Avoid test for AIDS, Toronto group warns", *The Globe and Mail*, March 4, 1985, p. P13.

Lord, Cathy, "Risks remote, victims told," *The Calgary Herald*, April 23, 1994, p. A3.

MacKenzie, Hilary, "Ottawa starts simple blood tests to screen for exposure to AIDS", *The Globe and Mail*, Aug. 27, 1984, p. M6.

Mickleburgh, Rod, "Red Cross delay led to AIDS, report says: 55 infected when screening not ready", *The Globe and Mail*, Nov. 5, 1992, page A1.

"Safe transfusions aim of AIDS tests", *The Globe and Mail*, Jan. 9, 1985, p. M2.

Solomon, Howard, "Blackie teen gets five years", *The Calgary Herald*, June 13, 1985, p. A4.

"Transfusions can pose AIDS risk doctor says", *The Gazette*, May 13, 1985, p. A3.

Zucchelli, Helen, testimony at the Commission of Inquiry on the Blood System in Canada, Vol. 35, Edmonton, April 22, 1994.

9: THROUGH THE LOOKING-GLASS

Blackwell, Tom, "Youth's life became 'hell' after HIV-tainted transfusion", Canadian Press (published in *The Citizen*), Feb. 22, 1994, p. A3.

Buskard, Noël, testimony at Commission of Inquiry on the Blood System in Canada, Vol. 28-30, Vancouver, April 6-8, 1994.

Davey, Martin, "AIDS, blood transfusions", *The Globe and Mail*, letter to the editor, June 4, 1987, p. A6.

DeMara, Bruce, "Lawsuit fears didn't halt HIV survey, probe told", *Toronto Star*, March 11, 1994, p. A5.

——, "A sacred trust betrayed: Recipients of tainted blood ask why they weren't told of the risk", *Toronto Star*, March 4, 1994, p. A21.

——, "Sick Kids can't trace 16 units of bad blood", *Toronto Star*, March 17, 1994, p. A1.

Drew, Joan, testimony at the Commission of Inquiry on the Blood System in Canada, Vol. 26, Vancouver, March 31, 1994.

"The Epidemiology of Transfusion-Associated HIV Infection in Canada, 1978-1985" (a report to Health Canada), Division of HIV/AIDS Epidemiology, Laboratory Centre for Disease Control, Aug. 1994.

Fagan, Drew, "U.S. blood-transfer bulletin not alarming, Canada told", *The Globe and Mail*, March 18, 1987, p. A12.

King, Susan, "Results of the HIV Information Project", Hospital for Sick Children, Toronto, Nov. 24, 1993.

——, testimony at the Commission of Inquiry on the Blood System in Canada, Toronto, Vol. 13-14, March 9-10, 1994.

Mickleburgh, Rod, "AIDS memorial a sad data base: Red Cross has traced fate of some blood donors through names on columns", *The Globe and Mail*, Feb. 19, 1994, p. A7.

——, "Anger, tears as victims tell of blood horror: Inquiry witnesses decry lack of warnings about HIV risk", *The Globe and Mail*, Feb. 22, 1994, p. A1.

——, "Sick Kids study finds 1 in 100 heart-surgery patients have HIV: Testing urged for all transfusion recipients 1980-85", *The Globe and Mail*, Nov. 25, 1993, p. A5.

Picard, André, "Asked to tell 40 children of AIDS risk, MDs refused: Alberta group initially balked, blood researcher testifies", *The Globe and Mail*, March 11, 1994, p. A8.

——, "The future of Canada's blood system: Restoring faith in the safety net," *The Globe and Mail*, Sept. 4, 1993, p. A1.

——, "Hundreds unknowingly infected, HIV experts say: Testing urged for thousands who received blood before '86", *The Globe and Mail*, May 19, 1993, p. A6.

——, "Study adds fears to blood recipients: Number who got HIV in 1978-85 may be three times higher than estimated", *The Globe and Mail*, Aug. 31, 1994, p. A3.

Picard, André, and Henry Hess, "Find tainted-blood victims, Ottawa told: Many may not know they are infected with AIDS virus, report by MPs says", *The Globe and Mail*, May 18, 1993, p. A1.

Rémis R.S., and G. Delage, "Estimate of HIV incidence among repeat blood donors in Montreal: A pilot study", paper presented at Ninth International Conference on AIDS, Berlin, June 6-11, 1993.

Robinson, Colonel Neville, "Summary of Suspect Post-Transfusion AIDS Cases (Operation 300)", The Canadian Red Cross Society, Vancouver BTS, Jan. 16, 1986.

10: MONEY CAN'T BUY ME LIFE

"AIDS: A Perspective For Canadians, Summary Report and Recommendations", Dr. Michel Chrétien, chairman, Royal Society of Canada, 1988.

Arenson, Kenneth, "Update on litigation and the MPTAP: Memorandum to all HIV clients", Feb. 8, 1994.

——, "Update on MPTAP and delay in suing: Memorandum to all HIV clients", March 8, 1994.

"Beatty announces assistance to persons infected with HIV from blood transfusions or blood products" (press release, with attachments), Health and Welfare Canada, Ottawa, Dec. 14, 1989.

Breckenridge, Joan, "Hemophiliacs with AIDS ask compensation," *The Globe and Mail*, Nov. 27, 1987, p. A1.

Cernetig, Miro, Rod Mickleburgh, Martin Mittlestaedt, André Picard, "Tainted blood deal offered: $139-million for the afflicted", *The Globe and Mail*, Sept. 16, 1993, p. A1.

Cox, Kevin, "Hemophiliac pleads for redress: Compensation for AIDS infection from blood products expires April 1", *The Globe and Mail*, Feb. 12, 1993, p. A3.

——, "Took AIDS fight public, family honoured in N.S.: Couple sought quality in their lives beyond staying alive," *The Globe and Mail*, Oct. 30, 1993, p. A12.

"EAP II up-date: Memorandum to Inter-provincial Task Force of the Canadian Hemophilia Society", The Canadian Hemophilia Society, Dec. 6, 1993.

Fischer, Doug, "Blood-product firms sweeten offers to AIDS victims", Southam News (published in *The Citizen*), Dec. 1, 1993, p. A3.

Gibson, Robert, *et al.*, *Archival Study*, Canadian Hemophilia Society, 1986.

Gooderham, Mary, "Some AIDS victims to be compensated", *The Globe and Mail*, Dec. 15, 1989, p. A1.

"Hemophilia Catastrophe Relief: An Urgent Request to the Government of Canada", Canadian Hemophilia Society, submitted August 1988.

"Hemophiliacs with AIDS seek money from Ottawa", Canadian Press (published in *The Globe and Mail*), March 23, 1989, p. A5.

"HIV Infection Assistance Package Finalized, Announced by Canadian Blood Agency", press release (with attachments), Canadian Blood Agency, Dec. 1, 1993.

Mackinnon, Martha, and Horace Krever, "Legal and Societal Aspects of AIDS in Canada", Royal Society of Canada, 1988.

Mickleburgh, Rod, "Blood package angers lawyers: Object to signing 'no duress' release", *The Globe and Mail*, March 1, 1994, p. A5.

——, "Grier to urge pay for victims of tainted blood: Breaks with past government policy as Alberta pushes for co-ordinated plan", *The Globe and Mail*, June 9, 1993, p. A8.

——, "Multimillion dollar deal rejected by hemophiliacs: Provinces told package is inadequate", *The Globe and Mail*, Aug. 10, 1993, p. A1.

——, "N.S. to compensate victims of AIDS-tainted blood: 'I did this because I felt it was right,' minister says as Nova Scotia breaks ranks with other provinces", *The Globe and Mail*, p. A4.

Moulton, Donalee, "N.S. under pressure to compensate HIV-infected hemophiliacs", *The Medical Post*, March 2, 1993, p. 8.

Picard, André, "Federal payments ending for hemophiliacs with AIDS", *The Globe and Mail*, April 1, 1993, p. A1.

——, "Provinces seek deal in blood scandal: Victims dying at rate of three a week", *The Globe and Mail*, Aug. 9, 1993, p. A1.

——, "Tainted blood lawsuits to continue", *The Globe and Mail*, March 16, 1994, p. A3.

Prichard, J. Robert S., "Liability and Compensation in Health Care: A Report to the Conference of Deputy Ministers of Health of the Federal/Provincial/Territorial Review on Liability and Compensation Issues in Health Care", University of Toronto Press, June 1, 1990.

"Scrap the blood deadline", editorial, *The Citizen*, March 9, 1994, p. A10.

11: UNDER THE MICROSCOPE

Boisseau, Peter, "Tainted-blood inquiry 'not a witch-hunt,' judge warns", Canadian Press (published in *The Citizen*), Feb. 15, 1994, p. A3.

Cernetig, Miro, and André Picard, "Tainted blood probe launched: Provinces back inquiry, but Quebec has questions", *The Globe and Mail*, Sept. 17, 1993, p. A1.

Evenson, Brad, "Red Cross enlists PR firm to revive image", *The Citizen*, Aug. 11, 1993, p. A3.

Fine, Sean, "A tough judge for a complex job: The man who will probe the HIV scandal faces a daunting task, but those who know Mr. Justice Horace Krever say he's up to it", *The Globe and Mail*, Oct. 12, 1993, p. A5.

Mickleburgh, Rod, "Bad Blood: A death sentence, Delay in testing for AIDS cost lives: High-risk donors not screened out", *The Globe and Mail*, Nov. 19, 1992, p. A1.

——, "Blood victims will have their say: The judge vows that all people infected through transfusions can testify", *The Globe and Mail*, Feb. 15, 1994, p. A4.

——, "Lobby firm hired to help Red Cross: Tainted blood affair cited," *The Globe and Mail*, Aug. 12, 1993, p. A12.

Noël, André, "Des centaines d'hémophiles contaminés à cause de la négligence des autorités: La Société de l'hémophilie parle d'un scandale canadien du sang contaminé", *La Presse*, Nov. 4, 1992, p. A1.

——, "La Croix-Rouge avoue que du sang contaminé a été distribué", *La Presse*, Nov. 6, 1992, p. A1.

Picard, André, "Bad Blood: A life sentence, Hemophiliacs pay a deadly price", *The Globe and Mail*, Nov. 18, 1992, p. A1.

——, "Inquiry's scope remains unresolved", *The Globe and Mail*, Sept. 6, 1993, p. A4.

——, "Tainted blood inquiry called: Public shaken, Bouchard admits", *The Globe and Mail*, May 26, 1993, p. A4.

Picard, André, and Henry Hess, "Find tainted-blood victims, Ottawa told: Many may not know they are infected with AIDS virus, report by MPs says", *The Globe and Mail*, May 18, 1993, p. A1.

Picard, André, and Geoffrey York, "No need for inquiry now, says Bouchard: Idea still open 'if it would help'", *The Globe and Mail*, Nov. 19, 1992, p. A21.

Pole, Ken, "Inquiry into blood supply a job for Solomon and Job", *The Medical Post*, Nov. 12, 1993, p. 16.

"Starting the ripple in the AIDS pond", editorial, *The Medical Post*, Aug. 20, 1985, p. 10.

Struzik, Ed, "Governments to probe tainted blood scandal: Inquiry seeks answers for 1,000 victims", *The Edmonton Journal* (published in *The Citizen*), Sept. 17, 1993, p. A1.

Todd, Dave, "Tories considered internal probe of blood scandal", Southam News (published in *The Gazette*), Nov. 24, 1993, p. B1.

12: GLOBAL CONNECTIONS

Baele, G., *et al.*, "Haemophilia, HIV Infection and blood transfusion in Belgium," *Acta Clinica Belgica* 43:2, 1988, pp. 95-100.

Casteret, Anne-Marie, *L'Affaire du sang*, Éditions La Découverte, Paris, 1992, pp. 284.

Guisnel, Jean (ed.), "Le sang contaminé: Un énorme scandale médical et politique", *Libération* No. 11, May 1993, pp. 68.

Jones, Peter, "AIDS: The African Connection?" *British Medical Journal*, Vol. 290, March 23, 1985, p. 932.

Lemonick, Michael D., "Over and over again: HIV-infected blood supplies have turned up all too often", *Time*, Nov. 15, 1993, pp. 40-43.

"MD links blood trade to AIDS", Reuters News Agency (published in *The Globe and Mail*), March 23, 1985, p. P17.

Nullis, Clare, "Tainted blood supplies spread AIDS fear from Europe to Third World", Associated Press, Nov. 5, 1993.

Picard, André, "France makes an example of misdeeds: A finding of guilt against four officials over tainted blood satisfied the desire for revenge and led to a major reform of the supply system", *The Globe and Mail*, Sept. 7, 1993, p. A4.

——, "Plight of hemophiliacs worse in Third World: Treatment, blood screening almost unknown," *The Globe and Mail*, Sept. 7, 1993, p. A4.

Rouzioux, Charles, *et al.*, "Immunoglobulin G antibodies to lymphadenopathy-associated virus in differently-treated French and Belgian Hemophiliacs", *Annals of Internal Medicine*, 1985, 102:476-79.

Simons, Marlise, "Swiss Red Cross faces AIDS probe: 3rd nation in Europe is hit by blood supply scandal", *The New York Times*, May 22, 1994, p. A1.

13: CALL TO ACTION

"AIDS, Blood and Politics", "Frontline", PBS, broadcast Nov. 30, 1993.

Callwood, June, "A Date With AIDS", *Saturday Night*, March 1995, pp. 53-58, 93.

Coutts, Jane, "Blood agency, Red Cross sign deal: Funding body gets policy power", *The Globe and Mail*, April 11, 1995, p. A1.

———, "Experts warn of trivial fixes in blood system: Panel says profound, immediate change is needed to preserve safety," *The Globe and Mail*, Dec. 8, 1994, p. A1.

———, "Single national body urged to run blood system: Public health association report says new setup could react more quickly to a crisis," *The Globe and Mail*, Nov. 25, 1994, p. A2.

Evenson, Brad, "Blood disaster possible again, experts say: System riddled with deficiencies, foreign panel says", *The Citizen*, Dec. 8, 1994, p. A1.

———, "Solving Canada's blood feud: Agreement expected 'within months'", *The Citizen*, Dec. 10, 1994, p. A1.

"Exotic Dangerous Communicable Diseases: Principles and Practices of Management. The Canadian Contingency Plan", report by Health and Welfare Canada, Ottawa, 1978.

Garrett, Laurie, *The Coming Plague: Newly Emerging Diseases in a World Out of Balance*, Farrar, Straus and Giroux, New York, 1994, pp. 750.

Krever, Horace, "Interim Report," Commission of Inquiry on the Blood System in Canada, Feb. 24, 1995, pp. 485.

McDougall, Deborah, "25 per cent would refuse transfusion: poll", Canadian Press (published in *The Gazette*), Nov. 4, 1994, p. B1.

Mickleburgh, Rod, "Blood plant wasted millions: Winnipeg fractionation lab was sold for nothing, document says," *The Globe and Mail*, Feb. 16, 1994, p. A1.

———, "Delay in testing for AIDS cost lives: High-risk donors not screened out", *The Globe and Mail*, Nov. 19, 1992, p. A1.

Picard, André, "Krever urges tainted blood warning: Interim report calls on hospitals to notify 3.5 million transfusion recipients of AIDS, hepatitis risk", *The Globe and Mail*, Feb. 25, 1995, p. A1.

Prichard, J. Robert S., "Liability and Compensation in Health Care: A Report to the Conference of Deputy Ministers of Health of the Federal/Provincial/Territorial Review on Liability and Compensation Issues in Health Care", University of Toronto Press, June 1, 1990.

Wigod, Rebecca, "Bad Blood: Who's To Blame? A judge must decide why our system failed", *Vancouver Sun*, April 9, 1994, p. B1.

———, "Disease control boss defends non-reporting of HIV cases", *Vancouver Sun*, April 6, 1994, p. A3.

EPILOGUE

Z., Mr. and Mrs., testimony at the Commission of Inquiry on the Blood System in Canada, Vol. 15A, Toronto, March 11, 1994.

APPENDIX

Use of Blood Products by Canadian Hemophiliacs

The increased use of factor concentrate coincided with the advent of AIDS, and the use of cryoprecipitate increased only marginally after public health officials recognized that AIDS was blood-borne in late 1982.

	1978	1979	1980	1981	1982	1983	1984
Factor VIII	289,030	20.4M	30.7M	33.7M	41.9M	43.2M	43.4M
cryo	303,184	216,512	151,114	151,504	141,599	164,549	192,935
Factor IX	4.7M	6.0M	9.4M	8.7M	10.9M	11.3M	11.6M

Source: Canadian Red Cross Society

Reasons for Transfusion

More than 400 Canadians were infected with HIV through transfusion between 1978 and 1985. A study of 261 of those people, all of whom received payments from the Extraordinary Assistance Plan, revealed they were given blood for the following underlying medical conditions:

Reason	Women (%)	Men (%)
Pregnancy and birth	29	—
Heart surgery	15	36
Accidents	—	10
Anemia	9	—
Hysterectomy	8	—
Gastrointestinal bleeding	5	8
Kidney-related	5	3
Orthopedic surgery	5	3
Post-operative bleeding	5	6
Cancer therapy	5	6
Coagulation disorders *	—	4
Ulcer-related bleeding	—	3
Miscellaneous surgery	3	11
Other reasons	10	10

Source: Health Canada (research conducted by Jack McDonald, Gerald Devins and Man-Chiu Poon)
* Disorders other than hemophilia.

Year of transfusion, diagnosis and death

An analysis of the medical records of 261 HIV-positive transfusion recipients who received payments from the Extraordinary Assistance Plan shows how the risk of infection grew over the years, and how doctors were slow to diagnose former transfusion patients with AIDS.

Year	% Transfusion	% Diagnosis	% Death
1978	1		
1979	0		
1980	2		
1981	3		
1982	17		
1983	20	1	1
1984	21	1	2
1985	34	7	4
1986	1	12	8
1987	1	28	19
1988		16	13
1989		10	17
1990		16	19
1991		8	16
1992		1	1
Total	100	100	100
	184 people*	261 people	135 people**

Source: Health Canada (research conducted by Jack McDonald, Gerald Devins and Man-Chiu Poon)
* In 55 cases, the date of transfusion was not recorded.
** The number of dead in 1992.

Analysis of blood donations testing positive for AIDS —Nov. 1, 1985, to Dec. 31, 1986

The first 13 months of testing blood showed that AIDS was far more prevalent in some parts of the country than others, for example, Quebec, and that self-deferral measures promoted in some provinces, such as B.C. and Newfoundland, reduced the number of high-risk donors.

	Donations	ELISA test		Western Blot *	
		# reactive	%	# positive	per thousand
B.C.	144,461	449	0.3	12	8
Alberta	130,622	409	0.3	20	15
Saskatchewan	51,192	156	0.3	4	8
Manitoba	73,603	252	0.3	2	3
Ontario	461,556	1,539	0.3	62	13
Quebec	257,415	937	0.4	117	45
New Brunswick	38,282	114	0.3	4	10
Nova Scotia/PEI	68,186	258	0.4	3	4
Newfoundland	32,991	131	0.4	1	3
NATIONAL**	1,258,308	4,245	0.3	225	18

Source: Canadian Red Cross Society
* The ELISA test allows mass screening but often gives false positives so blood is not considered infected unless antibodies are detected in a confirmatory test, in this case Western Blot.
** In testing statistics, PEI and Nova Scotia are combined, and the Territories are included in B.C. and Alberta.

Extraordinary Assistance Plan:
Approved Applications By Province
as of Aug. 17, 1993

Although EAP compensation was available to those who received blood transfusions as well as hemophiliacs who used blood products, the majority of those who received the money were hemophiliacs. Their risk of infection was greater because the products were made from pooled plasma and many infected transfusion recipients likely died without knowing they were infected with HIV.

Province	Hemophiliacs	# transfused	Total	% hemophiliacs
Newfoundland	15	4	19	79
P.E.I.	5	0	5	100
Nova Scotia	8	9	17	47
New Brunswick	51	5	56	91
Quebec	188	76	264	71
Ontario	264	111	375	70
Manitoba	23	2	25	92
Saskatchewan	26	3	29	90
Alberta	32	29	61	52
B.C.	64	38	102	63
Yukon/NWT	0	1		
TOTAL	676	278	954 *	71

Source: Health Canada, Canadian Hemophilia Society
* There are now more than 1,100 EAP registrants, but Health Canada refuses to release a detailed breakdown by province.

Age distribution for HIV-infected hemophiliacs

In making the case for compensation, hemophiliacs argued that AIDS hit hardest people who were in the prime of their working lives.

Age	%
0-9	5
10-19	22
20-29	25
30-39	32
40 +	16

Source: Canadian Hemophilia Society

INDEX

Schwarze, Pamela, 68-69
Screening of donors, 24, 31, 32, 34, 48
    for AIDS, 61, 64-65, 70-81, 95, 235
    in Belgium, 203, 204
    civil rights concerns, 70, 74, 75, 78, 128
    CRC drops plans (1983), 73-74
    infected repeat donors, 136
    recommendations from MSAC (Feb/83), 72
Self-donation, 227
Self-sufficiency
    in manufacturing. *See* Fractionation
    in plasma supply, 47-48, 65, 86, 89, 95,
        99, 204-205, 219, 220
Sharpe, Bud, 151-52, 184
Shilts, Randy, 80-81
Shumak, Dr. Kenneth, 227
Stanbury, Dr. Stuart, 26-27, 29-30, 214, 216
Steliga, Kama, 36-37
Steliga, Lyle, 36-37
Storage of blood products, 126, 135, 225
Strawczynski, Dr. Hanna, 94, 98, 99
Surrogate testing, 64-65, 70, 71, 123-24
    for Hepatitis C, 138
Swann, Antonia, 102-103
Sweden, 204
Switzerland, criminal charges, 202-203

T
T4 count, 57
Tainted blood. *See* Blood-borne AIDS
"Tainted tuna" affair, 134, 155
Taylor, Chris, 100
T-cell lymphotropic virus type V, 231
Testing of blood, 24, 31
    current (1995) testing of donations, 229-30
    for Hepatitis, 33-34, 47, 70, 71, 229
    for Hepatitis C, 138
    for HIV, 10, 128-35, 147, 161, 183, 229
        delays in, 128-31, 132-35, 159, 170,
            171, 223
        and infection rates, 198
        mandatory in Canada (Nov/85), 134, 226
        problems with, 137
        two-step procedure, 129, 132, 137
Thompson, Grace, 181
Timbrell, Dennis, 88, 154
Toronto Hospital, 11, 13, 14, 149-50, 227
Trace-back, 142-44, 145, 146, 183
    poor state of, 155-56
Transfusion AIDS, 55, 62, 63, 64, 126-27,
    131, 133-41, 185-86, 233-37
    deaths lead to traceback efforts, 141
    in the developing world, 205-207
    HIV Information Project at Hospital for
        Sick Children, 152-53

infection of babies of tainted-blood
    recipients, 170-71
number of cases, 136, 145, 147-48, 153-54
poor trace-back and look-back system, 141-56
sexual partners and children at risk, 144
Transfusion Canada (proposed new agency),
    216-21
Travenol, 108, 118
Tsoukas, Dr. Christos, 57, 58, 94, 98, 120-21
Tylenol scare, 93, 155

U
UB Plasma, 193, 202
U.S. Centers for Disease Control (CDC), 52,
    55, 56-57, 63, 64, 65, 66, 67, 105, 128, 226
    safety recommendations, 59, 73
    statistics on AIDS (1984), 106
U.S. Food and Drug Administration (FDA),
    101, 113, 123, 129, 205
U.S. House of Representatives, investigates
    AIDS crisis, 63-64
U.S. National Cancer Institute, 65-66

V
"Vampire shops", 48, 55, 193, 205
Vancouver, 141-44, 145
Varin, Claude, 166
Verreau, Bob, 228
Voluntary blood donation, 8-9, 23-24, 168-
    69, 221
Von Willebrand's disease, 38, 95

W
"Wait-and-see approach", 81, 112, 124, 144-45
Waiver of right to sue, 167, 168, 174, 175,
    176, 177
Wastage of blood donations, 98
Weber, George, 187-88, 189
Western Blot test, 129, 132, 137
Wet-heat treatment, 122, 123
Wilbee, Dr. Stan, 188
Willoughby, Dr. Brian, 76-77
Window period, 137
Winnipeg Plasma Laboratory, 90, 93, 97, 114, 122
Withdrawals of blood products, 123, 231
Women
    with AIDS, 61, 65, 125-26
    as donors, 65
World Health Organization, 63, 207

Y
Yersiniosis, 231

Z
Zucchelli, Tony, 126, 127, 129, 131, 138-39, 148